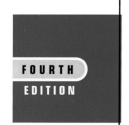

FOURTH EDITION

COMMUNICATION AND EDUCATION Skills for *Dietetics* PROFESSIONALS

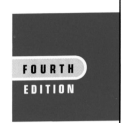

FOURTH EDITION

COMMUNICATION AND EDUCATION Skills for *Dietetics* PROFESSIONALS

Betsy B. Holli, EdD, RD, LD
Professor
Department of Nutrition Sciences
Dominican University
River Forest, Illinois

Richard J. Calabrese, PhD
Director
Master of Science in Organization Management
Dominican University
River Forest, Illinois

Julie O'Sullivan Maillet, PhD, RD, FADA
Associate Dean Academic Affairs and Research
University of Medicine & Dentistry of New Jersey
School of Health Related Professions
Newark, New Jersey

WITH A CONTRIBUTION BY:
Diane Rigassio Radler, MS, RD, CDE
Assistant Professor
University of Medicine & Dentistry of New Jersey
School of Health Related Professions
Newark, New Jersey

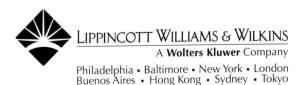

LIPPINCOTT WILLIAMS & WILKINS
A **Wolters Kluwer** Company
Philadelphia • Baltimore • New York • London
Buenos Aires • Hong Kong • Sydney • Tokyo

Editor: David B. Troy
Managing Editor: Matthew J. Hauber
Marketing Manager: Paul Jarecha
Project Editor: Caroline Define

Designer: Doug Smock
Compositor: LWW
Printer: R R Donnelly

Library of Congress Cataloging-in-Publication Data

Holli, Betsy B.
  Communication and education skills for dietetics professionals / Betsy B. Holli, Richard J. Calabrese, Jule O'Sullivan Maillet, with a contribution by Ann B. Williams.-- 4th ed.
    p. cm.
  Includes bibliographical references and index.
  ISBN 0-7817-3740-0
  1. Communication in diet therapy. 2. Patient education. 3. Interpersonal communication.
  I. Calabrese, Richard J. II. Maillet, Julie O'Sullivan. III. Title.
RM214.3.H65 2003
  615.8'54--dc21   2002043461

The publishers have made every effort to trace the copyright holders for borrowed material. If they have inadvertently overlooked any, they will be pleased to make the necessary arrangements at the first opportunity.

Photographs on pages 3 [unfig 1-3], 114 [unfig 6-2], 165 [unfig 8-1], 170 [unfig 8-2], 181 [unfig 8-5], 190 [unfig 9-1], 215 [unfig 10-2], and 223 [unfig10-4] taken from the United States Department of Agriculture Online Photography Service (Ken Hammond, photographer).

To purchase additional copies of this book call our customer service department at **(800) 638-3030** or fax orders to **(301) 824-7390**. International customers should call **(301) 714-2324**.

Visit Lippincott Williams & Wilkins on the Internet: http://www.lww.com. Lippincott Williams & Wilkins customer service representatives are available from 8:30 am to 6:00 pm, EST, Monday through Friday, for telephone access.

2 3 4 5 6 7 8 9 10

To Holli and Alexander Swinford.
BBH

To my son, Christopher; my daughter, Leslie; my son-in-law,
Todd; and my grandsons, Calen and Andrew.
RJC

To all the dietetics professionals I have known
who contribute to the health of the public by
translating the science of nutrition/dietetics
to the foods we eat through effective communications.
And to my children
Katie and Chris and husband Michael,
who teach me that communication is
a continuous process.
JOM

Dietetics professionals need the knowledge, skills, and competencies to succeed in a changing world and competitive environment. The 21st century practitioner will continue to see changes in information technology, the demographic composition of the United States, personal lifestyles, and health care delivery systems. Effective communication skills are essential for competent dietetics practice.

The United States is facing a public health crisis. Obesity is at an all-time high, physical activity levels need improving, and the eating practices of many people do not match the recommendations for optimal health. Dietetics professionals working with individuals must understand their needs, wants, and perceptions within the total environment. While motivating people to change their behavior is a challenge, providing them with the information they need is just one part of the solution. Many individuals know how to select a healthful diet, but they do not do it. To be effective, the dietetics professional must be able to apply the theories and models from the behavioral and social sciences in developing intervention strategies that help people examine the complex interaction of factors that determine personal choices of food and nutrition behaviors and, ultimately, result in decisions toward lifestyle change.

The Fourth Edition of *Communication and Education Skills for Dietetics Professionals* reviews the literature on individual, social, and cultural factors that influence behavior change and applies them to dietetics practice. There is no one gold standard theory or intervention strategy. A number of theories and models are presented as a basis for communicating to achieve changes in healthful food behaviors. Because no single theory or model has been found to be effective, the counselor must integrate those appropriate to the individual client. Included, among others, are the Transtheoretical Model of Behavior Change (Stages of Change), Health Belief Model, motivational interviewing, goal setting, behavior modification, cognitive restructuring, enhancing self-efficacy, self-management, relapse prevention, andragogy, and nutrition education.

The Commission on Accreditation for Dietetics Education (CADE) is responsible for the American Dietetic Association (ADA) accrediting functions. The 2002 CADE knowledge and skills for dietetics education that pertain to communication and education are included in the chapters. The purpose of the book is to prepare professionals with these skills to improve their communication with patients, clients, employees, and others, thus improving one's professional practice.

Dietetics professionals face many challenges in working with today's clients and employees. Women working outside of the home and single-parent households have a lack of time. Consumers want convenience in food products, so a steady diet of fast food, take out, and microwave meals is common in some families. A large proportion of family food expenditures is for foods eaten away from home. There are alternative therapies, use of nutritional supplements, herbal remedies, and functional foods.

Demographic trends include a larger number of seniors, changing socioeconomic status and lifestyles, and increasing cultural diversity. Food security remains an issue, especially in lower-income households. These issues present a challenge to nutrition professionals working to promote more healthful eating practices with individuals and groups.

Almost 100 million self-reliant United States adults use the Internet to find health-related information, both accurate and inaccurate. The consumer can visit the Web for BMI calculators, body weight calculators, self-nutritional assessment, and much more. Some clients arrive for counseling well versed about their medical problems and nutrition. The Internet expands the choices available for dietetics professionals to market and deliver services to clients and consumers. Already, some practitioners in business have web sites or are practicing over the Internet. This edition has added web site addresses where one may find additional information on chapter topics as well as materials to use with clients.

Dietetics professionals in management positions face challenges in dealing with a diverse work force with different cultural and ethnic backgrounds and values, ages, and educational levels. Managers use their communication skills in developing interpersonal relationships, interviewing and counseling employees, and providing training and education. The basic communication and education theories and skills used by clinical and community professionals also apply to managers, although they are used with a different audience. The chapters in this book apply many of the theories and principles to the manager's role.

There are a number of changes in this edition. The literature was searched carefully and references were updated, providing the reader with resources for further reading. Several chapters are substantially rewritten and each chapter now has learning objectives. Review questions and learning activities are also included, so that one can practice and apply the information in the chapters. Self-assessments and additional case studies are added to assist with applying chapter materials. Selected Internet sites provide sources of additional information or materials and resources professionals may wish to use with clients. Those at government sites are usually free.

With the fourth edition, we welcome a new co-author, Julie O'Sullivan Maillet, PhD, RD, FADA. She comes with vast experience as a registered dietitian and in dietetic association activities, serving as American Dietetic Association president in 2002–2003. We also welcome as a contributor Diane Rigassio Radler, MS, RD, CDE from the School of Health Related Professions at the University of Medicine and Dentistry of New Jersey.

Instructor's Manual

For faculty adopting the book, the *Instructor's Manual and Answer Guide* is available through a regional Lippincott Williams & Wilkins sales representatives (go to http://www.lww.com/replocator/map/ to locate an LWW representative in your region) or directly from the publisher (educsales@lww.com). The instructor's manual can be accessed at http://connection.lww.com/go/holli.

Acknowledgments

Anonymous reviewers made suggestions for changes in this new edition. We are grateful for their input and that of Matt Hauber, senior managing editor at Lippincott Williams & Wilkins. We also wish to thank The School of Health Related Professions at the University of Medicine and Dentistry of New Jersey for many of the photographs; the United States Department of Agriculture Online Photography Service; and Spencer Phippen for sketches.

Betsy B. Holli
Richard J. Calabrese
Julie O'Sullivan Maillet

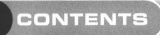

CONTENTS

CHAPTER **5** Nutrition Counseling

CHAPTER **6** Counseling for Behavior Modification
Diane Rigassio Radler, MS, RD, CDE

CHAPTER **7** Counseling for Cognitive Change

CHAPTER **8** Cross-Cultural and Life-Span Counseling

CHAPTER **9** Motivating Clients and Employees

CHAPTER 10 Principles and Theories of Learning

CHAPTER 11 Planning Learning

CHAPTER 12 Implementing and Evaluating Learning

CHAPTER 13 Group Facilitation and Dynamics

CHAPTER **14** Delivering Oral Presentations and Conducting Workshops

CHAPTER **15** Planning, Selecting, and Using Instructional Media

Challenges for Dietetics Professionals

After reading this chapter, you will be able to

1. discuss the origins of people's food habits or behaviors.
2. evaluate the problem of dietary adherence and suggest ways to improve it.
3. define selected American Dietetic Association (ADA) competencies needed for practice.
4. recognize ADA dietetic practice groups.

ood selection is a part of a complex behavioral system that is shaped by a vast array of variables. Food is essential for life. It is a powerful symbol of cultural identity as noted in the book, *You Eat What You Are: People, Culture and Food Traditions*,(1) a ritual object, and a product to be purchased. The pleasures of eating may coexist with feelings of guilt from eating something we perceive as "forbidden."(2) Dietary patterns affect our health and are important factors in the risk for several major chronic diseases.(3) Successful nutrition counseling requires you to understand why clients eat the way they do and then to use this knowledge to develop appropriate interventions.

This chapter discusses the origins of people's food habits, often described as food behaviors. Dietetics practitioners work with people to successfully make changes in their food habits as measured by dietary adherence, using strategies to motivate and improve people's success at change. The American Dietetic Association (ADA) and its Commission on Accreditation of Dietetics Education have defined the knowledge and skills needed for successful professional practice. Those that pertain to topics in this book are described.

How much do people already know about food and nutrition? How do nutrition knowledge, attitudes, and thoughts about food affect one's food choices? What behaviors are people willing to change? What are their beliefs about the relationship of food and health? These are some of the questions that must be answered before dietetics professionals can understand individuals well enough to begin talking with them about the challenges of changing their food choices. The goal of nutrition counseling and education is to help individuals change their food and eating behaviors so that they select healthful choices. The more knowledge that you have about people and their personal needs and practices, the more effective your counseling intervention will be. The goal of this book is to enhance your level of success in communicating with, counseling, and educating others.

Where does the public get their nutrition information? In a nationwide public opinion survey, 48% said they got the information from television, and 47% listed magazines as their primary sources of nutrition information.(4) The media have reported, for example, that fiber protects against colon cancer, that fiber does not protect against colon cancer, that fiber is helpful in type I diabetes mellitus, that margarine is better than butter, and that butter is better than margarine. Contradictory advice is even given in best-selling books. No wonder people are confused.

ORIGINS OF FOOD HABITS OR BEHAVIORS

Why do people eat the way they do? In physiological response to hunger, of course, but food choices and eating are far more complex. Cultural, social, economic, and other factors are involved in food selection in addition to individual choice, patterns, and personal taste. Understanding people's food choices is essential before planning an appropriate nutrition intervention.

The goal of nutrition counseling and education is to help clients modify and manage food choices and eating behaviors so that individuals improve their health. However, psychologists tell us that food and language are the "cultural traits humans learn first, and the ones that they change with the greatest reluctance."(5) A major influence is the food eaten during childhood that forever defines what is familiar and brings comfort. Food preferences from childhood continue to be exhibited by adults showing the profound role that early family experiences have in shaping food habits. Changing one's dietary choices is possible but not easily accomplished, and some intervention strategies are more effective than others.(3)

Every culture has its own definition of a meal.(6) Culture is the sum total of a group's learned and shared behavior. It is acquired by people living their everyday lives and provides a sense of identity, order, and security. As a group phenomenon, culture is learned from others and transmitted formally and informally to the next generation.

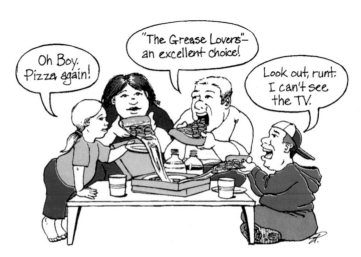

Food habits come from family habits and cultural groups.

These learned traditions are not static; they are dynamic with some changes accepted over time. All groups, including cultural and ethnic minorities, sustain their identities, in part, through their food practices, values, and beliefs. Family and culture determine what foods are appropriate and inappropriate. This makes it especially important to develop good food habits in the ho me for the sake of children.(7)

Does the person eat tortillas, croissants, cornbread, bagels or bread; hamburgers, sushi, moussaka, curry, bratwurst, pierogies, tacos, lasagna, or pizza; potato, rice, or pasta? Asian diets use rice as a staple, whereas Italians use pasta, for example. American children enjoy a peanut butter-and-jelly sandwich, whereas children from other cultures may have never heard of it. Americans, however, experiment with foods and mix the foods from a variety of cultural traditions, thus making eating practices a diverse cultural smorgasbord. Regional areas of the United States, such as Tex-Mex, New England, the Midwest, and the Southwest also may affect one's food choices. Examples of regional foods are New England clam chowder, Boston baked beans, Southern grits, New Orleans jambalaya, Texas chili, California sour dough bread, and a Wisconsin fish boil.

Over one third of calories come from food eaten away from home, where restaurants (including fast-food restaurants) serve large portions of food.(8) Small food portions are sometimes available, but many people choose medium, large, or king-sized portions. All-you-can eat buffets are popular. The media expose us to dozens of daily ads marketing fast foods, soft drinks, burgers, fries, pizza, and ice cream. Foods high in fat are widely available and frequently advertised. Have you seen any ads for grapes, apples, low-fat dairy products, whole wheat breads, or green and yellow vegetables? The United States food industry is the second largest advertiser (the auto industry is number one) with a huge financial investment. Rather than marketing food based on nutritional value, food is portrayed as a dream, a lifestyle, a source of emotional fulfillment and pleasure, a convenience, and a status symbol.(7)

No culture promotes eating alone.(9) Eating is a social activity. We eat with family and friends, but the actual number of shared family meals is diminishing. The family meal is still a symbol of family, although concerns have been raised about its demise.(6) Eating is a learned activity, and children's early experiences contribute to their food preferences. Children do not eat what they do not like. In the social setting at home or out, siblings, parents, and others can serve as role models to influence food choices, either good or bad. If the parental diet is poor or if food is used as a reward, the child's learning may not include enough healthy foods. The support of significant others—family, friends, and the health counselor—helps people make changes in food selection.

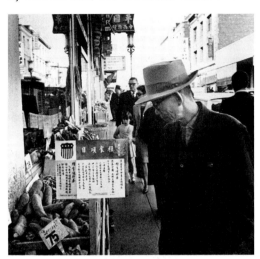

Counseling ethnic groups requires a knowledge of their foods.

Social changes are determining what, where, when, and why people eat. Lifestyles are less formal. There are single-parent homes, for example, and homes in which both parents work. Our social occasions, parties, birthdays, holidays, and anniversaries center around food.(10) Eating in restaurants, eating while grocery shopping, eating during weekend activities, and eating while traveling add challenges to our selection of healthful food choices. Preplanning for these circumstances helps. Food expresses friendship and hospitality, shows concern, and is a status symbol. Prestige is indicated by using expensive meats, fine wines, caviar, and exotic foods along with taking an exotic vacation, eating in a trendy restaurant, and having an expensive car.(7)

We give social and emotional meanings to food, such as feminine or masculine, good or bad, healthy or nonhealthy, sophisticated or common, virtuous or sinful, and a comfort or not. Foods such as chocolate may be perceived to have a sensuous nature. But luscious candy may be considered fattening or sinful by those worried about their weight.(11) Thus, mood may affect the food chosen and consumed.(12)

Studies show that people are very concerned about the taste of food. If food does not taste good, it is not likely to be eaten or enjoyed.(13) In eating, we stimulate all the senses at about the same time. We notice the appearance (vision), the flavor and aroma (taste and smell), the texture (tactile), temperature (thermal), and sound (hearing) as we chew crisp foods.(14)

Other influences on food selection include the price of food, religious rituals and customs, such as fasting, feasting, and food taboos, peer influences, availability of cooking facilities at home, skills of the consumer in food preparation, personal preferences and tolerances, and amount of time available. According to an environmental scan, "consumers are demanding convenience in products and services."(15) The range of convenience foods is steadily expanding. There is a shift to highly processed foods that have been prewashed, cut, prepared, and combined into ready-to-heat and ready-to-eat foods and meals.(16) Food preparation and cooking are now optional activities to a great extent. People use more convenience foods, have less time to cook, eat out more often, or bring food in.

A person's beliefs about his or her health may also influence food choices. The Health Belief Model postulates that a person's beliefs about health are determinants of the likelihood of an individual making lifestyle changes.(17,18) The three key factors are (a) the belief that a person is "susceptible" to contracting a specific disease, "has the disease" now, or is "resusceptible" in the case of an illness from which a person has recovered; (b) that the disease or its consequences are having a serious, negative effect on one's life; and (c) that there are benefits from changing health behaviors in terms of reducing susceptibility to or severity of the disease compared with the psychological cost and barriers to making changes. A person who has had a heart attack, for example, may be more ready to make dietary changes at least in the near term than a person with hypertension who has no symptoms.

Having positive rather than negative cognitions or thoughts helps a person to make changes. There is a big difference between "Nutrition is important and this is worth the effort for my health" and "It's too much trouble and I feel ok anyway." One study found that some women linked the word "diet" to losing weight, whereas men disliked the word. "Food choices" or "choose a meal" were suggested as alternatives.(19) Cognitions may be influenced by attitudes and feelings (discussed in detail in a later chapter). Therefore, attitudes are thought to influence peoples' decisions and actions. People may eat not only for physiological reasons such as hunger, but for psychological reasons,

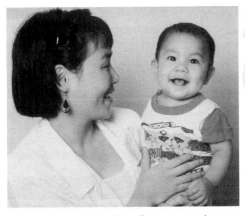

Children learn food preferences at home.

such as anxiety, depression, loneliness, stress, and boredom as well as from positive emotional states, such as happiness and celebrations. Food may assuage guilt as well as lead to guilt feelings.(7)

Knowledge of what to eat is certainly a first step in influencing healthful food choices, but it is probably overrated. There are individuals who know what to eat and do not do it. When people do not eat properly, some counselors redouble their efforts in educating as if the problem is lack of knowledge. The relationship between what people know about food and nutrition and what they eat is a very weak one. Other factors may be taking precedence and need to be explored. Knowledge helps only when people are willing and motivated to change.

Thus, there are many influences on food choices, including cognitive, sociocultural, physical, and geographical factors. The nutrition counselor needs to explore all of them to understand the client, the client's motivation for change, and the appropriate intervention to use. Figure 1-1 summarizes some of the variables motivating changes in people's food choices and health behaviors. Discussion of variables continues in chapters that follow.

DIETARY ADHERENCE

Changing food choices sounds easy, but it is actually a very complex problem. The characteristics of the dietary regimen are the most important factors in adherence. Adherence is defined as the extent to which the individual's food choices and behaviors coincide with dietary recommendations. Complexity is the most significant factor and has been negatively associated with adherence, perhaps because of the difficulty of fitting the regimen into a person's daily routine.(20)

Dietary changes encompass many of the factors associated with a higher incidence of nonadherence. They include required changes in lifestyle, which tend to be restrictive, last a long duration or for a lifetime, and interfere with customary family habits and practices. If other barriers exist, such as high cost of the foods, lack of access to the proper foods, or extra effort, time, and skill required to prepare the meals, the likelihood of nonadherence increases.

To change food behaviors, the counselor and the client must have good rapport, with the counselor taking into consideration the person's lifestyle, concerns, and expectations. Adherence may be more satisfactory if the client sees the same counselor at each visit and if clear-cut communication occurs based on what the client is willing to do. The client should set the goals for change, or select from alternatives suggested by the counselor if the client is unable to define any. A warm and caring environment and prompt scheduling of appointments puts the client in a good frame of mind. Long waiting periods at an appointment does not.

In patients with diabetes mellitus, dietitians reported the following barriers to

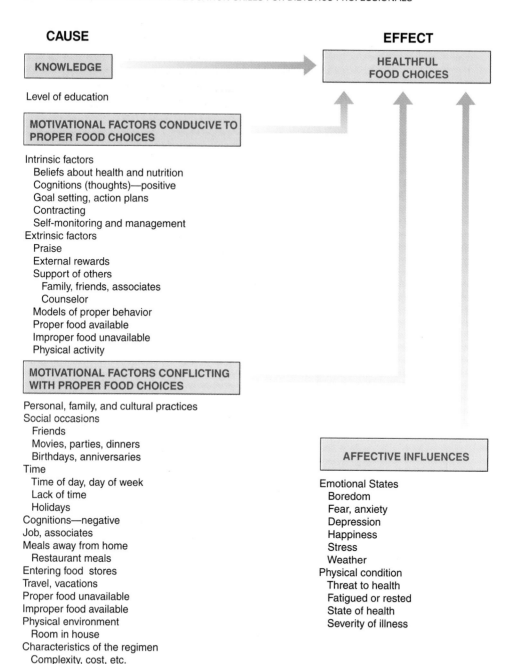

CAUSE

EFFECT

KNOWLEDGE

HEALTHFUL
FOOD CHOICES

Level of education

MOTIVATIONAL FACTORS CONDUCIVE TO
PROPER FOOD CHOICES

Intrinsic factors
  Beliefs about health and nutrition
  Cognitions (thoughts)—positive
  Goal setting, action plans
  Contracting
  Self-monitoring and management
Extrinsic factors
  Praise
  External rewards
  Support of others
    Family, friends, associates
    Counselor
  Models of proper behavior
  Proper food available
  Improper food unavailable
  Physical activity

MOTIVATIONAL FACTORS CONFLICTING
WITH PROPER FOOD CHOICES

Personal, family, and cultural practices
Social occasions
  Friends
  Movies, parties, dinners
  Birthdays, anniversaries
Time
  Time of day, day of week
  Lack of time
  Holidays
Cognitions—negative
Job, associates
Meals away from home
  Restaurant meals
Entering food stores
Travel, vacations
Proper food unavailable
Improper food available
Physical environment
  Room in house
Characteristics of the regimen
  Complexity, cost, etc.

AFFECTIVE INFLUENCES

Emotional States
  Boredom
  Fear, anxiety
  Depression
  Happiness
  Stress
  Weather
Physical condition
  Threat to health
  Fatigued or rested
  State of health
  Severity of illness

Figure 1-1 Variables motivating change in food choices and health behavior.

dietary adherence: lack of time, lack of health symptoms, lack of education, poor self-esteem, lack of empowerment, and misinformation from family, friends, and others with the same disease. To overcome these barriers, dietitians recommend individualizing meal plans, teaching patients to plan ahead, teaching about medical complications from lack of adherence, and setting obtainable goals.(21)

The Modification of Diet in Renal Disease (MDRD) study found that the most effective element of intervention that produced dietary adherence to goals was the process of "self-monitoring" of daily protein intake. It enhanced patient self-management by allowing individuals to identify targeted nutrient sources in their diets and then to develop daily strategies for modifying their eating behaviors to achieve desired goals.(22)

Nutrition counselors are concerned with the success or failure of people to make healthier food choices. The United States population, for example, eats excess calories to the extent that more than half of American adults (54%) are overweight, and children are following in the footsteps of their parents.(8) In spite of problems associated with changing food behaviors, some people do change. People today are consuming less red meat and eggs than previously, for example.

Measures of dietary adherence are examined frequently. As clients return for follow-up appointments, discussions may focus on what worked and what went well, as well as what did not work, to define the extent to which the person's food choices and behaviors coincide with the goals developed or the physician's dietary prescription. This information is useful in setting additional goals for change with the client.

It is unrealistic to expect 100% adherence 24 hours a day and 7 days a week. Travel, parties, holidays, and other events may be times when people relax their diet for a limited period of time. The short-term pleasure of a piece of chocolate cake or apple pie, for example, may take precedence temporarily over the dietary regimen. In the Dietary Approaches to Stop Hypertension (DASH) trial, lack of food variety and unappetizing foods contributed to noncompliance with the DASH diet for hypertension.(23)

Professionals may become frustrated with a client's lack of adherence. Remember that people do not like their food choices to be restricted. When something is forbidden, it may produce an obsession with that food or binge eating. The flexibility to allow a desired food occasionally in moderation may make for a more compliant client.(24)

How is adherence measured? Dietary adherence is often evaluated based on oral and written self-reports of foods and beverages consumed, both subjective measures. Daily self-monitoring records of food intake, interviews such as diet histories and 24-hour recalls, and the professional's subjective judgment are used to collect data. These methods depend on the client's honesty and accuracy in reporting.(23)

The challenge for health professionals is to be sensitive cross-culturally and to help clients change their food choices in ways in which the sociocultural functions of food are not disturbed. For dietary changes to succeed, a combination of approaches including behavioral and cognitive interventions, self-efficacy, relapse prevention, self monitoring, stages of change, social support, and educational strategies may be necessary to assist people to make changes in food choices. Strategies for promoting change and for working with clients to improve adherence are found in other chapters in the book.

MANAGEMENT PRACTICE IN DIETETICS

Many dietetics professionals have management roles. Some start their careers in management, whereas others take on managerial duties through promotion to upper level positions later in their careers. Management positions are available in a number of settings, including food services in hospitals and nursing homes, schools from daycare to universities, prisons, department stores, and other commercial establishments. Dietitians may be promoted to clinical nutrition manager, chief clinical dietitian, or direct a food service. A dietetic technician may supervise employees or manage a food service department.(25)

Public health and community nutritionists work in governmental agencies, private nonprofit agencies, and for-profit agencies. They plan and manage nutrition programs or agencies in community settings.(26) Other professionals enter private practice, are self-employed, and manage their own businesses or become entrepreneurs.

All professionals and especially managers need the ability to communicate and work effectively with their employees, with others on their same level, with superiors who are in authority, and with customers and clients. Dietetics professionals communicate to both individuals and to groups in meetings and classes. Managers interview and hire, supervise, train, and counsel employees, for example. They are involved in motivation and discipline and in conducting performance appraisals. The basic principles of communication in the following chapters apply in all practice settings, although the details of application may differ.

AMERICAN DIETETIC ASSOCIATION KNOWLEDGE AND SKILL REQUIREMENTS

The mission of the ADA is to promote optimal nutrition and well-being for all people by advocating for its members. Members are the leading source of food and nutrition services. The ADA has defined those competencies necessary for professional practice for both registered dietitians (RD) and dietetic technicians registered (DTR).(27) The aims of the book are to assist in the development of these specific knowledge and skills related to oral communication.

For Entry-Level Dietitians

The ADA requirements for entry-level dietitians include the following.

Foundation knowledge and skills:
Negotiation techniques
Media presentations
Interpersonal communication skills
Counseling theory and methods
Interviewing techniques
Educational theory and techniques
Concepts of human and group dynamics
Public speaking

Graduates will have demonstrated the ability to:
Use oral and written communications in presenting an educational session for a group
Counsel individuals on nutrition

On completion of the supervised practice component, graduates will be able to:

Provide dietetics education in supervised practice settings

Supervise counseling, education, and/or other interventions in health promotion/disease prevention for patient/clients needing medical nutrition therapy for uncomplicated instances of common conditions, such as hypertension, obesity, diabetes, and diverticular disease

Supervise education and training for target groups

For Dietetic Technicians

The ADA requirements for dietetic technicians include the following.

Foundation knowledge and skills:

Counseling theory and methods

Methods of teaching

Concepts of human and group dynamics

Interpersonal communication skills

Interviewing techniques

Graduates will have demonstrated the ability to:

Use oral and written communication in presenting an educational session for target groups

On completion of the supervised practice component, graduates will be able to:

Provide dietetics education in supervised practice settings

Educate patient/clients in disease prevention and health promotion and medical nutrition therapy for uncomplicated instances of common conditions, such as hypertension, obesity, diabetes, and diverticular disease

Conduct education and training for target groups

Knowledge of sociocultural and ethnic food consumption, the educational needs of diverse populations, and the influences of socioeconomic, cultural, and psychological factors on food and nutrition behavior is also expected.

DIETETIC PRACTICE GROUPS

One of the top-rated benefits of membership in ADA is the opportunity to affiliate with a dietetic practice group (DPG). Specialty practice groups provide networking, professional development and leadership opportunities, mentoring, and information sharing in newsletters and meetings by areas of interest and professional expertise.(28) At the time of publication, the following practice groups with available web addresses existed.

Clinical Nutrition Management

Consultant Dietitians in Health-Care Facilities: www.cdhcf.org

Diabetes Care and Education: www.dce.org

Dietetic Educators of Practitioners

Dietetic Technicians in Practice

Dietetics in Developmental and Psychiatric Disorders

Dietetics in Physical Medicine and Rehabilitation

Dietitians in Business and Communications: www.dbconline.org

Dietitians in General Clinical Practice

Dietitians in Nutrition Support

Food and Culinary Professionals

Gerontological Nutritionists: http://trc.ucdavis.edu/gerinutr

HIV/AIDS: www.hivaidsdpg.org

Hunger and Environmental Nutrition

Management in Food and Nutrition Systems: www.rdmanager.org

Nutrition Education for the Public: www.dietetics.com/nepdpg

Nutrition Educators of Health Professionals

Nutrition Entrepreneurs

Nutrition in Complementary Care: www.complementarynutrition.org

Oncology Nutrition

Pediatric Nutrition

Public Health/Community Nutrition

Renal Dietitians

Research

School Nutrition Services

Sports, Cardiovascular, and Wellness Nutritionists: www.nutrifit.org

Vegetarian Nutrition

Weight Management

Women and Reproductive Nutrition

REVIEW AND DISCUSSION QUESTIONS

1. How do dietetics professionals use communication skills?
2. List the influences on people's food habits or behaviors.
3. What factors influence dietary adherence?
4. What strategies can be used to help people make dietary changes and promote better dietary adherence?
5. What dietetics practice groups are of interest to you?

> **CASE STUDY 1**
>
> Karen, a 35-year-old married woman, made an appointment with a regis-
> tered dietitian in private practice to get counseling for weight loss and main-
> tenance. Karen works full-time as a secretary at a bank, often going out to
> lunch with coworkers. Her husband is in computer sales. They have three
> children ranging in age from 6 to 10 years, and all are in school. Karen's
> mother comes to watch the children after school until she arrives home.
>
> Karen is 5 feet 5 inches tall and weighs 170 pounds. She weighed 135
> when she was married 12 years ago.
>
> Karen described her daily schedule. She gets up early to make breakfast
> and help the children get ready for school. After work, she is tired and the
> children are hungry and clamoring for dinner, so she describes dinner as a
> "rush job" or something brought in. After cleaning up, she helps the children
> with homework, does laundry or other housework, attends evening activities
> at the school, runs errands, gets the children to bed, and then retires herself.
>
> 1. What lifestyle factors may help or hinder Karen in adhering to different
>   food choices so that she can lose weight?
> 2. What suggestions or alternatives can you give Karen to overcome any
>   problems identified in question one?

SUGGESTED ACTIVITIES

1. From the dietetic practice groups mentioned, select a subspecialty area of practice
   and interview a dietitian or nutritionist about his or her responsibilities, stressing
   the use of communication and education skills. Share this information with peers.
2. With someone trying to make changes in food choices, discuss the changes and the
   factors influencing the changes, including any opportunities, challenges, or barriers. What are the factors influencing the person's adherence?
3. Select a dietary regimen, such as increased fiber, restricted sodium, reduced calorie, or reduced fat and cholesterol, and follow it yourself for 7 days. Keep a daily
   record of all foods eaten. How easy or difficult was it to comply with the dietary
   change for a week? What factors helped or hindered your adherence?
4. Write down what you would eat in these situations if you were following the same
   dietary regimen: birthday, wedding, holidays such as Christmas or Easter. How are
   decisions made on food choices for these events?
5. Think about your own food practices. What influences them? To what extent are
   social and cultural factors involved?
6. Visit the American Dietetic Association (ADA) web site at www.eatright.org. Or
   visit the site of a dietetic practice group. Some state dietetic associations also have
   web addresses on the ADA site.
7. Watch three hours of television or examine three current magazines. What food
   products are advertised? How do these ads influence food choices? Compare with
   peers.
8. Discuss with peers the family and cultural origins of your food habits.

9. In your culture, what foods are served on special occasions, such as weddings and holidays. Compare with peers.
10. Interview a person from a different cultural or ethnic group to determine what they eat on a daily basis and on holidays.

WEB SITES

www.eatright.org/bibethnic.html / The American Dietetic Association ethnic bibliography

http://oregonstate.edu/dept/ehe/nu_diverse.htm / cultural aspects of foods with links to other sites

REFERENCES

1. Barer-Stein TB. You eat what you are: people, culture and food traditions. Willowdale, Ontario, Canada: Firefly Books, 1999.
2. Germov J, Williams L. Introducing the social appetite. In: Germov J, Williams L, eds. A sociology of food and nutrition: the social appetite. New York: Oxford University Press, 1999.
3. Brownell KD, Cohen LR. Adherence to dietary regimens 1: an overview of research. Behav Med 1995;20:149.
4. Americans' Food and Nutrition Attitudes and Behaviors—American Dietetic Association's Nutrition and You: Trends 2000. Press release Jan. 3, 2000. Available at www.eatright.org/pr/2000/01300a.html. Accessed 2/13/2002.
5. Gabaccia DR. We are what we eat. Cambridge, MA: Harvard University Press, 1998.
6. Makela J. Cultural definitions of the meal. In: HL Meiselman, ed. Dimensions of the meal: the science, culture, business, and art of eating. Gaithersburg, MD: Aspen Publishers, 2000.
7. Fieldhouse P. Food and nutrition: customs and culture, 2nd ed. London: Chapman & Hall, 1995.
8. Diet & health: ten megatrends. Nutrition Action Healthletter 2001;28:3.
9. Ikeda JP. Culture, food, and nutrition in increasingly culturally diverse societies. In Germov J, Williams L. A sociology of food and nutrition: the social appetite. New York: Oxford University Press, 1999.
10. McIntosh EN. American food habits in historical perspective. Westport, CT: Praeger, 1995.
11. Rozin P. Sociocultural influences on human food selection. In: Capaldi ED, ed. Why we eat what we eat: the psychology of eating. Washington, DC: American Psychology Association, 1996.
12. Social differentiation: food consumption and identity. In: Germov J, Williams L, eds. A sociology of food and nutrition: the social appetite. New York: Oxford University Press, 1999.
13. Hess MA. Taste: the neglected nutrition factor. Top Clin Nutr 1992;7:1.
14. Lawless HT. Sensory combinations in the meal. In: Meiselman HL, ed. Dimensions of the meal: the science culture, business, and art of eating. Gaithersburg, MD: Aspen Publishers, 2000.
15. Bezol C, Kang J. Looking to the future—the role of the ADA environmental scan. J Am Diet Assoc 1999;99:989.
16. Marshall DW. British meals and food choices. In: Meiselman, HL, ed. Dimensions of the meal: the science, culture, business, and art of eating. Gaithersburg, MD: Aspen Publishers, 2000.
17. Meichenbaum D, Turk DC. Facilitating treatment adherence: a practitioner's guidebook. New York: Plenum, 1987.

18. Brownell KD, Cohen LR. Adherence to dietary regimens 2: components of effective interventions. Behav Med 1995;20:155.
19. Kennedy E, Davis CA. Dietary Guidelines 2000—the opportunity and challenges for reaching the consumer. J Am Diet Assoc 2000;100:1462.
20. McCann BS, Retzlaff BM, Dowdy AA, et al. Promoting adherence to low-fat, low cholesterol diets. Review and recommendations. J Am Diet Assoc 1990;90:1408.
21. Williamson AR, Hunt AE, Pope JF, Tolman NM. Recommendations of dietitians for overcoming barriers to dietary adherence in individuals with diabetes. Diabetes Educator 2000;26:272.
22. Snetselaar L. New directions in nutrition for the renal patient. Perspect Appl Nutr 1994;4:3.
23. Windhauser MM, Evans MA, McCullough ML, et al. Dietary adherence in the dietary approaches to stop hypertension trial. J Am Diet Assoc 1999;99S:S76.
24. Karali M. The psychology of eating. Contemporary Dialysis & Nephrology 1999;20:33.
25. Hudson NL. Management practice in dietetics. Belmont, CA: Wadsworth, 2000.
26. Johnson DB, Eaton DL, Wahl PW, Gleason C. Public health nutrition practice in the United States. J Am Diet Assoc 2001;101:529.
27. Bruening KS, Mitchell BE, Pfeiffer MM. 2002 accreditation standards for dietetics education. J Am Diet Assoc 2002;102:566.
28. Indorato DA. Getting the most from your DPGs. Today's Dietitian 2001;3:40.

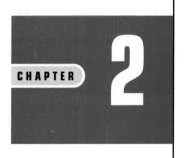

CHAPTER 2

Communication

After reading this chapter, you will be able to

1. define operationally effective communication.
2. list the components of the communication model.
3. discuss ways to make verbal communication effective.
4. relate ways to improve listening skills.
5. list communication barriers and how to overcome them.
6. describe the communication process.
7. list behaviors related to effective active listening.

There is no pleasure to me without communication: there is not so much as a sprightly thought comes into my mind that it does not grieve me to have produced alone, and that I have no one to tell it to.

Michel de Montaigne (1553—1592)

Well-developed communication skills increase the likelihood of the health care professional's success with clients and staff. The level of trust, cooperation, and confidence among those being "helped" is positively related to their subjective perceptions of the helpers' positive regard toward them. During the last few years, many studies confirmed the importance of the communication variable as it relates to the myriad other variables in the health care environment.(1–6) Research suggests that both employers and dietetics professionals ranked communication skills as being absolutely essential to success in both business and industry positions.(7,8)

EFFECTIVE COMMUNICATION OPERATIONALLY DEFINED

Effective communication can be operationally defined for dietetics practitioners as the ability to use language that is appropriate to the client's and staff's level of understanding, the ability to develop a relationship between themselves and their clients and staff, the ability to talk to them in a way that relieves anxiety, the ability to communicate to them in a way that ensures their being able to recall information actively, and the ability to provide them with feedback.

This chapter discusses communication as a process, examines its components, and points out applications for practitioners. A model of the communication process is presented and discussed, followed by an explanation of the implications of the process for the verbal, nonverbal, and listening behaviors of the dietetics practitioner. The chapter concludes with a discussion of negotiating and communicating skills to use with legislators.

Possessing only an intellectual appreciation of the various communication skills is of little use. Being able to pass a test by explaining how you ought to interact with clients and staff, how to defuse their hostility, and how to create a supportive communication climate is not the same as actually being able to do it. Putting the principles into practice requires a conscious effort, repeated attempts, and many trials. With practice, in a relatively short time, you will notice a difference in the way others respond to you. Honing the skills, however, is an ongoing process and begins with an understanding of the many elements included in the interpersonal communication exchange.

INTERPERSONAL COMMUNICATION MODEL

Complicated processes are easier to grasp when they can be visualized in a model. A model, however, is not the same as the actual phenomenon; rather, it is a graphic depiction to aid understanding. The elements included in the human communication model are the following: sender, receiver, the message itself—verbal and nonverbal, feedback, and interference. They are depicted graphically in Figure **2-1**.

Components of the Communication Model

Sender
Senders of the messages speak first. They initiate the communication.

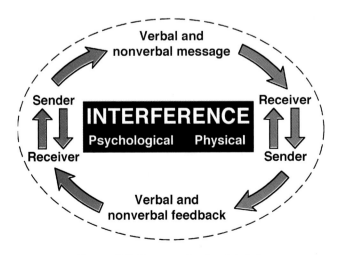

Figure 2-1 Communication Model.

Receiver

Receivers of the message—listeners—usually interpret and transmit simultaneously. They may be listening to what is being said and thinking about what they are going to say when the senders stop talking. Even when silent, it is impossible for receivers in a two-way communication transaction not to communicate. They may be reacting physiologically with a flushed face or trembling hands, or in some other way, depending on their inferences from the message. Senders make inferences based on the receivers' appearance and demeanor and adjust subsequent communication accordingly.

Message

The receiver interprets two messages simultaneously: the actual verbal message and the nonverbal message inferred from the sender and the environment. Nonverbal inferences arise from the perceived emotional tone of the sender's voice, facial expression, dress, choice of words, diction, and pronunciation, as well as from the communication environment.

Feedback

The term "feedback" refers to the process of responding to messages after interpreting them for oneself. It is the key ingredient that distinguishes two-way from one-way communication. In two-way, face-to-face communication, the sender is talking while looking at the other person. The other person's reactions to the sender's message, whether agreement, surprise, boredom, or hostility, are examples of feedback. Unless the communication channel is kept clear for feedback, distortion occurs, leaving the sender unable to detect accurately how the message is received.(8,9)

In written communication, writers cannot clarify for readers because they do not see them. Even when writers carefully select words for the benefit of their intended readers, written communication is generally less effective than one-to-one verbal communication because of its inability to re-explain and adjust language in response to the feedback from receivers.

Interpersonal communication, after the first few seconds, becomes a simultaneous two-way sending-and-receiving process. While senders are talking, they are receiving nonverbal reactions from receivers. Based on these reactions they may change their tone, speak louder, use simpler language, or in some other way adjust their communication so that their message is better understood.

Interference

This term denotes the many factors inherent in the communicators (sender and receiver) and their environment that may affect the interpretation of messages. These factors include the unique attributes inherent in each of them; the room size, shape, and color; temperature; furniture arrangement; and the physiological state of each communicator at the moment. The sophisticated communicator needs to understand these dynamics and compensate or safeguard accordingly, so that the intended message is the one received.

A crying baby, the sound of thunder, and low-flying planes, for example, not only can hinder the receiver in hearing the sender's message, but also can generate messages and interpretations in the receiver that were never intended by the sender. Another source of interference is the physiological state of the communicators at the moment. No two bodies are exactly alike. Because no one has shared in the exact life experience of another, no two people understand language in precisely the same way.

Today's "Americans," more than ever, originate from a wide variety of cultural and ethic backgrounds. This increases the likelihood of a miscommunication in a verbal exchange with people from outside their group. Distortions can stem from psychological interference as well, including bias, prejudice, and closed-mindedness. Psychological interference in health care patients is often due to fear of illness and its consequences. The job of senders is to generate in receivers those meanings for language that are closest to the senders' own. Because meanings are not universal, they can be affected by external as well as internal influences. Communication environment, cultural differences, the distance between speakers, lighting, temperature, and colors are a few of the variables that can affect meanings ascribed to a message. These variables can be sources of interference and account for the difficulty in generating in others the meanings people intend.

VERBAL AND NONVERBAL COMMUNICATION

Verbal communication includes the actual words selected by the sender and the way in which these symbols are arranged into thought units. Nonverbal communication includes the communication environment, the manner and style in which the communication is delivered, and the internal qualities inherent in the sender and receiver that influence their interpretation of external stimuli. Although both verbal communication and nonverbal communication occur simultaneously during interaction, they are discussed separately here in the context of their influence on the communication process. The salient point to remember is that the lack of clear communication, particularly regarding the work expectations used for appraisal by the dietetics practitioner is the most common cause of poor employee performance. Conscious and clear communication is the key to a congruent relationship with both clients and staff.

Verbal Communication

To keep the communication channel open between the client or employee and the dietitian or dietetic technician, the professional needs to know how to create a supportive climate. A supportive climate is one in which as one person speaks, the other listens, attending to the message rather than to his or her own internal thoughts and feelings. A defensive climate, which occurs when the other person is feeling threatened, creates the opposite effect, with the listener "shutting down." When this happens, there is little point in continuing the interaction because the message is no longer penetrating. Although maintaining a supportive climate is always a concern, it becomes especially crucial when the professional is attempting either to discuss a topic viewed differently or to resolve conflict and de-fuse anger.

Although accurate communication exchanges have the best chance of being understood when the conditions of a supportive climate are present, sustaining a supportive climate is imperative when attempting to resolve conflict. Conflict can be positive and act as the catalyst to move a relationship forward. Contemporary organizational theory, in fact, states that conflict is essential for organizational development or is sometimes encouraged.(10–13)

The verbal guidelines for creating a supportive communication climate are to 1) discuss problems descriptively rather than evaluatively; 2) describe situations with a problem orientation rather than in a manipulative way; 3) offer alternatives provisionally rather than dogmatically; 4) treat clients as equals; and 5) be empathic rather than neutral or self-centered.

Descriptive Rather than Evaluative

Ordinarily, when approaching topics that tend to provoke defensiveness in clients, professionals should think through the discussion before engaging the client, so that the problem area is exposed descriptively rather than evaluatively. Whenever people feel as if others are judging their attitudes, behavior, or the quality of their work, they show an increased tendency to become defensive. Such comments as "You don't seem to be trying," "You don't care about cooperating," or "You are selfish" are based on inferences rather than facts. So when the other's response is "I do care," "I am too trying," or "I am not selfish," the framework for an argument is set, with no way of proving objectively who is right or wrong. Instead of making judgments regarding another's attitudes, the safest and least offensive way of dealing with a touchy issue is to describe the facts as objectively as possible. For example, when the professional tells a client descriptively that his or her continuing to eat chocolate several times each day is frustrating to her as the client's counselor, she is confronting the problem honestly and objectively without being evaluative. The client can then address the topic rather than argue about the professional's negative evaluation of his or her poor attitude, lack of concern, or noncooperativeness.

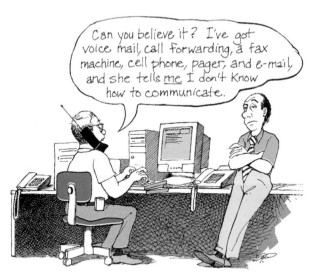

Good communication skills must be developed.

In a work-related situation, accusing an employee who has arrived late several mornings of being "irresponsible" and "uncaring" is likely to provoke a hostile refutation or cold silence. The employee may believe that being late does not warrant a reprimand. There may, in fact, be a reasonable explanation about which you should inquire. Describing how being late is causing problems to those who depend on him or her and causing work to back up is honest and descriptive and allows for nondefensive dialogue.

Problem-Oriented Rather than Manipulative

Orienting a person to a problem rather than manipulating him or her promotes a supportive communication climate. Frequently, when people want others to appreciate their point of view, they lead them through a series of questions until the other reaches the "appropriate" insight. This is a form of manipulation and provokes defensiveness as soon as respondents realize they are being channeled to share the other's vision.

> **EXAMPLE:** *"Several weeks ago you agreed that you were going to stop eating chocolate; however, each week you continue to acknowledge eating chocolate candy bars. About a month ago, you agreed to switch to fresh fruit as a snack, but that has not occurred. Last week you suggested that you were willing to eat a high-fiber cereal for breakfast, and today you acknowledge that you haven't followed through on that. If you were dealing with a client like yourself, would you begin to get the feeling that this person is playing games with you?"*

A discussion with the client would probably be more productive if the practitioner took a direct problem-oriented approach.

> **EXAMPLE:** *"In 6 weeks you have gained 3 pounds. I am certain that you should have had a weight loss of 4 to 5 pounds while on the diet on which we agreed. There seems to be a problem here. Let's discuss what possibilities might explain the weight gain."*

Employees and clients respect the professional when they believe the professional is being straightforward and authentic. A slick, manipulative style ordinarily can be seen through immediately and causes others to become disdainful.

Although as the practitioner you should plan opening remarks descriptively rather than evaluatively, after making such remarks you should allow for spontaneous problem solving without preplanned solutions. Creative, superior, and long-lasting solutions are more likely to occur when each person hears out the other fully and is heard in return and when the client comes up with the solution. When a practitioner is intent on "selling" a solution, there is a natural disposition on the part of the other to block out conflicting opinions. The problem-solving process is discussed in detail in other chapters.

In the previous examples, the practitioner's subsequent remarks depend on how the client or employee responds to the directive to explain the underlying problem. The professional needs to give the client time to think; this often means waiting for an answer. Providing excuses or putting words into the other's mouth is a mistake. The practitioner needs to learn the discipline of sitting through the tension of silence supportively until the client or employee responds. Frequently, the first explanations are those that people believe will not upset or shock the professional. The "real" reasons, however, may not be revealed until the client or staff member feels secure enough to risk shocking the professional without fear of being humiliated or embarrassed. In other words, after the first explanations are offered, dietitians or dietetics technicians would do best simply to repeat in their own words what they have understood. Only when the clients or employees are comfortable enough, will they be able to express their authentic reactions, questions, or answers, these ordinarily being less logical, more emotional, and more risky to expose.

Provisional Rather than Dogmatic

When offering advice to clients or helping them to solve problems, the professional should give advice provisionally rather than dogmatically. "Provisionally" implies the possibility of the practitioner changing his or her options, provided that additional facts emerge. It keeps the door open for clients to add information. When advice is offered in a dogmatic way, it becomes threatening for clients or employees to challenge or to add their own information. A dogmatic prescription might be, "This is what you must do. I know this is the way to solve your problem." A provisional prescription might be, "Here are several alternative things you might consider," or "There may be other ways of handling this problem; perhaps you have some ideas too, but here are things you might consider."

Egalitarian Rather than Superior

In discussing issues, clients and professionals should regard each other as equals. Whenever the possibility of defensiveness exists, even between persons of equal rank, any verbal or nonverbal behavior that the other interprets as an attempt to emphasize superiority generates a defensive response. In the relationship between professionals and clients or managers and employees, the dietetics practitioners' tendencies to emphasize status or rank may arise unconsciously from a desire to convince the other to accept their recommendations. Comments such as the following may cause the other to feel inferior, hurt, or angry: "As a lay person, you may find this difficult to understand, but it works," or "Just do what I recommend; I've been doing this for 10 years." Certainly, there is nothing wrong with professionals letting clients know that they are educated and competent. In fact, clients often need and appreciate the reassurance. The manner in which it is done is crucial, however. A more effective and subtle way to solve problems with a client is to say, "I have studied this problem and dealt with other clients who have similar symptoms. I am interested, however, in incorporating your own insights and plans into the solution. You must be satisfied and willing to try the diet, so please express your views, too. We will continue to modify over time."

An employee making a recommendation to a manager that the manager had tried unsuccessfully many years ago, might be told, "If I were in your shoes, I would think the same thing. Someday when you are more experienced, you'll know why it won't work." The subtle underscoring of the inferior relative status of the subordinate could be enough to cause a defensive battle. The professional would have done far better with a comment such as "I can understand why you say that. I have thought the same myself, but when I tried, it was not successful." Here, the employee is left feeling reinforced and appreciated rather than humiliated. Showing respect for the client's and employee's intelligence and life experiences and recognizing their human dignity facilitates cooperation.

In conflict resolution, problem solving, and the discussion of any issues that may be threatening to the client or employee, collaboration is far more effective than trying to persuade the person to act according to the dictates of the professional. Collaboration has other virtues as well. People feel more obligation to uphold solu-

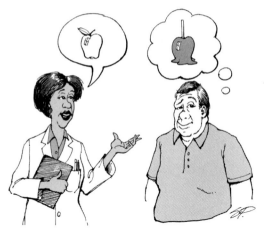

To determine whether or not the receiver has the correct message, feedback is necessary.

tions that they themselves have participated in designing. If clients are trying the professional's solution, they may feel little satisfaction in proving that he or she was right; however, if the solution is one that was arrived at through collaboration, there is genuine satisfaction in proving its validity. An additional reason for practitioners to involve others in problem solving is that often a valid solution that is superior to any that the individual or professional would have discovered alone can be arrived at through collaboration. Two people sharing insights, knowledge, experience, and feelings can generate creative thought processes in each other, which in turn generate other ideas that would not otherwise have emerged.

Empathic Rather than "Neutral"

Another verbal skill essential to maintaining a supportive climate is the ability to put yourself in the other's shoes. For a helping professional, however, this is not enough. To be effective in working with clients and employees, dietetics practitioners must be able to demonstrate in some way their desire to understand what it is those they are helping are feeling. This "demonstration" might be an empathic response to their comments. In an empathic response, the listener tells the other that he or she is attempting to understand not only the speaker's content, but also the underlying feelings. For example, a client might say, "For my entire life I have eaten spicy foods; they are a part of my culture. I don't know what my life will be like without them." The professional might then respond, "You seem to be worried that the quality of your life will change because of the dietary changes."

If the professional is accurate in his or her empathic remarks, the client will acknowledge it and probably go on talking, assured that the helper listens. If the professional is wrong, however, the client will clarify the judgment and continue to talk, assured that the helper cares. Thus, the dietetics practitioner need not be accurate in inferring the other's feelings as long as he or she is willing to try to understand them. In addition, empathic responses allow the professional to respond without giving advice, focusing instead on the individual's need to talk and to express feelings and concerns. Before clients or employees can listen to the professional, they must express their concerns; otherwise, while the practitioner is talking, the clients or employees are thinking about what they will say when the practitioner stops talking.

An employee who has asked to be released from work on a busy weekend to attend a family gathering out of town might receive the following neutral response: "No offense, but a rule is a rule. If I make an exception for you; others will expect it too. Have you asked anyone to trade days off with you?" Alternatively, the employee would still feel sad about working but would feel less antagonistic toward the supervisor if he or she were to receive the following empathic response: "I realize how badly you feel about not being able to attend the family gathering. I feel terrible myself having to refuse your request. I am truly sorry, but I can't afford to let you off." The supervisor, by letting the subordinate know that he or she has understood the subordinate's underlying feelings and is sympathetic, uses the most effective means of de-fusing the subordinate's anger or antagonism. There is additional discussion of empathy in other chapters of this text.

Paraphrasing, a Critical Skill for Dietetics Professionals

Most people have not incorporated the skill of paraphrasing into their communication repertoire. Even after people realize how vital this step is and begin to practice it, they may feel uncomfortable. Often the person just beginning to use paraphrasing in interactions feels self-conscious and fears others may be insulted or think he is "showing off" professional communication skills. A hint for the professional feeling awkward about asking clients and staff to paraphrase would be to ask for the paraphrase by acknowledging your own need to verify that what was heard is what the other intended.

> **E X A M P L E :** *"I know that I don't always explain as well as I should, and that frequently, people have questions. The topic is complicated. Just to be sure I clearly covered the instructions, would you mind explaining in your own words how you will plan your meals?"*

Of course, it takes less time to ask, "Do you understand?" Asking this question is less effective, however. Because of the perceived status distinction between the helper and the person being helped, the latter may be ashamed to admit that he or she has not understood. Perhaps the person being helped is thinking that he or she can read about it later or ask the patient in the next bed for an explanation after the professional leaves the room. When persons of perceived higher status ask others if they "understand," almost always the answer is, "yes." This phenomenon is particularly likely when working within certain ethnic groups, such as the Japanese. Another possibility is that the client or staff member honestly believes that he or she has understood, and for that reason has answered, "yes." The understanding, however, may include some alteration of the original message, in the form of substitution, distortion, addition, or subtraction. The skill of paraphrasing needs to become second nature and automatic for the dietetics practitioner to verify important instructions and significant client/staff disclosures.

Because of the anxiety attached to being in the presence of another of perceived higher status, the client or staff member may be less articulate than usual when describing symptoms or explaining a problem. The dietetics practitioner should paraphrase to verify that he or she understands the message as the "sender" intends. The professional should try to avoid sounding too clinical with such comments as "What I hear you saying is . . ." or "Let me repeat what you just said"; rather, keep the language clear, simple, and natural. A comment such as "I want to make sure I am understanding this; let me repeat what you are saying in my own words" is more natural.

Two points need to be emphasized regarding paraphrasing: (1) Not everything the other person says needs paraphrasing. It would become a distraction if, after every sentence, the professional interrupted with a request to paraphrase. Paraphrasing is essential only when the discussion is centered on critical information that must be understood. (2) Paraphrasing often leads to additional disclosure and therefore tends to cause longer interaction sessions. People are so accustomed to being with others who do not really listen that when they are with someone who proves he or she has been paying attention by repeating the content of what has been said, they usually want to talk more. For the dietetics professional, this additional information can be valuable. Another benefit is that after the client or staff member has expressed all questions and concerns and has cleared his or her mental agenda, he or she is psychologically ready to sit back and listen or to solve problems. By talking too much or too soon, the professional may not be able to convey all of the message to the other, who may be using the difference in time between how fast the professional speaks and how fast the professional's own mind processes information (the human mind operates five to eight times faster than human speech) to rehearse what he is going to say next.

SELF ASSESSMENT—Paraphrase the following:

1. Client: "I've been overweight most of my life. I've tried many different diets; I lose a few pounds, and gain it all back."

2. Employee: "I don't know why you want to keep changing things around here. Our old manager was satisfied with our procedures."

Nonverbal Communication

Of the two messages received simultaneously by receivers—verbal and nonverbal— ordinarily the nonverbal is more influential. As receivers of messages, people learn to trust their interpretations of nonverbal behavior more than the verbal word choices consciously selected by the sender. Intuitively, they know that control of nonverbal behavior is generally unconscious, whereas control of verbal messages is usually deliberate.

Communication experts and social scientists feel that the image that a person projects accounts for over half of the total message conveyed to another person at a first meeting. Personal appearance, including clothing, hairstyle, and accessories, is one of the most important elements of the image. Personal space variables should be experimented with to determine where a person feels most comfortable and how that distance makes others feel.

The chief nonverbal vehicles inherent in communicators are facial expression, tone of voice, eye contact, gesture, and touch, with meanings varying across cultures; see Figure 2-2. Receivers of communication perceive nonverbal behavior in clusters. Ordinarily, do not notice posture, eye contact, or facial expression isolated from the other nonverbal channels. For this reason, professionals need to monitor all nonverbal communication vehicles so that together the clusters are congruent with one another as well as with the verbal messages.

Facial expression is usually the first nonverbal trait noticed in interaction. A relaxed face with pleasant expression is congruent with a supportive climate. A supportive tone of voice is one that is calm, controlled, energetic, and enthusiastic. Supportive eye contact includes gazing at the other person in a way that allows the communicator to encounter the other visually—to the extent of being able to notice the other's facial and bodily messages. Besides being an excellent vehicle for feedback, eye contact also ensures the other person of the dietetics professional's interest and desire to communicate. Attending to the other visually allows inferences of interest, concern,

Fingers Crossed
•Protection
•Friendship
•Copulation
•Go to the
  bathroom

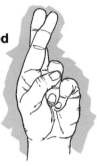

V Sign
•Horns
•Victory
•Two
•Sexual insult

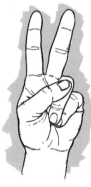

Ear Touch
•Effeminate
•Warning
•Good
•Informer
•Protection
•Disbelief
•Has no
  meaning

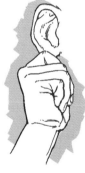

Thumbs Up
•Okay
•One
•Sexual insult
•Hitchhike
•Direction
•Patron
•Boss
•Husband

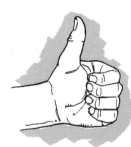

Vertical Horn Sign
•Cuckold
•General insult
•Protection
•Curse
•Two

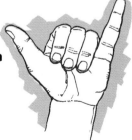

Figure 2-2 Meaning varies across cultures (Based on Klopf DW. Intercultural encounters, 4th ed. Englewood, CO: Morton Publishing Company, 1998.)

and respect. The professional's posture is best when leaning somewhat toward the person rather than away from the person. Large expansive gestures may be interpreted as a show of power and generally should be avoided.

Like eye contact, touch can work positively in two ways: (1) Through a gentle touch, a pat, or a squeeze of the hand, one can communicate instantly a desire to solve a problem without offending the other. Touch can communicate affection, concern, and interest faster than these messages can be generated verbally. (2) Like eye contact, touch is a vehicle for feedback. Although an individual may look calm, controlled, and totally at ease, a touch can reveal nervousness and insecurity. These clues, when monitored by the dietetics practitioner, often provide insight. The practitioner reacts to them by spending more time putting the person at ease; he or she has the individual paraphrase to make sure information is being understood and makes an effort to alter the communication style to be more overt in support. People usually respond positively to touch, whether or not they are consciously aware of it.

Although the content preceding is valid for most of the contemporary American public, remember that variations among ethnic groups may require professionals to adapt their nonverbal behavior, as seen in the example here. If the client shows any sign of resisting or objecting to the professional's eye contact or touch, for example, the professional should immediately desist.

Inappropriate Nonverbal Messages According to Various Ethnic Groups

Bulgaria	A nod means "no"; a shake of the head "yes."
Australia	Winking at women is improper.
Fiji	Folding one's arms shows disrespect.
Finland	Folding one's arms shows arrogance and pride.
Egypt	Tapping fingers together means, "Would you like to sleep together?"
Greece	Waving is an insult.
Brazil	A-OK means the same as flipping the middle finger in the USA.
Parts of Europe	Gucci loafers are considered bedroom slippers.
Japan	Only an occasional glance into the other person's face is polite. An uncovered neck in women is considered sensuous; keep covered.
Romania	Eating with your napkin on your lap is taboo.
England	Shouting in public is frowned on.
Hungary	Saying "bus" means fornication.
Brazil	Thumb between index and middle finger is an obscenity.
Philippines	Women dressed in trousers, blouse, and braless is taboo.
China	A formal, dark suit with beige loafers at an important meeting is taboo.

Dietetics Professionals Must Be Alert to Nonverbal Signals Emanating from the Other

Besides the professional's concerns with the environment and his or her own verbal and nonverbal behavior in an attempt to create a trusting climate, the professional must also be sensitive to nonverbal cues in other people. Even though the practitioner is being open, natural, caring, and attending to his or her own behavior and the environment, the internal anxiety, confusion, nervousness, or fear in people may be causing them to misunderstand or to react inappropriately. Two requirements for effective interpersonal communication are to observe the nonverbal cues in others and then respond to them in an affirming way.

If the client or employee is nodding the head to suggest understanding but looks puzzled, the professional needs to verify understanding by having the person paraphrase important instructions or dietary recommendations. If the patient is flushed, has trembling hands, or tears rolling down the cheeks, the professional may need to deal directly with relieving anxiety before communicating instructions or explanations. Until the patient is relaxed enough to concentrate, optimal two-way communication is unlikely.

After talking with one another for only a few minutes, both the dietetics practitioner and the client can sense the "warmness" or "coldness" of the other, as well as the degree of the other's concern. Each person tends to generalize these impressions, while inferring additional traits. If the speaker has a gentle touch, pleasant expression, and looks directly into the eyes of the listener as he or she talks, he or she might be generating inferences in the listener of being a caring spouse, supportive community member, or loving parent. After the initial positive impression has been created, the impression tends to spread into other areas not directly related to the originally observed behavior. The process can work in reverse as well. If the professional does not look at the client as he or she talks or touches the client too firmly and has an unpleasant facial expression, the inferences being created now may be negative—arrogance, lack of concern, indifference, and "coldness." Even though these initial reactions, both positive and negative, may be inaccurate, faulty first impressions are common. The helping professional might not be given a second chance to win the client's trust and cooperation; the client's inferences regarding the professional's concern and positive regard need to be anticipated and begun at the initial encounter.

Positive Affect Must Be Consistent

Seeing clients/employees regularly gives practitioners (or managers) an opportunity to reinforce or alter the perceptions the other person has of them. If you are cold, aloof, and uncaring on a daily basis, and, suddenly, because it is time to conduct a performance appraisal or counseling session with an employee, you act differently, you will not be believed. Practitioners need to be consistent in adding positive inferences to the impressions of their staff and clients. Dietetics professionals must make a total commitment to the word-of-mouth process by listening and questioning effectively, taking appropriate action, focusing on a subordinate/client orientation, delivering on promises, and teaching people—both employees and clients—how to seek information efficiently.

Not only is it important to attempt to generate concern through your own nonverbal behavior, manner, and disposition, it is also essential to control, whenever possible, the communication environment so that it, too, leads to positive inferences with a minimum of "interference." Attractive offices, pastel-colored rooms, soft lighting, comfortable and private space for counseling, and comfortable furniture all can add to the client's or staff member's collective perception, promoting inferences that you as a professional are concerned. Empirical studies, for example, reported that because so much of the professional's counseling takes place in a clinical setting, more attention must be given to creating an inviting educational atmosphere within this environment and attending closely to nonverbal cues.(14–15)

Related indirectly to effective communication are the actual dress and physical appearance of the professional. Dress and appearance are usually consciously selected, and they are nonverbal communication vehicles. The female dietetics practitioner who is overly made up or too strongly scented or the male practitioner who is wearing a nose ring or open shirt revealing a hairy chest may be well-meaning and competent. However, by their dress they risk offending a more conservative person. Professionals communicate their image best when they are clean and wearing clean and pressed clothing and only a mildly scented cologne. Because any ostentatious show of material wealth or status tends to provoke a defense reaction in others, items such as expensive jewelry and other valuable possessions should not be worn.

Another aspect of effective communication is conflict management. In the workplace, the way to win an argument is to stop it as quickly as possible by settling the dispute rationally. This is not easy to do because generally people are programmed to respond to aggression in one of three ways: fighting back, running away, or becoming immobilized. Sometimes, when dealing with a hostile client or employee, the professional may want to remain calm and supportive, but the body may refuse to cooperate. The face may turn red, hands may begin to shake, and voices may become loud and threatening. If this occurs, acknowledge that although you had wished to resolve the problem with the individual, you are feeling defensive and realize that this might be upsetting the person. Because the individual sees the physical manifestations of the professional's defensiveness, the dietetics professional should acknowledge the reaction rather than attempt to feign control. Under these circumstances, avoid further immediate communication and schedule another appointment after regaining composure.

Among the requirements for effective interpersonal communication is the need for the dietetics practitioner to send verbal and nonverbal messages that are congruent with one another. A client may hear a practitioner say, "I want to help you; I'm concerned about your health and the possible recurrence of your heart problem as a result of your food choices." But if, at the same time, the client sees the practitioner making no attempt to connect physically through handshake and looking down at notes or checking his or her watch rather than looking at the client, the contradictory second message of impersonality or impatience will be more intense than the stated message of concern. The professional may have said all the "right" words but is judged as insincere.

Helping professionals and managers who do not genuinely like working with people are destined ultimately to fail; often, however, professionals who do like people and care for their clients and employees fail as well. To be

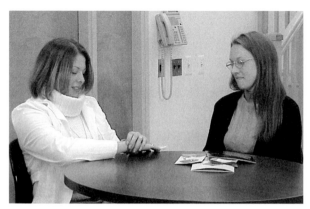

Clients are aware of the professional's nonverbal behavior.

successful in working with others, the professional must develop congruent verbal and nonverbal communication skills. A person can develop all the appropriate verbal skills and still be unsuccessful in calming a hostile employee or in securing a client's agreement to the dietary plan. Only when the professional treats others with respect, soliciting their opinions and responding to them, can an environment of trust and openness be created.(16)

> *Communication is a continual balancing act, juggling the conflicting needs for intimacy and independence. To survive in the world, we have to act in concert with others, but to survive as ourselves, rather than simply as cogs in a wheel, we have to act alone.*
>
> **Deborah Tannen (20th century)**

LISTENING SKILLS

Well-developed listening skills are an essential requirement for effective interpersonal communication between health practitioners and their clients and staff.(17–25) An individual with average intelligence can process information at speeds of approximately five times that of human speech. The higher the intelligence, the faster the mind tends to process information. Some individuals can think at speeds of eight to ten times the rate of human speech. Thus, while practitioners are listening to their clients or staff members talk, they have time to be thinking about other things simultaneously. Everyone has had the experience of listening to a speaker and thinking about what that person might be like at home or of letting the mind wander to other topics. From the speaker's clothes, shoes, jewelry, diction, and speech patterns, people tend to fill in details and develop an elaborate scenario while they listen, more or less, to the presentation. The process of good listening involves learning to harness your attention so that you are able to concentrate totally on the speaker's message, both verbal and nonverbal. Development of these skills is not difficult, but it does require a conscious effort and perseverance.

Listening is taught as an academic subject in the department of communication studies in most colleges and universities; in fact, people have earned PhD degrees studying the subject. The bottom line, however, is that listening ability can be enriched only when the person desires such enrichment and is willing to follow the training with practice. The following list of four of the most common issues related to poor listening is an excellent starting place for readers who desire to practice improving listening skills:

1. Most people have a limited and undeveloped attention span.
2. People tend to stop listening when they have decided that the material is uninteresting and tend to pay attention only to material they "like" or see an immediate benefit in knowing.
3. Listeners tend to trust their intuition regarding the speaker's credibility, basing their judgments more on the speaker's nonverbal behavior than on the content of the message.
4. Listeners tend to attach too much credibility to messages heard on electronic media, such as radio, television, movies, tapes, and so forth.

Listening can be improved with practice. The most important step in such improvement is resolving to listen more efficiently. Simply being motivated to listen causes one to be more alert and active as a receiver. The following are specific suggestions for improving listening:

1. Before engaging in the communication transaction, listeners should remind themselves of their intent to listen carefully.
2. The communication situation should be approached with the attitude of objectivity, with an open mind, and with a spirit of inquiry.
3. Listeners need to watch for clues. Just as one uses bold type and italics in writing, speakers use physical arrangement, program outlines, voice inflection, rate, emphasis, voice quality, and bodily actions as aids to help the listener determine the meaning of what is being said and what the speaker believes is most important.
4. Listeners need to make use of the thinking-speaking time difference and to remind themselves to concentrate on the speaker's message. They must use the extra time to think critically about the message, to relate it to what they already know, to consider the logic of the arguments, and to notice the accompanying nonverbal behavior—all simultaneously.
5. Listeners need to look beyond the actual words to determine what the speaker means, and to determine whether the clusters of accompanying nonverbal behavior are congruent with the verbal message.
6. Listeners need to provide feedback to the speaker, either indirectly through nonverbal reactions or directly through paraphrasing, to verify that what is being understood by the listener is what the speaker intends.

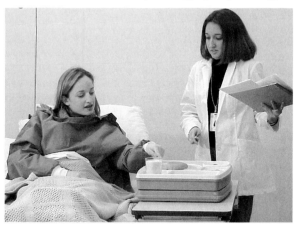
Listening is an essential skill.

Giving accurate feedback is the best way to prove that another person's message has been heard and understood. Ultimately, the most valuable listening skill is ongoing practice. Those who want to improve their listening must put themselves in difficult listening situations, must concentrate, and must practice good listening.

NEGOTIATION

Negotiation permeates human interaction; everyone needs to negotiate. Negotiation can be defined as a process in which two or more parties exchange goods or services and attempt to agree on the exchange rate for them. Negotiating with clients refers to the exchange of alternatives for dietary change between the dietetics professional and the client. The purpose of this section of text is to introduce dietetics practitioners to the concept and to reference them to more detailed accounts.(26–32)

Before actually engaging in the negotiating process, people need to take time to assess their own goals, consider the other party's goals and interests, and develop a strategy. Generally, the process is considered to consist of five stages: preparation and planning, definition of ground rules, clarification and justification of one another's positions, the actual bargaining and problem-solving discussion, and, finally, closure and implementation. Negotiating with clients involves discussing several alternative dietary changes, involving the client in the selection of the alternative being considered, and modifying the options until they are acceptable.

The following suggestions can improve your negotiating skills in the workplace:

Begin with a positive overture. Concessions tend to be reciprocated and lead to agreements. Even a small concession is perceived as a positive overture and stimulates a reciprocal give and take climate.

Address problems, not personalities. There is little value in focusing on the personal characteristics of the other. Negotiators understand that what is important is the other's ideas or position, and those can be disagreed with, not the individual personally. Separating the people from the problem and not personalizing differences characterize the seasoned negotiator.

Pay attention to initial discussions and offers. Everyone has to have an initial position, and it should be thought of as merely a point of departure. When initial offers are extreme and idealistic, the sophisticated negotiator remains calm and nonjudgmental and counters with a more realistic option or options.

Emphasize win-win solutions. Inexperienced negotiators often assume that any gain must come at the expense of the other party. When a person is patient and willing to tolerate the uncertainty and ambiguity that accompanies what seems like a deadlocked situation, creative thinking is most likely to occur with solutions that allow both people to be satisfied and conclude with win-win solutions. When you enter into the process assuming a zero-sum game in which one can only win if the other loses, missed opportunities for trade-offs that could benefit both sides occur. When conditions are supportive and options are framed in terms of the opponent's interests, synergetic solutions are most likely to surface in negotiations.

Create an open and trusting climate. To negotiate well, the negotiator needs well-honed communication skills, especially the skill of listening. Skilled negotiators ask more questions, focus their alternatives more directly, are less defensive, and have learned to avoid words and phrases that can irritate others. They know how to create an open and trusting climate, the kind of climate so critical for an integrative settlement.

Although there appears to be no significant direct relationship between an individual's personality and negotiation style, cultural background is relevant. The contemporary practitioner/negotiator benefits from an understanding of the other's cultural context. For example, the French tend to like conflict and tend to take a long time in negotiating agreement, not being particularly concerned about whether their opponents like or dislike them. The Chinese, too, tend to draw out negotiations, but they believe negotiations never end and are always willing to start over. Americans, however, are known for their impatience and desire to be liked. Many astute international negotiators turn these characteristics to their advantage with Americans by dragging out negotiations and withholding friendship as conditional on the final settlement.

Negotiating skills improve with time and experience. You need to understand the principles and look for opportunities to practice them. Dietetics practitioners need not wait for differences to begin learning. Practicing in your private/personal life is often less threatening and can provide an excellent training field.

COMMUNICATING WITH LEGISLATORS

Knowledge of how to communicate with legislators has become another skill critical for health care professionals generally and dietetics professionals specifically. Thousands of voices compete for congressional attention as laws are written and money is provided for everything from health care to weapons.(33–37)

Lobbying can be both effective and ethical. In a democratic society, where government is designed to represent and protect the interests of all citizens and all parties, talking with legislators is exactly what people should do to ensure that decisions and legislation reflect a consensus and take into consideration the interests of all parties affected. Besides using the services of professional lobbyists, organizations such as the American Dietetic Association benefit from the networking and contacts made by the members of the profession. One of the most effective ways to make legislators aware of issues is at the grassroots level. It is naive to assume that government officials know everything they need to know about the dietetics profession. It becomes the members' responsibility to talk with elected representatives, get to know them and their staff, get on a first-name basis with them, and earn their trust and respect. The time to get networked with public officials, making sure they appreciate the point of view from the perspective of dietetics practitioners, is before they start considering legislation that might be of interest to the dietetics profession. Some of the ways to get the message across include working with the profession's national association, writing letters, making phone calls, meeting with congressman or senators in the home district, developing a relationship with the district administrative assistant, and developing a relationship with health staffers who handle the issues relating to the dietetics profession.

Individuals, organizations, and professional associations can influence the way laws are made and enforced. The contemporary dietetics professional should consider the task of communicating with legislators as another professional responsibility. The professional, by the way, who learns how to communicate with legislators and develops a network of political connections becomes invaluable to the organization and develops increased power and prestige as a result.

This chapter has presented numerous suggestions for improving the dietitian's and dietetic technician's communication competence with clients and staff. One can, however, read and reread this chapter, pass a quiz on the material with a grade of A+, and still be ineffective in practicing communication skills. To develop communication skills, readers must begin immediately to put into practice what has been read. Do not be discouraged because practice is necessary. Generally, months of conscious attention to these skills are needed before they become a part of your natural approach to clients and staff.

CASE STUDY 1

Joan Stivers, RD, noted on the medical record that her patient, John Jones, age 63, was 5'11" tall and weighed 250 pounds. A retiree, he was just diagnosed with type II diabetes mellitus. Joan stopped by his hospital room, introduced herself, and told him that the purpose of her visit was to discuss his current food intake. During the conversation, Mr. Jones and his roommate were watching a baseball game on television and periodically commented briefly on the plays and players. Finally, Mr. Jones said, "You need to talk to my wife, not me. She does the cooking." Just then, the physician came by to make rounds.

1. Identify the barriers to communication.
2. What should the dietetics professional do to overcome the barriers?

CASE STUDY 2

John is a new employee in the kitchen. He was hired as an assistant cook 2 months ago. Although his skills are good, the manager noticed that his attendance could be better. In the past 2 weeks, he has been late for work 3 times, ranging from 10 to 35 minutes. Today he is late again, and the manager asks him to come into the office.

1. What should the manager do to create a supportive communication climate?
2. What should the manager say to John?

Nothing is as frightening to humans as the fear of uncertainty and ambiguity. When people have the opportunity to try out new communication behavior, forces within them tend to pull them toward their past behavior. Even when the old strategies are unsuccessful, they generally tend to be repeated because the probable outcomes are predictable.

The professional who is serious about increasing communication competence needs to swallow hard and stretch, forcing him- or herself to attempt the new behavior. The time to begin is now. You do not need to have access to clients or staff. You can exercise these skills just as effectively in your personal as in your professional life. Despite all the problems, improved communication is possible, and the professional who is aware of the problems and the recommended safeguards to minimize them is going to be more effective.

REVIEW AND DISCUSSION QUESTIONS

1. In the helping professions, what conveys the professional's effectiveness with clients and staff?
2. What are the common elements of the definition of communication?
3. What are the components of the communication model?

4. What are the verbal guidelines for creating a supportive communication climate?
5. Of the two messages received simultaneously by receivers, which is more influential, verbal or nonverbal?
6. What are the four most common poor listening habits?
7. What are some specific suggestions for improving listening?

SUGGESTED ACTIVITIES

1. After filling out the questions below, join with classmates in groups of three to share and discuss your responses with one another.

   A. What types of nonverbal signals from your instructor or supervisor indicate to you that he or she is unhappy?

      a.
      b.
      c.

   B. What nonverbal cues indicate that you are getting angry?

      a.
      b.
      c.

   C. List some of the nonverbal signals that you send when you are talking and some-one interrupts you.

      a.
      b.
      c.

   D. List some of the nonverbal signals you send when you want to signal confidence or approval of the other person.

      a.
      b.
      c.

   E. List changes you might make in the room where you are reading to alter its climate positively.

      a.
      b.
      c.

2. Write a two-paragraph description of a current interpersonal conflict you are experiencing. Be sure to indicate: (1) the behavior on the part of the other that has caused you a problem and (2) what "feelings" you are experiencing as a result of that behavior. Do not sign your name unless you want to be acknowledged. After the instructor has collected the descriptions, he or she may read them and either invite students to participate in role-playing of the situations using the guidelines for supportive verbal and nonverbal behavior or engage the class in a case study discussion of how the communication skills might be used to resolve the conflict.

3. You can increase your knowledge of nonverbal behavior by viewing others talking but not hearing what they are saying. Turn the television to a soap opera or talk show; turn off the volume, watch the nonverbal behavior, and try to interpret it.

After 3 to 5 minutes, turn the volume up. Then again, turn off the volume. Do this several times and attempt to grasp the verbal messages without the sound by merely interpreting the nonverbal behavior. Take notes and be prepared to share your experience in class.

4. As an in-class exercise, silently jot down your general "meanings" for the nonverbal behaviors listed below. Compare answers with classmates. Is there general agreement on all, or is there a range of answers? Where answers vary, discuss the possible reasons why.

   a. lack of sustained eye contact
   b. lowering of eyes/looking away
   c. furrow on brow
   d. tight lips
   e. biting lip or quivering of lower lip
   f. nodding head up and down
   g. hanging head down
   h. shaking head right to left
   i. folding arms across chest
   j. unfolded arms
   k. leaning forward
   l. slouching, leaning back
   m. trembling hands
   n. flushed face
   o. holding hands tightly
   p. tapping foot continuously
   q. sitting behind a desk
   r. sitting nearby without any intervening objects

5. The following is an exercise that you might try with friends. The first person expresses the message to the second person, who in turn expresses it to the third, and so on, until six people have heard it. Ordinarily, the message is audiotaped and played back. This allows the participants to see the many ways in which messages are altered as they pass from person to person.

> **MESSAGE:** *A child has hurt herself at the pool, and I must report it to the police. It is necessary, however, for me to get to the hospital as soon as possible. She was walking up the diving board and getting reading to jump, when someone in a blue bathing suit pushed ahead. A boy in a red suit tried to stop her, but she fell off and landed on her back. The boy claims it was the young girl's fault, but she blames him.*

WEB SITES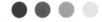

COMMUNICATING WITH LEGISLATORS

http://www.cahsah.org/rootfind.asp / communicating with legislators

LISTENING SKILLS

http://www.advanceforot.com/pastarticles/oct25_00feature4.html / practitioners' listening skills

VERBAL AND NONVERBAL COMMUNICATION

http://www.psych.ucr.edu/faculty/friedman/journal.html / nonverbal communication between patients and medical practitioners

MOTIVATION AND SELF-ESTEEM

http://www.humanlinks.com/manres/articles/self_esteem.htm / self-esteem and employees

REFERENCES

1. Benzold C, Kang J. Looking to the future: the role of the ADA environmental scan. J Am Diet Assoc 1999;99:989.
2. Patterson R, Satia J, Kristal A, et al. Is there a consumer backlash against the diet and health message? J Am Diet Assoc 2001;101:37.
3. Hunt A, Hilgenkamp K, Farley R. Skills and competencies of dietitians practicing in wellness settings. J Am Diet Assoc 2000;100:1537.
4. Dodds J, Polhamus B. Self-perceived competence of advanced public health nutritionists in the United States. J Am Diet Assoc 1999;99:807.
5. Clark N. Identifying the educational needs of aspiring sports nutritionists. J Am Diet Assoc 2000;100:1622.
6. ADA Reports. Practice report of the American Dietetic Association: home care: an emerging practice area for dietetics. J Am Diet Assoc 2000;100:1453.
7. Kirk D, Shanklin C, Gorman, MA. Attributes and qualifications that employers seek when hiring dietitians in business and industry. J Am Diet Assoc 1989:89:494.
8. Fielden JS. Why can't managers communicate? Business 1989;39:41.
9. Tindall WN, Beardsley RS, Kimberlin CW. Communication in pharmacy practice, 3rd ed. Baltimore: Lippincott Williams & Wilkins, 1994.
10. Valentine P. Management of conflict. J Adv Nurs (England) 1995;22:1.
11. Fritchie R. Conflict and its management. Brit J Hosp Med (England) 1995;53:9.
12. Littlefield V. Conflict resolution. J Prof Nurs 1995;11:1.
13. Picus SS. Evaluation of the nutrition-counseling environment of hospitalized patients. J Am Diet Assoc 1989;89:403.
14. Giannini A. Measurement of nonverbal receptive abilities in medical students. Perceptual and Motor Skills 2000;90:1145.
15. Langton S. The mutual influence of gaze and head orientation in the analysis of social attention direction. Quart J Exp Psych 2000;53:825.
16. Field L, Knowles L. Can we talk? The key to a productive management pattern. Canadian Mgr 1989;14:21.
17. Wachs J. Listening. AAOHN Journal (Official Journal of the American Association of Occupational Health Nurses) 1995;43:11.
18. Giron M, Manjon-Arce P. Clinical interview skills and identification of emotional disorders in primary care. Am J Psychiatr 1998;155:530.
19. Mechanic D, Meyer S. Concepts of trust among patients with serious illness. Soc Sci Med 2000;51:651.
20. Doescher M, Saver B, Franks P, Fiscella K. Racial and ethnic disparities in perceptions of physician style and trust. Arch Fam Med 2000;9:1156.

21. Pechham S. Big ears goes to work. Nurs Times 1997;93:22.
22. Hagevik S. Just listening. J Environ Health 2001;62:46.
23. Donahue M. How active is your listening? Current Health 1999;223:27.
24. Muchnick J. The listening challenge. Parents Mag 1999;74:179.
25. Giordano J. Effective communication and counseling with older adults. Int J Aging Hum Dev 2000;51:315.
26. Adelman S. Physicians for responsible negotiations will be heard. Western J Med 1999;22:298.
27. Bragg T. The manager as negotiator. Occupational Hazards 2000;62:53.
28. Frings C. How to negotiate effectively. Med Lab Observer 2000;32:38.
29. Allen D, Ch'ien A, et al. Employment contracts, negotiation strategies and the nurse practitioner. Nurs Pract 2000;25:18.
30. Mangan D. Shape a contract you'll be glad you signed. Med Econ 2000;78:79.
31. Hagevick S. Negotiating your way to success. J Environ Health 2000;62:34.
32. Mandel J. Top 10 tips for negotiation. Med Meetings 2000;27:106.
33. White J, Hughes B. Influencing legislators. J Am Diet Assoc 2001;101:172.
34. Landers S. Ashwini S. How do physicians lobby their members of congress? Arch Intern Med 2000;160:3248.
35. Lindgren J. Dr. Smith goes to Washington: 20 tips for effective lobbying. Am Fam Physician 1997;56:291.
36. Hofford R. Seven tips for effecting legislative change. Fam Pract Mgt 2001;8:35.
37. Stoil M. Be prepared for the new lobbying. Nurs Homes 1998;47:8.

CHAPTER 3 Interviewing

After reading this chapter, you will be able to

1. discuss the purposes of different kinds of interviews, such as a nutrition interview and a pre-employment interview.
2. explain the conditions necessary for effective interviewing.
3. identify the parts of an interview and what should be included in each.
4. discuss the advantages and disadvantages of various types of questions.
5. develop a list of appropriate questions for a nutrition interview and sequence them.
6. identify the different types of responses to an interviewee's remarks.
7. use techniques of interviewing and conduct a nutrition interview.

Professional: "What did you have to eat yesterday?"
Client: "Yesterday? I don't remember."

Although the client may not be able to answer the above question on the spur of the moment, recall can be improved with some prompting from a good interviewer. The client may be reminded of the day of the week, where he or she spent the day, whether meals were eaten at home or at a restaurant, whether others were present, and so on.

Before a dietetics professional can begin to counsel people about their nutritional needs or food choices, it is important to determine what they are eating now. Using interviewing techniques, the practitioner questions the client to complete an assessment of current eating practices and their nutritional adequacy.

Interviewing skills are equally as important in management positions. They are used to screen potential new employees, to obtain information from current employees, and to explore solutions to problems.

This chapter covers the basics of interviewing skills. Included are the principles and process of interviews, the conditions facilitating interviews, the three parts of an interview, the use of different types of questions, and the types of interviewer responses. The interview is a complex process with many interacting variables. One must be aware of the impact of the environment, verbal and nonverbal communication interactions, perceptions and roles of the two parties, needs and interests, personalities, attitudes, beliefs and values, and feedback. To become a skilled interviewer takes time and practice until the principles and techniques come naturally.

Interviewing may be defined as a guided communication process between two people with the predetermined purpose of exchanging or obtaining specific information by questioning. The goal of the interview is to collect specific, accurate information from the respondent while maintaining an interpersonal environment conducive to disclosure.

An effective interviewer must be a good listener. The interviewer concentrates on both the verbal responses and the nonverbal behavior, or body language, of the respondent. To discover what is important to the client, listen not only for facts, but also for emotions, attitudes, feelings, and values. A person newly diagnosed with diabetes mellitus, for example, may be upset, anxious, or fearful. These emotions need to be recognized and dealt with before counseling is begun.

To illustrate the interviewing principles and process, two examples of interviews are presented in this chapter—the nutrition interview and the pre-employment interview. Although a full explanation of the content of these types of interviews is beyond the scope of this book, a brief explanation of each follows. For more detailed information on content, other sources should be examined.(1–7)

NUTRITION INTERVIEWS

A nutrition interview is an account of a person's food habits, preferences, eating behaviors, and other factors influencing food choices discussed in Chapter 1. An initial nutritional assessment interview serves one or more purposes:

- Makes counselor and client aware of client's dietary practices and their origins, influential lifestyle factors, and related information.
- Contributes to accurately defining the nutritional status of the client in conjunction with other data.
- Defines problems and issues so that realistic goals can be set.
- Helps the counselor identify possible alternatives to suggest for change.
- Continues to develop rapport and a good relationship with the client.
- Discovers any nutritional problems and screens for malnutrition so that an appropriate nutrition care plan is developed.
- Provides baseline data against which one monitors changes.

Currently, there is no gold standard method for obtaining information about a person's dietary intake, but approaches used frequently are the 24-hour recall, the record of usual daily food intake, and the food frequency checklist; the situation guides the selection. All forms of dietary assessment have inherent inaccuracies.(7–9)

In the 24-hour recall, the interviewer asks the client to recount the types and amounts of foods and beverages consumed in the previous 24-hour period. The second method, the usual daily food intake, asks clients to explain the types and amounts of foods and beverages that they *usually* consume during one day's time. In both approaches, the portion sizes, the methods of food preparation (frying versus roasting), the between-meal snacks, the times of day food is consumed, the condiments, the use of vitamin and mineral supplements or alternative nutrition therapies, and any alcoholic beverages consumed require consideration.

No method is considered to have a high degree of accuracy in assessing the nutritional status of the client, and each has potential deficiencies.(4,8) For example:

- The previous 24-hour period may not have been typical.
- Weekends may differ from weekdays.
- There are seasonal variations.
- The person may be unable to judge portion sizes.
- The person may have memory lapses.
- There is underreporting.
- Certain food may be considered socially undesirable or unhealthy by the client, so he or she prefers not to reveal eating it.

To overcome the problem of judging portion sizes, counselors may use three-dimensional food models, food pictures, serving utensils, dishes, and beverage glasses. An 8-ounce glass is small, for example, compared with the large servings at convenience stores and fast-food restaurants. Portions of foods such as potato chips, French fries, and popcorn may be difficult to visualize. A selection of food packages may also be helpful.

Reports indicate that clients do not volunteer information about foods they consider that others think are less desirable. Examples of sensitive topics include chocolate, alcoholic beverages, certain snacks, butter/margarine, take-out foods, and others.(7,8) A skilled interviewer needs to inquire about these.

One way to increase the accuracy of the information is to use a food frequency checklist in addition. A food frequency determines the daily or weekly frequency of consuming basic foods, such as milk and dairy products, meats-fish-poultry, eggs, fruits and fruit juices, vegetables and salads, breads and cereals, desserts and sweets, butter-margarine-fats and oils, between-meal snacks, and beverages, including coffee, tea, colas, and alcoholic beverages. If the client responds about consumption of orange juice during the food frequency, for example, and it was not mentioned during the usual daily intake, the interviewer can prompt the client to recall where it fits into the daily pattern and in what amount. This improves the assessment of energy and nutrient intake.(4) The food frequency can be targeted to the dietary problem, such as emphasizing dietary sources of fat in heart disease, foods high in sodium in hypertension, or calcium and vitamin D in osteoporosis.

PRE-EMPLOYMENT INTERVIEWS

An example of an interview used by a management professional is the pre-employment interview with prospective employees. Several applicants may be interviewed for a position. A structured interview in which all questions are preplanned and each applicant is asked the same questions is recommended.(3,6) The same interviewing principles and techniques are used, but for a different purpose. In this case, the interviewer wants to find the applicant with the competencies and talents that best match the requirements of the job according to the job description. Because federal legislation outlaws discrimination based on race, color, religion, gender, national origin, age over 40, and disability, questions about any of these are not recommended and may lead to lawsuits. Those who need more information should consult additional resources.(3,6)

CONDITIONS FACILITATING INTERVIEWS

For best results, you need to increase your effectiveness as an interviewer(5,10) by including the following:

- Clearly defining the *purpose* of the interview to the interviewee.
- Attentiveness to verbal and nonverbal behavior by listening.
- Building rapport.
- Providing freedom from interruptions.
- Providing psychological privacy.
- Having appropriate physical surroundings.
- Having emotional objectivity.
- Considering the personal context of the respondent.
- Limiting note taking.

Purpose

When an interviewer is asking questions, the respondent may be wondering why the questions are important. Without knowing the answer, a person may be unwilling to respond. As a result, the interviewer needs to explain the purpose of the interview as described earlier. With clients, you can also stress that the interview is necessary to provide better assistance with problems, services, or health care recommendations. For example: "Let's do a careful evaluation of your food choices and see if we find any ways to enhance your choices." With job applicants, note that it is important to find an employee who will be satisfied with the company and the position. If the purpose is clear and understood, better cooperation from the interviewee may be anticipated.

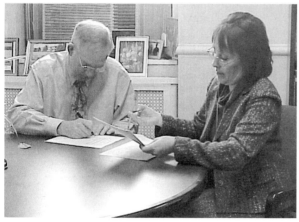

An informal setting improves an interview.

Attentiveness

Listening attentively helps to create a climate in which the interviewee can communicate easily. Dietetics professionals need to develop skills in listening, which is an active, not a passive, process and requires a great deal of concentration. Many interviewers tend to talk too much and focus on themselves. Instead, the interviewer should listen carefully and assist the respondents in communicating their thoughts and feelings. The message includes both verbal and nonverbal behaviors. Periodically paraphrasing or summarizing confirms that you are listening and trying to understand. Keep in mind that the interviewee is also observing the professional and making judgments. Frequent looking at one's watch, failure to maintain eye contact, sitting back in too relaxed a posture, frowning, yawning, and tone of voice all may convey a negative message and inhibit effective interviews. Attentiveness can be shown, for example, by appropriate nonverbal behaviors such as eye contact, interested facial expression, good posture, smiling, and nodding.

Building Rapport

Rapport should be established early in the interview and continue to be developed for a good interview climate. Rapport is the personal relationship established between the interviewer and the respondent. It is necessary to build a warm and supportive climate, to release stress, to put the person at ease, and to be nonjudgmental no matter what the person says.

The relationship between the two parties develops over time. The interviewer strives to create an environment of respect and trust by arranging conditions in which individuals perceive themselves as accepted, warmly received, valued, and understood. Trust must be earned; without it vital self-disclosure on the part of the respondent may be limited. People will not give personal information unless they trust the other person. The client's self-disclosure must be treated with respect. Avoid labeling individual's responses as "right" or "wrong," provide privacy and confidentiality, show concern and understanding through careful listening, and provide nonjudgmental verbal and nonverbal responses. Setting yourself up as the "expert" and the respondent as the "receiver of one's expertise" will inhibit the relationship. "I've had a lot of experience with this and will be able to tell you what to do," is not a helpful approach. Respondents may be overwhelmed by the professional's expertise and position, giving information they think is being sought instead of what is useful.

Rapport may be inhibited by addressing people by their first names, a practice common with close friends and family. This may be interpreted as too informal or a lack of respect by some people. A woman 72 years of age, for example, may not like being called "Martha" by someone who is 25 years old. When in doubt, use both names, such as "Martha Smith" or "Mrs. Smith" or a query "would you prefer to be addressed as Mrs. Smith or Martha?" The custom of the institution is a guide.

Freedom from Interruptions

To devote full attention to the interviewee, freedom from interruptions is needed.(5) The professional should arrange to have phone calls held; if a call must be answered, the call should be brief with apologies given. In the hospital setting, asking to turn off the television and selecting a time when staff and visitors are less likely to interrupt is advisable.

Psychological Privacy

Since private matters will be discussed, the interviewer and interviewee should be alone. A quiet office without interruption is preferable. At the patient's bedside in a hospital setting, however, others may be present in the room. Whenever possible, arrange the setting so that the interview cannot be overheard and is not interrupted; this promotes the giving of undivided attention.(5)

Assure the interviewee that information revealed will be treated confidentially and shared only with the pertinent health care providers. Anecdotes and stories should not be shared with others over coffee breaks, lunch, or social gatherings.

Physical Surroundings

A comfortable environment with proper furniture, lighting, temperature, ventilation, and pleasant surroundings can enhance an interview. A setting should be arranged in which eye contact can be maintained. Since standing over a patient lying in bed may trigger deferential behavior, it is preferable to be at the same head level. The optimum distance between people involved in an interview is 3 or 4 feet—about an arm's length—but cultural practices differ.(10) The most formal seating arrangement is for one person to sit across the desk from another, whereas a chair alongside the desk is less formal and makes people feel more equal in status.(5) Two parties seated without a table is informal, but when it is necessary to view materials, a round table is less formal than a square or rectangle because it prevents the head-of-the table position. In general, the fewer barriers to the line of sight, the better. A desk top with a computer, telephone, books, plants, and other materials between you and the client is a distraction.

Emotional Objectivity

The professional's personal feelings and preferences should be controlled and not revealed to the interviewee. The client should feel free to express all feelings, attitudes, and values and, in the process, may express some that are contrary to those of the professional. An attitude of acceptance and concern for the interviewee should be maintained, with a desire to understand behavior, rather than to pass judgment.

The professional relationship is most easily established with persons similar to ourselves whereas barriers may arise if there are differences. People from all socioeconomic groups, various cultural and ethnic groups, and ages from young to elderly participate differently in the professional relationship. A thorough understanding of the food choices and practices of other groups assists in the interview process.

Any expression of judgment or condemnation experienced by the interviewee blocks the progress. A raised eyebrow, look of shock, surprise, or amusement, or an incredulous follow-up questions (e.g., "You had three beers for lunch?" or "All you had for lunch was a box of cookies?") may cause an interviewee to change or end the story. One seeks to understand, not to pass judgment.

Interviewers should develop an awareness of their own conscious and unconscious values and prejudices. These include not only racial, ethnic, and religious preferences, but also exaggerated dislikes of people and their characteristics. Examples may include the poorly or weirdly dressed, uneducated, aggressive women, meek men, highly pitched voices, or weak handshakes. Identifying your own intolerances may help to control any expression of them through nonverbal behaviors.

Personal Context

Interviewees bring with them their own personal contexts or systems of beliefs, attitudes, feelings, and values that must be recognized. Concerns about perceived threats to health can be so frightening, for example, that they preoccupy thoughts and block conversation. You need to recognize the respondent's situation and the subjective and objective aspects of it. After a heart attack, for example, a man may feel fear, resentment, anger, anxiety, dependence, or regression, which may interfere with concentration and cooperation. An understanding of the psychological reactions to illness and ways of dealing with them is necessary. Show a sense of caring and concern to the client.

You may need to facilitate the venting of feelings and to acknowledge them before going on to the interview. A job applicant, for example, may have been laid off recently from a long-time position. The subjective way the person feels about the situation, however, is as important as the facts. Anxiety, nervousness, and depression may be evident. The professional should be alert to nonverbal and verbal clues about the person as they give a frame of reference for understanding. Interviewees may have many other things on their minds. Although the professional is focused on the task, to be effective the personal context of the respondent should not be ignored. The interviewee's thoughts and feelings come first.

Usually, the professional has some background information about the person in advance. In the hospital setting, the medical record is the source of information on the social and economic circumstances that may influence the goals for change and treatment: marital status, number in the household, age, occupation, religion, level of education, physical health, medications, weight and height, and medical history. In pre-employment interviews, the application form should be examined before the interview, since it contains information on education and previous work experience.

Cognitive approaches conceptualize four distinct stages that a person goes through in response to another's questions, each of which may lead to errors in responses—comprehension, retrieval, estimation/judgment, and response. Comprehension is the first stage in which the interviewee interprets the meaning of the question asked. In retrieval, the second stage, the respondent searches short-and long-term memory for an appropriate answer. Third, in estimation/judgment, the interviewee evaluates the relevance of the information from memory, decides whether or not it is appropriate, and possibly combines various bits of information. In the fourth and final stage, response, other factors may be weighed, such as how sensitive the information is, whether or not the answer is socially expected or desirable, the amount of accuracy to provide, and so forth. The person then provides a response to the question.(11)

Note Taking

Taking too many notes may hamper the flow of conversation, inhibit rapport between the two parties, and prevent the interviewer's concentration on the verbal and nonverbal answers of the respondent. In addition, the interviewee may be distracted or apprehensive about what is being written.(5)

The inexperienced interviewer, however, may find it necessary to take notes. If so, they should be as brief as possible. To avoid concern, the professional should ask the interviewee's permission to jot down a few notes and should explain why they are necessary and how they will be used. The practitioner may say, for example: "Is it all right if I take a few notes so that later, I can review what we said?"(6)

If writing, try to maintain eye contact as much as possible. You need to develop a few key words, phrases, or abbreviations to use. A breakfast of orange juice, cereal, toast and coffee with cream and sugar, for example, may be abbreviated, "OJ, cer, tst, C-C-S," while a pineapple-cottage cheese salad may be noted as "P/A-CC sld." This skill can be developed with time.

Comprehensive notes should be dictated or written immediately after the person has departed. Waiting 15 minutes or longer, seeing another client or job applicant, or accepting phone calls may cause the interviewer to forget essential information.

PARTS OF THE INTERVIEW

Each interview can be divided into three parts.

- Opening
- Exploration
- Closing

The beginning of the interview, or opening, involves introductions and establishing rapport, a process of creating trust and good will between the parties.(10) The exploration phase includes the use of questions to obtain information while maintaining the personal relationship, as the interviewer guides and directs the interview with responses. In the final phase, the interview is closed and any future contacts are planned. Table 3-1 summarizes the interview process.

TABLE 3-1   The Interview Process

Phases	Tasks
Opening	Introductions
	Establish rapport
	Discuss purpose
Exploration	Gather information with questions
	Explore problems
	Explore both thoughts and feelings
	Continue building rapport
Closing	Express appreciation
	Review purpose
	Ask for comments or questions
	Plan future contacts

OPENING

The opening sets the tone of the interview—friendly or unfriendly, professional or informal, relaxed or tense, leisurely or rushed—and influences how the interviewee perceives you. Interviewers should greet the client and state their name and job title, for example, "Good morning. I'm Judy Jones, a registered dietitian." A smile, eye contact, a handshake or placing a hand on the other's hand or arm, and a friendly face and tone of voice are supporting nonverbal behaviors.

In the hospital setting, the interviewer may ask, "Are you Mary Johnson?" If answered affirmatively, you may respond, "I'm glad to meet you. Do you prefer to be addressed as Mrs. Johnson or as Mary?" The professional may add how she prefers to be addressed, such as "Please call me Judy."

If the patient's physician has requested the contact, the interviewer may mention this. "Did Dr. Smith tell you that he asked me to visit you?" If the person answers "no," explain about the physician's request. A discussion of the nature and purpose of the interview may follow, along with how the interviewee will benefit from the interview. For example: "Dr. Smith mentioned that you have high blood pressure. He asked me to talk with you and see whether we can find a way to reduce the amount of salt and sodium in the foods you eat. This will help you control your blood pressure."

Before unleashing a barrage of questions, a few minutes may be spent on other topics to develop some rapport. Discussion of known information from the medical record or from the application form of job applicants may be appropriate. Alternatively, the weather, sporting events, holidays, a national or international event, traffic, parking, or any topic of joint interest may be helpful in opening the discussion. Small talk is important in developing and building the relationship between the two people. It should not be prolonged, however, or the interviewee may be wondering when the purpose will begin.

When interviewees initiate the appointment, it is preferable to let them state in their own words their problem or purpose for coming. The dietetics professional may ask, "What brought you to the Friendly Company to seek employment, Mr. Smithfield?" or 'How have things been going since your last appointment when we talked about your goals for change?" or "When we talked on the phone, Mrs. Jones, you mentioned that your doctor told you that you have borderline diabetes. How can I be of assistance?" When interviewees are given the chance to express themselves first, the interview begins with their agenda, or what they think is important. This is preferable.

Although it may be time-consuming for the busy professional, the opening exchange of either information or pleasantries is important and should not be omitted. Rapport, a degree of warmth, a supportive atmosphere, and a sense of mutual involvement are critical components in the interview. Willingness to disclose information about oneself is influenced by the level of trust established in the relationship, and cooperation and disclosure are crucial to the success of interviews. Interviewees quickly develop perceptions of the situation and make decisions about the amount and kind of information they will share. They form impressions of the interviewer just as the professional does of them. Before directing the conversation to the second stage, the purpose or nature of the interview should be clearly stated and understood so the person knows what to expect.

INTERVIEW OPENINGS SELF-ASSESSMENT

How satisfactory are the following openings? How can they be improved?

Employment Interview

1. "Come on in. I'm very busy today, but need to hire a new employee. Do you have any work experience?"

2. "Hi, I'm Steve Johnson (shaking hands). We're looking for a cook for early shift. Do you prefer early hours or late?"

Patient/Client Interview

1. "Hi, Mr. Jones. I'm Mary, a registered dietitian. Have you been on a diabetic diet before?"

2. Entering patient room: "Good morning, Julia. What's up? How are you guys doing today? I'm here to tell you what to eat on a sodium restricted diet."

EXPLORATION PHASE

In the second stage, the interviewee is asked a series of questions; these are the tools used by the interviewer to obtain information. A good interviewer has carefully pre-planned these questions in a prepared "interview guide," an outline of the information desired or topics to be covered that are relevant to the purpose of the interview. The guide should tell not only what questions will be asked, but also how questions will be phrased to gain the most information in the limited time available. With practice, a natural flow will occur.

Topics should be arranged in a definite sequence. In a nutrition or diet history, for example, the interviewer may desire information about beverages consumed, eating in restaurants, portion sizes, meals, methods of food preparation, and snacks. Put in sequence, the list includes meals, portion sizes, methods of food preparation, snacks, beverages, and eating in restaurants. See Table 3-2 for questions and directives for diet histories. In a pre-employment interview, the sequence may be previous work experience, career goals, education, present activities and interests that are job-related, and personal qualifications. Specific questions intended to gain information about the applicant's qualifications, compared with those in the job description, should be planned in advance.

Although it ensures that information is gathered in a systematic manner, the interview guide does not have to be followed strictly. When the interviewee brings up a topic or asks a question, this shows interest and should be pursued. The interviewer should be thoroughly familiar with the questions and not have to refer to them constantly. Knowing the purpose and significance of each question is important so that questions are not asked in a perfunctory manner and so the interviewer does not accept superficial or inadequate answers.

Asking a job applicant about offices held in organizations, for example, is an attempt to seek information about leadership ability and the acceptance of responsibil-

TABLE 3-2	Examples of Questions and Directives for Diet Histories

1. "Who plans and prepares the meals at home? Who does the grocery shopping?"
2. "Are you currently restricting your food choices in any way?" (because of allergy, religion, intolerance, etc.)
3. "Can you tell me about any questions or issues you have in making food choices; about the people in your family who eat together and any dietary problems they have."
4. "How physically active are you?"
5. "Now I will ask you to think of all the foods and beverages you consume in a typical day. Please tell me about the first food or drink you have after arising and the amount of that food."
6. "That's good. Now tell me about what you eat and drink next including the amount."
7. "And then, what would you eat or drink next?"
8. "What types of seasonings do you use in cooking? Tell me about them."
9. "Snacks and beverages are often forgotten. What do you have between each of your meals and during the evening or before bed?
10. "You haven't mentioned alcoholic beverages. What about them?"
11. "How often do you take a vitamin/mineral supplement or use herbs or alternative therapies? If yes, describe the kinds and amounts."
12. "What time of day are your meals?"
13. "How many times a week do you eat a meal away from home? What would you have?"
14. "Would you say that the amounts of foods you have described are typical, more than usual, or less than usual?
15. "To summarize what you have told me, can you tell me how many servings you eat daily or weekly of these foods?" (continue with a food frequency)

ity. Inquiring about career plans over the next 3 to 5 years is an attempt to learn about short- and long-range goals. See Table 3-3 for pre-employment interview questions. To answer fully, interviewees must see how the questions are relevant. With patients or clients, the dietetics professional can explain that the answers are a basis for nutritional assessment, counseling, or education.

Using Questions

Questions play a major role in interviews as tools of the trade. The wording of questions is as important as one's manner and tone of voice. A friendly approach in asking the questions communicates the desire to understand and be of assistance. The kind of questions asked should require the other person to talk 60% to 70% of the time. Questions that are highly specific or may be answered with one word, such as "yes" or "no" should be avoided initially, but may be necessary later to follow up on specific information.

TABLE 3-3 Sample Pre-employment Interview Questions

Permissible Questions and Their Significance

In general, questions asked in pre-employment interviews should be job-related or predictive of success on the job. They should elicit information to compare the individual's qualifications and interests with those of the job description for the vacant position. Depending on the applicant and the job opening, the following are examples with their significance:

1. "Now I would like to ask you some questions about yourself and your previous work experience." Introduces the questioning.
2. "Tell me about your previous work experience and how it relates to the job you are interested in." Gives general impressions of whether the person is qualified.
3. "Please describe for me one or two important accomplishments in your previous job." Tells abilities.
4. "What were your responsibilities on your previous job?" Gives knowledge, skills, and abilities.
5. "What would you say are your greatest strengths as a worker? Areas to improve?" Gives skills and abilities.
6. "What kind of work interests you?" Tells interest and motivation.
7. "What subjects in school did you like most? Least?" Shows interests.
8. "What was your grade point average? Class rank?" Shows mental ability and motivation.
9. "While in school, what extracurricular activities did you participate in that have a bearing on this job?" Shows diversity of interest, interpersonal skills, and teamwork.
10. "What organizations do you belong to that are relevant to the job you are applying for?" Shows interests and interpersonal skills.
11. "What offices have you held?" Shows leadership ability and acceptance of responsibility.
12. "What are your career goals? Where do you see yourself in three to five years?" Shows whether or not the person plans ahead and what their plans are as well as whether or not they are congruent with those of the company.
13. "What hours do you prefer to work? How much flexibility do you have with your schedule?" Tells availability various hours of the day and days of the week.
14. "What brought you to our company to apply for work? Why would you like to work for us?" Tells whether the person is knowledgeable about the company and interests.
15. "Do you prefer to work alone or in a group?" Tells if would be good in a team environment or not.
16. "What questions do you have?"

Questions That Should Not Be Asked

Certain subjects can be the basis for complaints of discrimination on the basis of race, color, gender, marital status, national origin, religion, age, and disability. For this reason, the following questions are examples of ones that should be avoided in pre-employment interviews.

TABLE 3-3	Sample Pre-employment Interview Questions

1. "Are you a citizen of another country?"
2. "What is your religious faith?"
3. "Are your married? Single? Divorced?"
4. "What is your maiden name?"
5 "Where does your spouse work? What does he/she think of your working?"
6. "Who will baby-sit for you?"
7. "Do you have a family or plans to start a family?"
8. "What is your date of birth? Date of graduation from school?"

Knowledge of the kinds of questions to use and skill in using them are important for successful interviewing as well as for counseling others. Questions may be classified in three ways: open or closed, primary or secondary, and neutral or leading.(10)

Open and Closed Questions
Open questions are broad and give the interviewee great freedom in deciding what to say while giving the professional an opportunity to listen and observe. Examples of open questions are:

"Can you tell me a little about yourself?"

"What are some foods you like to eat?"

At the beginning of an interview, open questions are less threatening and communicate more interest and trust; answers reveal what the interviewee thinks is most important. Disadvantages are that they may involve a greater amount of time, the collection of unnecessary information, and lengthy, disorganized answers.(5)

Additional examples of open questions, but with moderate restrictions, are:

"Can you tell me about your meals?"

"What did the doctor tell you about your diet?"

"What were your job responsibilities in your previous position?"

"How did you became interested in this position?"

"What skills do you have that are important for this job?"

In follow-up visits, open questions should be broad to allow the client to determine the focus of the interview. Examples are, "How are your food goals progressing?" or "What progress have you made since we last talked?" The professional should begin discussion with whatever is of current concern to the client. For opening questions, the interviewer should also refer to the records regarding the client's background, problems, and previous counseling.

Closed questions are more restrictive; that is, they limit answers. Some closed questions are more limiting than others, such as:

"Who cooks the food at home?"

"Do you salt your food?"

"Can you tell me about any snacks you eat between meals?"

"What special diet or food restrictions do you follow?"

Closed questions give the interviewer more control, require less effort from the interviewee, and are less time consuming, which is of value when only a short screening is needed. Disadvantages include the inhibition of communication, which might result if the interviewer shows little interest in the answers, taking more questions to obtain the same information, and getting answers that may not reveal why the respondent feels as he or she does. Table 3-4 summarizes the advantages and disadvantages of the different kinds of questions.

Primary and Secondary Questions

Questions may also be classified as primary or secondary. Primary questions are used to introduce topics or new areas of discussion. The following are examples:

"Now that we have discussed your most recent position, can you tell me about your former job with Smith & Company?"

"Now that we have discussed the foods you eat at home, tell me about what you eat when you go to restaurants."

Note that mentioning what was just said shows that you have been listening.

Secondary questions attempt to obtain further information or explanation that primary questions have failed to elicit. They are also referred to as "follow-up" questions. Interviewees may have given an inadequate response for many reasons, including poor memory, misunderstanding of the question or amount of detail needed, and the feeling that the question is too personal or irrelevant, or that the professional would not understand the response. Specific follow-up questions, such as the following, may be asked:

"How much orange juice do you drink?"

TABLE 3-4	Advantages and Disadvantages of Questions	
Type of Question	**Advantages**	**Disadvantages**
Open	Gives interviewee control Communicates trust/interest Less threatening Tells what the person thinks is important	Time-consuming Gets unneeded information
Closed	Gives interviewer control Provides quick answers	Gets incomplete answers Short answers force more questions
Primary	Introduces new topics	
Secondary	Elicits further information	
Leading		Reveals bias of interviewer Directs person's answer
Neutral	More accurate answers	

"What do you put in your coffee?"

"In your previous position, how many people did you supervise?"

Neutral and Leading Questions

Neutral questions are preferred to leading questions.(5) Leading questions direct the respondent toward one answer in preference to others, an effect that may be unintentional on the part of an inexperienced interviewer. Leading questions reveal a suggested or expected answer by the interviewer, which may not be realized. Listed below are examples:

"You drink milk, don't you?" "Yes, of course." Instead, ask: "What beverages do you drink?"

"You aren't going to eat desserts anymore, are you?" "No." Instead ask: "What will you have for dessert?"

"What do you eat for breakfast?" "Cereal." Instead ask: "What do you have to eat after you get up in the morning?"

One of these questions assumes the client eats breakfast, and in these instances people probably answer as they think they are expected to, even if they usually omit the meal. Clients may change their answers on the basis of a nonverbal appearance of the dietetics professional of surprise, disgust, dislike, or disagreement with what clients are saying. To receive uninhibited responses from clients, the interviewer should try to avoid these appearances.

SELF-ASSESSMENT

Identify the following questions as open, closed, primary, secondary, or leading.

1. "You mentioned that the only meal you eat at home is dinner. Can you tell me where you eat your breakfast and lunch and what you are likely to have?"
2. "Do you put catsup on your hamburger?"
3. "What do you put on your salad?"
4. "How do you cook your meats?"

The practitioner's language and wording must be understood by the client if successful communication is to take place. You do not need to impress people with medical and dietetic vocabulary. Complex terminology should be avoided or used sparingly, and only when you are sure that the client understands. The following is a statement likely to be misunderstood in a conversation: "People with hyperlipidemia should avoid eating foods containing saturated fatty acids and emphasize monounsaturates and polyunsaturates instead. This can help lower your low-density lipoproteins."

Directives

When you as the interviewer sense that too many questions are being asked and the respondent may be developing a feeling of interrogation, you may introduce some questions as a statement or directive. For example: "How has your diet been going?" may be changed to "I'd be interested in hearing how your diet has been going." "How did you become interested in this position?" may be changed to "I'd be interested in some of the reasons you decided to apply for this position." This makes the interview more conversational. Questions should be asked one at a time and the interviewer should concentrate on listening carefully to the answers rather than thinking ahead to the next questions to be asked.

Sequencing Questions

Questions can be arranged in a "funnel" sequence.(10) A funnel sequence begins with broad, open questions and proceeds to more restrictive ones.

> **E X A M P L E :** *"Tell me about the foods you eat during a day's time."*
> *"What do you have for snacks between meals?"*
> *"We haven't discussed alcoholic beverages—what do you like to drink?"*

Beginning the interview with open-ended questions poses the least threat to the client and induces a response. The person then volunteers much information, making it unnecessary to ask additional questions. At times, an inverted funnel sequence may be preferable. In pre-employment interviews, for example, applicants may feel more comfortable dealing with a specific question than with a broad, open one, such as "Tell me about yourself," when they are apprehensive and unsure of what to say or what the interviewer expects.

In taking a diet history, questions or statements starting with "What" or "Tell me about" elicit better responses than "Do you. . .?" See diet history examples. Questions that do not require a sufficient answer or may be answered with one word or "yes" or "no" are less productive, such as in the example:

> **E X A M P L E :** *"Do you eat breakfast?" "Yes."*
> *"Do you like milk?" "No."*
> *"How often do you eat meat?" "Once a day."*

A series of short, sequential, dead-end questions from the professional's list of information to be gathered prevents people from telling their stories their way, and information may be omitted as a result. Instead, ask as follows:

> **E X A M P L E :** *"Please tell me about your first meal of the day, what you eat, and the amount."*

"Why" Questions

Some recommend avoiding questions beginning with "why."(9) Although asking "why" may seek information, it may also indicate disapproval, displeasure, or mistrust, and it appears to ask the person to justify or explain behavior, for example:

"Why don't you follow your diet more closely?"

"Why don't you eat breakfast?"

"Why did you resign from your job?"

"Why don't you exercise more often?"

Clients may react defensively or explain their behavior in a manner they believe is acceptable to the interviewer.

"I don't follow my diet because I don't like it. You wouldn't like it either."

"I can eat breakfast if you think I should."

"I resigned because there was no chance for advancement."

"I don't exercise because I don't have time. Do you exercise?"

If threatened by a "why" question and unwilling to reveal the answer, the individual may answer in an evasive manner, in which case nothing is gained.

RESPONSES

In the verbal interaction of interviews, interviewer responses may be divided into several categories:

1. Understanding
2. Probing
3. Confrontation
4. Evaluative
5. Hostile
6. Reassuring

Understanding Responses

The understanding response is one of the best choices. With it, interviewers try to understand the person's message and re-create it within their own frame of reference. People have more rapport with those who try to understand them rather than judge them. This may lead to more cooperation on the part of the client.

> **EXAMPLE:** *Mrs. Jones: "I haven't lost any weight this week. I ate just a few cookies. The diet doesn't work."*
> *Counselor: "You are* feeling concerned *because you haven't lost any weight, Mrs. Jones, and you are wondering if it was something you ate, or a problem with the diet?"*

The paraphrase in this understanding response helps the person feel accepted even if her behavior has not been perfect. The client will feel safe in expressing her sentiments and exploring them further. The client who finds an understanding counselor may cooperate more fully in solving problems.

Note that the professional should focus on Mrs. Jones's feelings and attitudes, rather than only on the content of what she said. She may be *feeling* concerned or disappointed with the diet or with herself. She may feel guilty. She may be frustrated with trying to change her food choices. The counselor has guessed "concerned" and if this is incorrect, Mrs. Jones will correct the mistaken impression. This gives even more information.

The understanding response is most helpful in assisting the clients to recognize problems and to devise their own solutions. The client may progress from initial negative feelings to more neutral ones and finally to more positive attitudes and solutions.

In the case of information about death, prolonged illness, discomforts, or other problems, expressions of sincere sympathy may assist in building bridges in personal relationships. A quick response can be "Oh my, I'm sorry!" or "I'm very sorry to hear that."

It is necessary to differentiate and understand both the content and the feelings of the client's remarks. To determine the *content*, you may ask yourself, "What is this person telling me or thinking?" *Feelings* may be classified as positive, negative, or ambivalent, and these may change as the interview progresses.(9) In identifying feelings, ask, "What is this person feeling, and why is he feeling that way?"

You may use the following sentence in paraphrasing the person's statement to verify your understanding. The answer may be inserted into a format.

> **E X A M P L E :**   *"I think I hear you saying that you* feel . . . *because . . ."*

Although one may have an incorrect impression, such as a feeling that a person is concerned when the person actually is tired, the interviewee usually provides the correct interpretation, thereby furthering the interviewer's understanding. This process demonstrates that one is trying to understand the other.

To avoid overuse of the same phrase and to avoid sounding mechanistic, the phrase can be varied.

> **E X A M P L E :**   *"Do I understand correctly that you feel . . .?"*
> *"You seem to be saying that you are feeling . . ."*
> *"I gather that . . ."*
> *"You sound . . ."*
> *"In other words, you are feeling . . . "*

Interviewee responses that suggest feelings about an event may provide an important key to the person's behavior. How patients or clients feel about their lifestyle, food habits or choices, or their health is critical to dietary adherence. Food behaviors may be influenced by psychological, cultural, and environmental variables that are important to understand.

Job applicants may also express feelings about previous work experience, relationships with superiors and subordinates, and activities and interests. Preceding a statement with "I think . . .," "I feel . . .," or "I believe. . ." gives a signal that the statement expresses opinions, beliefs, attitudes, or values. Possible follow-up probes are in the following examples:

> **E X A M P L E :**   *"Can you explain more about your feelings?"*
> *"What do YOU think about that?"*
> *"What do you think causes that?"*

Probing Responses

The probing response is helpful in clarifying or in gaining additional information as respondents recall details. In dietary interviews, for example, details on food quantities, added ingredients, food preparation methods, and snacks are probed frequently.

Probing implies that the person should give more information so that the professional can understand.

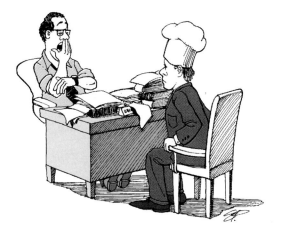

Things to avoid when communicating with another.

EXAMPLE: *Mrs. Jones: "I haven't lost any weight this week. I ate just a few cookies. The diet doesn't work."*
Counselor: "So you think the diet doesn't work, Mrs. Jones. I wonder if you could tell me a little more about that."

This helps the person to tell her story, and further information can be obtained.

There are many probing techniques, which may be used in addition to secondary or follow-up questions. They should be nondirective to avoid leading people to specific answers, nonthreatening, and nonjudgmental. A brief silence may be effective, as may repetition of the last phrase spoken by the client or a summary sentence. Probing further in the case of superficial and vague responses, as well as probing for feelings about events, is suggested in the following paragraphs.

When a more detailed response is desired in the case of superficial answers, the following may be asked:

EXAMPLE: *"Can you tell me more about that?"*
"What do you do next?"
"Please explain a little more about . . ."
"What else?"

To obtain clarification if the answer is vague, you may respond:

EXAMPLE: *"Could you clarify for me what you meant by . . .?" "I don't think I quite understand . . ."*

Paraphrasing is another technique to ensure that the information is clear and correct. By repeating, summarizing, or rewording what was said, interviewers show that they are trying to understand.

When the person seems hesitant to go on, the interviewer may remain silent, pausing for the respondent to gather his or her thoughts and continue. The professional should appear attentive, with perhaps a thoughtful or expectant look, but should avoid eye contact for the moment. The inexperienced interviewer may find silence uncomfortable and embarrassing and push on too quickly, but a more experienced interviewer realizes that too hasty a response may cause part of the story to remain untold or change what is disclosed. If the respondent does not go on within 30 to 60 seconds, however, he or she may perceive the silence as disinterest of disapproval; the interviewer should commence before such an impression occurs.

A technique useful in breaking a silence is to repeat or echo the last phrase or sentence the person has said, raising the tone of voice to a question.

> **EXAMPLE:** *"I follow my diet except when I eat out."*
> *"Except when you eat out?"*
> *"I especially enjoy doing special projects with coworkers."*
> *"Special projects with co-workers?"*

Repetition, however, should not be overdone, or it has a parrot-like effect. If this is noticed by the respondent, it will inhibit conversation.

A summary sentence stated as a question also elicits further elaboration.

> **EXAMPLE:** *"You say that you already know how to plan a diabetic diet?"*
> *"You think this company is the one you want to work for?"*

Other probes are the following:

> **EXAMPLE:** *"Go on."*
> *"I see."*
> *"I understand, Mrs. Jones. Please continue."*
> *"Uh huh."*
> *"Hmmm."*
> *"And next."*
> *"Oh?" or "Oh!"*
> *"Really?"*
> *"Very good!"*
> *"That's interesting."*

"I see," "I understand," and "that's interesting" may give a feeling of acceptance and encourage conversation or elaboration of a point of view. "Very good" gives the person a pat on the back and is another kind of acceptance comment. Nonverbal probes include giving a quizzical look, leaning forward in the chair, and nodding of the head occasionally.

Confrontation

Confrontation is an authority-laden response in which the interviewer tactfully and tentatively calls to the person's attention some inconsistency in his or her story, words, or actions, pointing out the discrepancy to the individual.(12)

EXAMPLE: *Mrs. Jones: "I haven't lost any weight this week I ate just a few cookies. The diet doesn't work."*
Counselor: "I'm a bit concerned. You say you want to lose weight and yet you have not lost any weight for a month. What do you think is the problem?

This response challenges and encourages the person to recognize and cope psychologically with some aspect of behavior that is self-defeating or to examine the consequences of some behavior. It should be said nonjudgmentally as discussion centers on resolution of problems.

Confrontation is an advanced level skill that should seldom be used by an inexperienced interviewer or when good rapport and a supportive atmosphere are missing. Otherwise, such responses can become threatening or appear punitive and will inhibit conversation.

During the interview, you can examine not only what the person says, but also what is not said. Are there gaps that the interviewer should be trying to fill? Also note nonverbal behaviors, such as tension, inability to maintain eye contact, hand movements, fidgeting, and facial expressions of discomfort, nervousness, anger, or lack of understanding. The nonverbal behaviors may be inconsistent with the verbal message, or may add to it.

Although interviewers adjust the pace of the interview to that of the respondent, they are also responsible for the direction of the interview. When the topics for discussion are inappropriate, the skilled interviewer brings the conversation back to appropriate topics. The patient talking about his wife or children, for example, must be brought gently back to the nutrition history. A job applicant discussing a recent visit to Spain must be brought back to relevant topics. People who are especially talkative may ramble frequently, requiring more direction and leadership on the part of the interviewer. In these cases, restating or emphasizing the last thing said that was pertinent to the interview and asking a related question can be helpful.

Evaluative Response

In the evaluative response, the interviewer makes a judgment about the person's feelings or responses or implies how the person ought to feel. The evaluative response leads to the offering of advice by the professional for the solution to the client's problem.

EXAMPLE: *Mrs. Jones: "I haven't lost any weight this week. I ate just a few cookies. The diet doesn't work."*
Counselor: "I suggest that you stop buying those cookies, Mrs. Jones."

Note that the evaluative response leads to giving advice, not information or problem solving. Little attempt is made to understand the psychological needs of the client or the reasons that the cookies were eaten. The recipient of the advice has the choice of following the advice or not. At times, some people ignore advice as a means of maintaining their independence. Responses should be nonjudgmental rather than evaluative.

Hostile Response

In the hostile response, the professional's anger or frustration is uncontrolled, and the response may lead to antagonism or humiliation of the client.

> **EXAMPLE:** *Mrs. Jones: "I haven't lost any weight this week. I ate just a few cookies. The diet doesn't work."*
> *Counselor: "You're not acting very mature, Mrs. Jones. I've told you before to avoid all sweets and desserts if you want to lose weight. You haven't lost any weight for a month! Why are you still buying cookies?"*

The hostile response may lead the client to a reply that retaliates.

> **EXAMPLE:** *Mrs. Jones: "How would you know about dieting? Look how thin you are."*

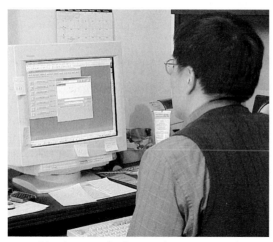

Nutrient analysis may be completed on a computer.

A vicious cycle of angry, hostile responses results, destroying the professional-client relationship. The fact that the client is anxious about the inability to follow the diet has been ignored. The interviewer who is frustrated by the client who is not following the diet should avoid responding in this manner.

Reassuring Response

With a reassuring response, the client is prevented from working through her feelings since the interviewer suggests that there is nothing to worry about. Frequently, a client's expressions of anxiety are followed by the professional's reassuring response that things will improve and that the person should not worry.

> **EXAMPLE:** *Mrs. Jones: "I haven't lost any weight this week even though I am trying."*
> *Counselor: "Don't worry, Mrs. Jones. It takes time to adjust to new eating patterns. You'll do better next week."*

This response suggests that the problem does not exist, or that the counselor does not want to discuss it. Such responses make it difficult to solve the client's problem or to discuss it further. Admission of failure with the diet may have been difficult for the client, but it indicated a desire to discuss the problem.

SELF-ASSESSMENT

Identify the following types of responses as understanding, probing, confrontation, evaluative, hostile, and reassuring.

1. "The food does taste different without salt. Let's see if we can find some substitutes that you can try."
2. "I know you can do it. It just takes time."
3. "How do you expect to lose weight if you continue to eat fast foods every day?"
4. "That's interesting. Tell me more about that."
5. "You say that you watch your food choices week days, but eat whatever you want on weekends. Do you think that is why you have not lost any weight?"
6. "When you are at a party, try to find someone to talk to instead of eating."

CLOSING THE INTERVIEW

The third part or closing of the interview takes the shortest amount of time, but should not be rushed or taken lightly. During the closing, a word of appreciation sincerely expressed, such as thanking the person for his or her time and cooperation, is appropriate. Another suggestion is to review the purpose of the interview and declare its completion. "That's all the questions I have. Thank you for your time and information." You may ask if there are any questions the client would like to ask or any other comments they want to make, which may elicit important new information for which adequate time should be available. For example: "What else would you like to ask or tell me about?" One may ask the client to summarize points agreed on.

The time, place, and purpose of future contacts should be mentioned. To a hospitalized patient, the professional may say, "I'll stop by to see you tomorrow to discuss your food choices with you." With a client, arrangements for a future appointment may be made: "When can we meet again to discuss your progress and answer questions?" To make sure that each has understood the other, plans may be paraphrased.

As a courtesy to job applicants, they should be told approximately when the employment decision will be made and how they will be notified if selected, as, for example, "We are interviewing additional candidates for this position, but if you are selected, you'll hear from human resources in about a week or two. Thank you for coming and for your interest in our company." For those not selected, a letter may be sent thanking them for their applications and interest in the company and telling them the position has been filled. This letter is a public relations effort that may be handled by the human resources department.(5,6) The applicant who hears nothing after an interview may react negatively or telephone again for information.

You may signal the close of the interview nonverbally by breaking eye contact, pushing back the chair, placing hands on the arms of the chair, standing up, offering to shake hands, smiling, and walking the interviewee to the door.

COMPETENCY: *Utilizes effective communication skills in the practice of dietetics.*

INTERVIEW SKILLS OR BEHAVIOR

Date:	3	2	1	COMMENTS

CLIMATE OF INTERVIEW

1. Observes initial social amenities.

2. Indicates mutual respect.

3. Responds positively to signs of anxiety.

4. Shows empathy.

USE OF QUESTIONS

5. Elicits comments about self and concerns about diet, medical condition, etc.
6. Uses non-leading (gives no clues to desired answer)

7. Uses non-directive (avoids yes/no, single word answers)
8. Uses open-ended (allows for elaboration)

9. Questions are easily understood

10. Demonstrates the use of clarification (e.g. paraphrasing)

LISTENING ABILITY

11. Identifies "clues" for further probing
12. Utilizes and understands information offered
13. Uses appropriate verbal & nonverbal clues to engage client response
14. Avoids unnecessary interruptions

15. Separates interviewing activities from counseling
16. Shows a nonjudgmental, noncritical attitude toward client's eating pattern and chosen lifestyle

LANGUAGE

17. Uses language appropriate to the situation
18. Provides explanation for each step in the process

Figure 3-1 Client interviewing/counseling evaluation form. (Courtesy of School of Health-Related Professions, University of Medicine and Dentistry of New Jersey.)

NAME OF INTERN: _____

COUNSELING SKILLS OR BEHAVIOR

Date:	3	2	1	COMMENTS

1. Elicits client's statement of purpose and objectives
2. States purposes and objectives of diet modification/counseling.
3. Provides accurate explanations and rationale including diet: health relationship
4. Answers client's questions about diet and/or disease clearly and accurately

5. Adjusts explanations to learning abilities, constraints of time, etc.

6. Assesses client's understanding by having client restate information in his/her own words
7. Enlists active participation of client in formulating goals and planning of diet
8. Encourages client identification of obstacles and helps client develop strategies
9. Uses visual and other teaching aids appropriately and provides educational resources
10. Demonstrates correct use of self-disclosure

11. Maintains rapport with client throughout
12. Summarizes principles of diet

13. Re-states client goals

14. Explains goals for next visit and establishes plan for follow-up
15. Presents counseling within reasonable time frame

EVALUATION KEY:
   3 = Consistently demonstrates skill
   2 = Adequately progressing with skill development
   1 = Needs greater emphasis

CLOSING SELF-ASSESSMENT

Directions: How satisfactory are these closings? How can they be improved?

Employment Interview:

Standing up, "I have another applicant waiting, so our time is up. Thanks for coming today." Shakes hands.

Client Interview:

"Well I have all the information I need. See ya' later."

In summary, interviewing is a skill. As with other skills, it takes practice to develop. The inexperienced interviewer needs to plan in writing what topics need to be covered. Various types of questions can be prepared in advance in an appropriate sequence for the three parts of the interview. Physical surroundings and freedom from interruption should be planned. These conditions put the professional in a better position to concentrate on the interviewee and on the process of developing rapport, noting the verbal and nonverbal responses, and providing understanding responses with empathy. The interview session should be followed by a self-evaluation to determine areas that went well, as well as those that could be improved for the next interview. Questions you may ask include the following:

"How effective was the atmosphere?" "Was it relaxed and informal with good rapport?"
"How effective was my interview opening?"
"How effective were my questions in obtaining information I needed?"
"How effective were my responses to the person's statements?"
"Was I nonjudgmental and empathic?"
"How effective was my interview closing?"
"How much time did I listen versus talk?"

Figure 3-1 presents a sample client interviewing/counseling evaluation form.

CASE STUDY 1

Josephine Brown is an applicant for a job as assistant cook at a school lunch program at Willard High School with an enrollment of 200 students. According to her application, her address is in the high school district, she is a high school graduate, and she has worked for the past year as a cook at a nursing home.

On greeting her, the interviewer notices that she appears to be 35 to 40 years old and wears a wedding ring.

1. How would you develop rapport with Mrs. Brown?
2. What is the purpose of the interview?
3. Make a list of questions you would ask her. Explain why each question is relevant.

CASE STUDY **2**

Delores Maynard is a 55-year-old woman who works in a corporate office. She visits the corporate wellness center and makes an appointment with Joan Stivers, a registered dietitian. D.M. is 5'2" tall and weighs 190 pounds. She has mild hypertension. She is married with two grown children.

Joan: "What brings you to this appointment? How can I help?"

D.M.: "Well, I need to lose some weight to help control my blood pressure."

Joan: "Can you tell me about any other times you have tried to lose weight?"

D.M.: "I wasn't overweight until after I was married and bringing up two kids. Then I gradually gained weight. Over the years, I've tried many different diets. I lose weight but gain it all back, and sometimes more."

1. What questions would you ask in obtaining D.M.'s nutrition history? Put them in sequence. Discuss the reason why each questions is important in assisting the client.
2. What related questions would you like to ask, such as questions about meal preparation, food shopping, vitamin-mineral supplements, family meal practices, snacks, eating in restaurants, and weekend meals?
3. What other questions would you explore related to D.M.'s family and lifestyle?

REVIEW AND DISCUSSION QUESTIONS

1. What are the possible purposes of a diet history or nutrition interview? Of a pre-employment interview?
2. What conditions facilitate an interview?
3. Explain the three parts of an interview. What occurs in each part?
4. Differentiate between the following types of questions: open and closed; primary and secondary; and neutral and leading.
5. Explain the six types of responses.

SUGGESTED ACTIVITIES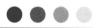

1. Watch an interview on television noting the parts of the interview, techniques used, and verbal and nonverbal responses. Write up your reactions and analysis.
2. Observe a television interview show. What types of questions are asked? What kinds of responses does the interviewer obtain? How was the rapport between the two parties?
3. Plan an interview guide specifying the content and sequence of questions. Write examples of various kinds of questions, such as open and closed, primary and secondary, neutral and leading. Which kinds of questions do you prefer to answer?

4. Divide into groups of two for role-playing, with each person interviewing the other in turn. Use various types of responses, such as probing, paraphrasing, and understanding. If three people are available, the third may serve as evaluator.

5. Make an audiotape of a simulated or actual interview, if the participant's permission is granted. Complete an evaluation.

6. Make a videotape of a simulated or actual interview, if the participant's permission is granted. This will show both the verbal and nonverbal behaviors as well as any personal idiosyncrasies. Complete an evaluation

7. Turn on the television set without the sound. Try to interpret the nonverbal behavior you are seeing.

8. Visit three offices and observe the physical surroundings. Which is most comfortable and conducive to communication? Why? Which is least comfortable? Why? Arrange the furniture in a room or office for an optimum interviewing setting.

9. Change the following technical words that are used by professionals into terms that will help a client to understand their meanings: fiber, nutrients, sodium, lipids, protein, serum glucose, carbohydrates, low-density lipoproteins, polyunsaturated fatty acids, saturated fatty acids, colitis, gastric ulcer, hypertension, fluid intake, osteoporosis.

10. Directions: Read the lettered statements below. Identify both the thought the person is expressing and the feelings the person may be experiencing. Write a paraphrased statement reflecting the thought or content of the message:

    A. "I've had diabetes for 6 years. They put me on a diet and insulin injections when I first found out about it, and I check my blood sugar sometimes. The diet isn't too bad."

    B. "I'm expecting my second baby. I never paid any attention to what I ate during my first pregnancy and my baby was healthy."

    C. "The doctor told me that I can go home tomorrow, but I live alone so I have no one to help me with a diet, and I'm in no hurry to leave."

    D. "Joan talks to people all day long and doesn't get her work done. The rest of us have to finish for her or we get yelled at."

    E. "I've been working here for 10 years. Now you come in as a new supervisor and want to change everything around. What's wrong with keeping things the way they are?"

    F. "How do you expect me to get all this work done? First, you tell me to do one thing, and then you tell me to do another."

    Directions: Write a second paraphrased statement reflecting the feelings in the above examples, such as:

    "You seem to be *feeling* (angry, depressed, lonely etc.) *because* . . . ."

    "It sounds like you *feel* . . . ."

    "I hear you saying that you *feel* . . . . Tell me if I'm understanding you accurately."

    Example: Client: "My friend and I are both dieting. She has lost weight, but I haven't even though I have been trying."

    Counselor: "You seem to be *feeling* upset *because* your friend has lost weight and you haven't."

    Discuss your paraphrases with others.

WEB SITES

http://safetynet.doleta.gov/intrview.htm / the US Dept. of Labor site for employee interviewing

http://riskfactor.cancer.gov/DHQ / the National Cancer Institute site with a self-administered food frequency questionnaire

http://depts.washington.edu/nwlrc/dietfis.html / the Northwest Lipid Research Clinic Fat Intake Scale

www.nutritiononestop.com/jobs/resource/questions.html / common employee interview questions

REFERENCES

1. Arthur D. Recruiting, interviewing, selecting & orienting new employees, 3rd ed. New York: American Management Association, 1998.
2. Dessler G. Human resource management, 8th ed. New Jersey: Prentice Hall, 2000.
3. Bohlander G, Snell S, Sherman A. Managing human resources, 12th ed. Cincinnati: South-Western, 2001.
4. Lee RD, Nieman DC. Nutritional assessment. Madison, WI: Brown & Benchmark Pub, 1993.
5. Hudson NL. Management practice in dietetics. Belmont, CA: Wadsworth, 2000.
6. McConnell CR. A working manager's guide to effective and legal employee selection interviewing. Supervisor 1999;17:77.
7. Thompson FE, Suber AF. Dietary assessment methodology. In: Coulston AM, Rock CL, Monsen ER, eds. Nutrition in the prevention and treatment of disease. San Diego: Academic Press, 2001.
8. Kubena KS. Accuracy in dietary assessment: on the road to good science. J Am Diet Assoc 2000;100:775.
9. Tassell LC, Breninger V, Barvard J. Applying conversation analysis to faster accurate reporting in the diet history interview. J Am Diet Assoc 2000;100:818.
10. Stewart CJ Cash WB. Interviewing principles and practices, 8th ed. Boston: McGraw Hill, 1997.
11. Jobe JB, Mingay DJ. Cognitive research improves questionnaires. Am J Public Health 1989;79:1053.
12. Evans DR, Hearn MT, Uhlemann MR, et al. Essential interviewing: a programmed approach to effective communication, 4th ed. Pacific Grove, CA: BrooksCole, 1993.

4 Counseling

After reading this chapter, you will be able to

1. discuss the dietetics practitioner's role in counseling clients and staff.
2. define counseling, its role, and the process of counseling.
3. identify the attributes of a successful counselor.
4. describe various theories of counseling.
5. explain the stages in the counseling process.
6. differentiate between directive and nondirective counseling approaches and their uses.
7. describe motivational interviewing as a form of counseling.

One of the key roles of the dietetics professional is to promote the optimal health of the public. The practitioner translates the science of nutrition into appropriate food and nutrient intake. To accomplish appropriate food intake, often behaviors and lifestyles must change. Nutrition counseling focuses on helping clients accomplish these changes. Counseling also comes into play in the managerial aspects of dietetics in the form of staff counseling for development or remediation.

The Commission on Accreditation for Dietetics Education of the American Dietetic Association requires that dietetics students have a working knowledge of counseling theories and methods and that they are able to counsel individuals on nutrition. Counseling is essential to the success of the dietetics practitioner, whether as a manager, an ambulatory care practitioner, or a practitioner in private practice. As health care intensifies its emphasis on outcomes, the results of counseling will be examined. If the intervention, whether assessment, education, or counseling, does not produce a change in knowledge, skills, behavior, or health outcome, the continuation of the intervention will appropriately be questioned.

Counseling may be defined as a process that assists people in learning about themselves, their environment, and the methods of handling their roles and relationships. It involves problem solving, identifying goals, and change. Counselors assist individuals with the decision-making process, resolving interpersonal concerns, and helping them learn new ways of dealing with and adjusting to life situations. Counseling is a science with a body of literature that assesses techniques and their effectiveness. It is also an art; the skills of the counselor allow the counselor to customize the counseling to the individual client.

66

This chapter is an overview of the counseling process as it applies to dietetics practitioners. Counseling is a process that involves the development of a trusting, helping relationship between counselor and client, evaluation of what the client issues are, and various techniques of problem solving. The approaches to counseling may be classified as nondirective or directive. The nondirective or "client-centered" approach is applied to the nutrition counseling of clients. Directive counseling is often applied to staff regarding job-related issues.

ROGERIAN CLIENT-CENTERED (NONDIRECTIVE) COUNSELING

The nondirective approach to counseling is often called "client-centered" and is best represented by the writings of its originator, Carl Ransom Rogers. Dr. Rogers' theory was first presented in his book, *Counseling and Psychotherapy* (1942) and was further refined in subsequent publications.(1,2) The theory is constantly developing, changing with experience and research; however the fundamental assumptions have not changed. The theory is one of the more detailed, integrated, and consistent theories currently existing and has led to, and is supported by, a greater amount of research than any other approach to counseling.(3)

A basic assumption in the client-centered point of view is that humans are basically rational, socialized, and realistic. Individuals, if their needs for positive regard from others and for positive self-regard are satisfied, possess an inherent tendency toward realizing their potential for growth and self-actualization. Counseling releases the potentials and capacities of the individual.

One of the most important characteristics of the Rogerian theory is the relationship it suggests between the counselor and the client. The underlying assumption is that the client cannot be helped simply by listening to the knowledge the counselor possesses or to the counselor's explanation of the client's personality or behavior. Prescribing "cures" and corrective behaviors are seen as being of little lasting value. The relationship that is most helpful to clients and that enables them to discover within themselves the capacity to use the relationship to change and grow is not a cognitive, intellectual one. Rogers states: "I believe the quality of my encounter is more important in the long run than is my scholarly knowledge, my professional training, my counseling orientation, the techniques I use in the interview."(4) There are four specific characteristics that Rogers suggests the counselor possess for the therapy relationship: acceptance, congruence, understanding, and the ability to communicate these to the client.

The counselor needs to be accepting of clients as individuals as they are, with their good and bad points, their conflicts and inconsistencies. Only after clients are convinced that they are accepted unconditionally and nonjudgmentally can they begin to trust the counselor. Research, moreover, has indicated that trust is not a nebulous feeling that people have about other individuals; rather, it is focused on predictability, genuine concern, and faithfulness.(5)

Exceptional counselors are characterized by congruence within the counseling relationship. They are unified, integrated, and consistent, with no contradictions between what they are and what they say. These counselors are able to express outwardly to their clients what they are feeling within themselves. Their verbal and nonverbal behaviors are consistent.

The counselor must experience an accurate, empathic understanding of the client's world as seen from the inside, sensing the client's world as if it were his or her own, but without losing the "as if" quality. This empathy is essential to nondirective therapy. The understanding enables clients to explore freely and deeply and develop a better comprehension of themselves.

It is of no value for the counselor to be accepting, congruent, and understanding if the client does not perceive or experience this. The acceptance, congruence, and understanding need to be communicated to the client verbally and nonverbally. Rogers is definite in his belief that these not be "techniques," but a genuine and spontaneous expression of the counselor's inner attitudes, having contact with people.(3)

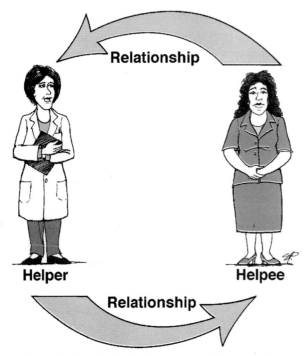

The relationship is key to successful counseling.

If the counselor has these characteristics and attitudes and is able to communicate them to the client, then a relationship develops that is experienced by the client as safe, secure, free from threat, and supportive. The counselor is perceived as dependable, trustworthy, and consistent. This requires being a good listener, having intuition, providing feedback on both data and feelings, and providing inspiration.(6) This is the type of relationship that supports behavioral change, whether you are working with clients or with staff.

COUNSELING PROCESSES

Various models describe the counseling process. Many have a Rogerian foundation and incorporate the client's readiness for change for transforming a behavior. Counseling is an individualized process that does not involve giving ready-made advice, but suggesting constructive alternatives based on what is important to and manageable for the client.(7,8) Counseling is an interactive process that goes well beyond education of the client. Several approaches are described in the following text, including motivational interviewing, The Transtheoretical Model or Stages of Change Model, Rollnick's framework for changing behavior, and a four-stage process of counseling.

Motivational interviewing is an approach designed to "help clients build commitment and reach a decision to change."(9) It combines directive and nondirective approaches to counseling. Motivational interviewing, the Transtheoretical Model described in detail in Chapter 5, and Rollnick's framework focus on the readiness of the client to change. The transtheoretical model identifies stages of change that individuals pass through including precontemplation, contemplation, preparation, action, and maintenance.(10) Integrating the change stage of the client with the four-stage process described below will improve the success of counseling sessions.

MOTIVATIONAL INTERVIEWING

Motivational interviewing was originally developed from work with "addictive behaviors," but the intervention approach can be used in a variety of situations. It offers an approach for increasing the client's readiness to change eating behaviors. Even if people are aware of damaging consequences of their behavior, such as overeating or non-nutritious choices, they may use "short-term gratification at the expense of long-term harm."(9)

Although the motivational approach draws on client-centered counseling, it is a directive client-centered approach. The counselor maintains a "sense of purpose and direction," actively intervening at the right moment, thus combining directive and nondirective approaches.(11) It can be integrated into Prochaska and DiClemente's Stages of Change Model in which people move from being unaware or unwilling to do anything about a problem, called *precontemplation*, to considering the possibility of change or contemplation, preparing to make a change or determination and finally taking action.(10) Since the client may be at any of several stages, the initial step is to assess where the client is.

Motivational interviewing strategies draw on principles of social, cognitive, and motivational psychology; on ambivalence, or the conflict between restraint and indulgence, which can be immobilizing; and on the theory of self-regulation. The approach works well with people who are reluctant to change. These people are the "precontemplators" and "contemplators."

What is motivational interviewing? It is "a particular way to help people recognize and do something about their present or potential problem."(9) It is especially useful with clients who are ambivalent about or reluctant to change. It helps to resolve the ambivalence and move the person toward change. Once unstuck from the conflicting motivations of whether or not to change that immobilize people, they can move toward a decision and a commitment to take action.

What is the role of the counselor? An authoritarian role that sends the message "I'm an expert and will tell you what to do" is counterproductive. The responsibility for change lies with the client. "It's up to you to decide what to do. It's your choice." The person is free to take our suggestions or ignore them. The goal is to "increase the client's motivation, so that change arises from within rather than imposed from without."(9) The client, not the counselor, needs to develop and say orally the arguments for change. One image of the counselor is that of a helper accompanying a person on a journey. The guide "needs the qualities of a companion and the skills of someone who knows the route," but acknowledges the client's personal responsibility for change and freedom of choice.(9)

While motivational interviewing incorporates some of Carl Rogers' nondirective and client-centered approach, it is also directive. The counselor sees clear goals (e.g., changing eating behaviors, cooking differently) and pursues strategies to reach an appropriate goal. Feedback and suggested changes are given. The counselor directs the client toward motivation to change.

Five general principles underlie this approach:

1. Express empathy.
2. Develop discrepancy.
3. Avoid argumentation.
4. Roll with resistance.
5. Support self-efficacy.(9)

Empathy suggests acceptance. The counselor seeks to understand the client's feelings and beliefs in a noncritical, nonjudgmental manner. The counselor listens carefully and respectfully. Empathy involves the counselor verbally reflecting what the client says to clarify and amplify the client's experience, feelings, and meanings, even if the counselor has not had a similar experience. Sharp attention to each client statement allows the counselor to hypothesize as to the meaning. The best guess as to the meaning is then reflected back to the client for verification. Ambivalence is considered normal. The client often considers continuing the current behavior desirable. The reasons must be explored, so attempts can be made to decrease or counterbalance them.

The counselor seeks to *develop discrepancy* between present behavior and a new behavior, that is, where the person is and where he or she wants to be. One approach is to examine the costs and benefits of the current course of behavior as well as the benefits and costs of change, determining the relative importance of each (Table 4-1). If the person has a conflict with an important goal, such as better health, self-image, or happiness, change is more likely. Motivation to change increases when people see a discrepancy between present behavior and goals that are important to them.

People who come for counseling on their own, as opposed to those referred by a health care provider, can be expected to perceive some discrepancy already. But they may be ambivalent, stuck between the conflict of whether or not to change. Then it is necessary to clarify the client's important goals and explore how present behavior conflicts with them. The goal is to increase the discrepancy until it overrides the attachment to the current behavior. Eventually, clients may see and articulate the arguments for change as their own. The client has more commitment to change when he or she makes the decision, thus increasing motivation.

A third principle is that the counselor *avoids arguments* and confrontation. When a counselor argues that the client needs to change, the client defends the opposite view

TABLE 4-1 Cost-Benefit Analysis			
Continue to Eat as Before		**Change Eating Behavior**	
Pros	**Cons**	**Pros**	**Cons**
Pleasurable	Damages health	Better health	Change is difficult
Comfortable	Bad example	Feels better	Can't party with
Easy	for family	Loses weight	friends
Decreases loneliness			Requires effort

and resists change. People assert their ability to do as they please and make their own decisions. Although the purpose of motivational interviewing is to increase awareness of a problem and the need to change, the counselor does not want to confront and thus increase resistance to change.

If the client is *resistant*, the counselor can acknowledge that reluctance to change and ambivalence are natural and understandable. The client may be offered new information or alternatives to consider. Or, rather than generating solutions, the counselor can ask the client for solutions to his or her problems. This involves the client in problem solving.

Self-efficacy refers to a person's belief in his or her ability to succeed with a specific task. It is a key to motivation for change. If a person does not believe he or she can change, little or no effort will be made. A client may be encouraged by the counselor's offer of help or by seeing the success of others in the same or similar situations (role models). The counselor needs to reinforce the client's hope, optimism, and self-efficacy.

How the counselor responds to what the client says is an important element of reflective listening. Reflective listening may be one of several types. The counselor may repeat part of what the person said or may rephrase slightly using different words. Paraphrasing is a more major restatement in which the counselor tries to determine the meaning in the statement and reflects back in new words adding to or extending the meaning. Finally, the deepest form of reflection is to reflect feelings in a paraphrase that searches for the client's emotions behind the statement. Thinking up a response to what the client is saying and offering it is *not* reflective listening. Nor is giving advice, making suggestions, criticizing, consoling, reassuring, sympathizing, probing, or telling clients what they "should" do.

> **EXAMPLE:** *Client: "I just don't know if I can lose weight, but I need to."*
> *(ambivalence)*
> *Counselor: "Of course you can." (reassuring)*
> *Client: "But it is so difficult."*
> *Counselor: "Yes, it is." (sympathizing)*
> *Client: "I never have eaten breakfast, because I don't have time."*
> *Counselor: "Just have some cereal and milk." (giving advice)*

In the above example, the counselor is not really listening or giving the client a chance to explore the problem. Instead, the reflective listener hears and decodes the message, makes a reasonable guess as to the meaning, and puts the guess into a responding statement. The statement is a declarative one and not phrased as a question, as follows:

> **EXAMPLE:** *Client: "I just don't know if I can lose weight, but I need to."*
> *(ambivalence)*
> *Counselor: "It sounds as if you are pulled in two ways. You want to lose weight. At the same time, you wonder if you can do it successfully." [Avoid: "You are concerned about losing weight?" as a question.]*
> *Client: "But it is so difficult."*
> *Counselor: "You found that your past efforts to change what you eat and lose weight were difficult. I think it's great that you want to try again."*
> *Client: "I never have eaten breakfast, because I don't have time."*
> *Counselor: "Your morning schedule must be a busy one."*

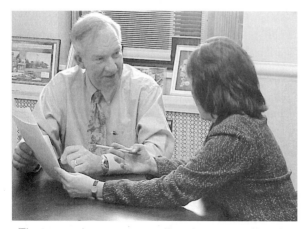

The counselor may use a directive or nondirective approach, or both.

Reflective listening and responding is a way of checking the meaning rather than assuming that you know exactly what is meant. It is a guess or hypothesis. This allows the client to keep moving in thought. Not every comment is reflected, however. The counselor decides what to emphasize and what to ignore.

In the early stage of the interview, open-ended questions allow individuals to explore the problems and help establish an atmosphere of trust and acceptance. The counselor may say: "In the time we have together, I want to get an understanding of any issues you have with your choices of foods. I'll be listening so I can understand your concerns. I'll also need to get some specific information from you. What do you see as the issues? What would you like to discuss first? What concerns you about your food intake?"

The client does more of the talking. The counselor may ask what problems concern the person or do the cost-and-benefit analysis. Follow up with the reflective listening. Periodic summaries move the interview along. You may summarize the client's statements about the problem, the client's ambivalence, self-motivational statements made by the client, and your assessment of the situation. Draw together the reasons for change. This helps clients make up their minds. It reinforces what they may already know to be true, but may be avoiding. Reflection is especially important after answers to open-ended questions and after self-motivational statements.

Motivation may be defined as "the probability that a person will enter into, continue, and adhere to a specific change strategy."(9) The counselor needs to increase the likelihood that the person will move toward change. The counselor wants to note and facilitate any self-motivational statements on the part of the client. There are several possible examples. First, the client recognizes that a problem exists. ("I guess my weight is a problem affecting my blood pressure.") Second, the client may express concern about the problem nonverbally, for example, by facial expression, sighing, tone of voice, or verbally ("I've got to make changes now and eat better for the sake of my health.") Finally, the client may feel positive about the change, thus reflecting self-efficacy. ("I'm sure I can start exercising this week.") Reflecting back these types of statements allows the client to hear the message for the second time and enhances self-motivation. Also, the counselor can reinforce nonverbally, such as by nodding the head.

The counselor may question the client to evoke self-motivational statements.

EXAMPLE: *For problem recognition: "What difficulties have you had in relation to your choices of foods?"*
For concern: "In what ways does choosing different foods or eating differently concern you?"

For intention to change: "What are the reasons you see for making a change?"
For optimism: "What encourages you to think that you can make this change?"

When clients reach the action stage of change, their questions can still be met with reflections. Here are possible questions to ask:

"What is the next step?"

"What do you plan to do?"

"Where do we go from here?"

"What good results will occur from this change?"

If the client asks the counselor for advice or information, one approach is to offer several alternatives rather than only one. For example: "I can give you several alternatives. Then you can tell me what you think will work for you." When the client selects an alternative, he or she is more likely to try it and adhere to it than if the counselor provides only one option. The client takes responsibility for a personal choice. In the case of only one alternative, the client may say: "That sounds good, but it won't work for me," thus rejecting the solution.(9)

Reaching a final plan requires setting clear goals. Having goals can facilitate change. Goals have been found to motivate because they set a standard against which the client can compare a current with a new behavior. They should be clearly stated, reasonable, and attainable. Selecting goals enhances personal choice and control, making it more likely that the person will succeed. Goals motivate change.

Lapse and relapse are a normal part of the change process. Effective counseling helps clients to identify and overcome any barriers to change. These may include, for example, lack of time, cost, family environment, lack of social support, nonsupportive friends, fear of adverse psychological or physiological consequences, and so forth.

Clients need feedback about the change to enhance motivation. It can be provided in many ways. Examples are self-monitoring records, results of improved medical laboratory tests, positive comments from friends, family, and the counselor, and the client's own positive self-talk ("I'm doing better").

When time is limited, brief interventions have been found to be effective. They commonly include six elements, summarized by the acronym FRAMES.

- Feedback
- Responsibility
- Advice
- Menu
- Empathy
- Self-efficacy(11)

After the counselor's initial assessment, *feedback* about relevant health information is given by the counselor. Personal *responsibility* for change is emphasized. "It's up to you to decide. You're the one who has to make changes in your food choices." Choices must be made freely and decisions to change are made only by the client. The client decides what, if anything to do with the feedback. Clear *advice* to change or make changes may be given as a *menu* of the variety of alternative ways that changes could be accomplished. Motivation can be enhanced when a person freely makes a decision and feels responsibility for the change. *Empathy* for the client is emphasized and expressed. Finally, attempts are included to strengthen the person's *self-efficacy* for change, to reinforce positive thoughts, and to reinforce the ability to succeed.

Brief motivational interventions were used with adolescents in the Dietary Intervention Study in Children (DISC). The purpose was to improve and renew motivation to adhere to a diet limited in fat to decrease low-density lipoprotein cholesterol in high-risk children. This intervention was successful with participants and appeared to renew and increase adherence to the DISC dietary plan. The intervention included establishing rapport, making an opening statement, assessing current eating behaviors and progress, giving feedback, assessment of readiness to change, and tailoring an intervention approach based on readiness to change.(12)

Motivational interviewing can overcome ambivalence and move the client from precontemplation to contemplation. It promotes the client's readiness to change and to try various courses of action. The client elaborates and the counselor reflects back again.

Rollnick's Framework

Rollnick suggests that you can assess readiness for change by asking two questions: How important is the change to you? How successful do you think you will be regarding the change?(8) Table 4-2 gives you a series of questions to assess these two areas with clients.(13) These questions assist in determining the stage of change.

COUNSELING AS A FOUR-STAGE PROCESS

Counseling is a customized interaction with the client. The process is an interactive one. The four-stage process is one approach to the session.(14) The development of rapport, empathy, and a trusting relationship is the first stage or "involving" stage. The three subsequent stages include "exploring," "resolving," and "concluding" the client's issues. Counseling deals simultaneously with both content and feelings. Trained counselors realize that only after the client's underlying feelings/beliefs have been identified and talked about can the content behind those feelings be discussed. Each stage requires special counseling skills that may have a particular usefulness and relevance at that stage.(14)

The goal of the first stage, involving, is to give clients clear expectations of the counseling process and a level of comfort and trust to enable an authentic and effective relationship. Concern and caring are often expressed in ways other than words. The old adage is valid: Actions speak louder than words. If the counselor seems uninterested, the client is likely to feel uncomfortable and confused. Attentive nonverbal behavior allows a person to infer caring and concern. Counselors need to be conscious of eye contact, body posture, hand and arm movements, facial expressions, and vocal quality, because these are the signals by which clients infer the degree of attentiveness, caring, and concern. A counselor's words equally make a difference. They can encourage openness or limit the client's disclosures. Look back at the questions and responses described under motivational interviewing.

TABLE 4-2 Assessing Importance and Confidence of the Patient

Useful Questions to Explore Importance	Useful Questions to Build Confidence
What would have to happen for it to become more important for you to change?	What would make you more confident about making these changes?
What would have to happen before you seriously considered changing?	Why have you given yourself such a high score on confidence?
Why have you given yourself such a high score on importance?	How could you move up higher, so that your score goes from . . . to . . .?
What would need to happen for your importance score to move up from . . . to . . .?	How can I help you succeed?
What stops you moving up from . . . to. . .?	Is there anything you found helpful in any previous attempts to change?
What are the good things (or things you like) about [current behavior]?	What have you learned from the way things went wrong last time you tried?
What are some of the less good things (or things you dislike) about . . . [current behavior]?	If you were to decide to change what might your options be? Are there any ways you know about that have worked for other people?
What concerns do you have about . . . [current behavior]?	What are some of the practical things you would need to do to achieve this goal? Do any of them sound achievable?
If you were to change, what would it be like?	Is there anything you can think of that would help you feel more confident?
Where does this leave you now? (When you want to ask about change in a neutral way).	

From Rollnick S, Mason P, Butler C. Health behavior change—A guide for practitioners. New York: Churchill Livingston, 1999.

Stages II, III, and IV relate more specifically to the recognition and initiation of specific behavior-change strategies. Exploring discusses the nature of the specific issue/problem in concrete terms. The goal is to encourage the client to identify the issues and provide details related to the problem. Resolving includes setting the client's goal to begin planning some corrective actions to resolve the problem. The counselor, mostly through the use of questions, attempts to collaborate, suggest alternatives, and serve as a resource. The final stage, concluding, is intended to verify for the client the plan for subsequent actions. The counselor may reinforce the client's plan, but the primary task is to make certain that the client can state the decisions made and the subsequent actions.

DIRECTIVE COUNSELING

The remainder of this chapter focuses on the general applications of directive counseling strategies as they might be used in nutrition counseling and in employee counseling. The discussion on nutrition counseling in Chapter 5 demonstrates the application of nondirective counseling. Directive counseling tends to be most appropriate when the counselor is aware of the problem and/or is concerned about the behavior of the client, but the client is unaware of the problem or is avoiding acknowledging it. Nondirective counseling tends to be most appropriate when the client has insight and calls on the counselor to assist in the problem solving. In practice, many counseling sessions use a composite of the two approaches such as in motivational interviewing.

In directive counseling, the counselor initiates discussion or approaches the client/staff member. In nondirective counseling, the client/staff member is aware of the problem and seeks help from the counselor. Clients/staff tend to be far more likely to become defensive and resist problem solving under the conditions of directive counseling. For this reason, counselors using this method need to be especially sensitive to all verbal and nonverbal behaviors and to be supportive while attempting to explore the issue at hand.

Directive counseling is most common in the manager-employee relationship rather than in the dietetics practitioner-client relationship. Directive counseling techniques are used for remedial counseling sessions to address poor employee performance when employees are unaware or unwilling to address it themselves. Nondirective counseling is ordinarily the preferred counseling method when dealing with clients who need to plan and set wellness goals or with employees who have sought out the help of their manager or supervisor. Frequently, counselors use a combination of both methods.

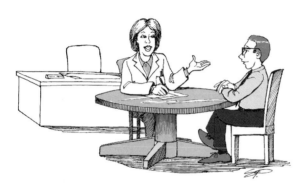

A casual setting creates a better rapport.

Applications of Directive Counseling

Managers have a skill set that is different from a clinician's skill set. Often, individuals who are extraordinary in their professional expertise or ability to perform a professional task are selected to manage others. Promoting technical professionals into management without first providing them with adequate training for the job is like sending individuals to bat with two strikes against them. Although all dietetics practitioners have a strong foundation regarding the competencies for being a supervisor or manager, additional continuing professional education in directive counseling or conflict resolution is often desirable.

Directive counseling is used for discussing unsatisfactory job performance. Counseling occurs after the manager has assessed that the employee knows his or her job description, has been trained for the position, and knows the performance expectation.(15) Directive counseling of employees is a form of discipline, and those administering it need to understand the concept. The root of the word "discipline" comes from Latin and means "to train" or "to mold." The attitude of the counselor needs to be that of a caring teacher who wishes to assist the other in improving. The objective of employee counseling is to change behaviors and develop productive members of the organization. After a manager has assembled and reviewed the facts surrounding a problem with sufficient detail, these must be shared and discussed with the employee. Next, the employee should be given options on how to correct the behavior and the consequences of failing to improve the behavior.

As pointed out earlier, clients/staff are far more likely to become hostile and defensive in directive counseling than in nondirective counseling, because they are "called in" rather than doing the "calling," and they may be more concerned with exonerating themselves of blame than with collaborating to solve the problem.

Employee Counseling   Employee counseling can be defined as the discussion of a work-related problem to eliminate or reduce it. Unless dietetics practitioners have advanced degrees with appropriate clinical counseling experience, counseling staff should be limited to the job-related concerns and should not include probing into personal problems such as depression, drug abuse, alcoholism, and mid-life crisis. For such personal problems, the dietetics practitioner should provide referrals to professional therapists or employee assistance programs. When employee counseling loses its problem-performance orientation, it runs the risk of being interpreted as meddling or an invasion of privacy.

Managers have an obligation to conduct work-related counseling sessions with employees. These should be held as often as necessary, assisting the staff in their professional development as well as dealing with career problems as they occur. The manager should not postpone employee counseling until the annual or semi-annual performance appraisal interviews. Allowing problems to accumulate and handling them all at one time is generally ineffective.

Guidelines for Directive Counseling

Involving Stage   In opening the discussion with the staff member, the counselor must be explicit in the desire to solve a problem rather than to punish. The aim is to improve the staff's performance. One way of keeping the conversation from becoming threatening is to keep remarks performance-centered rather than to make judgments about the staff member. It is more supportive and factual to say, "You have been late six times in the past 2 weeks," than to say, for example, "Lately you don't seem to care about your job; your attitude is poor." Inferences are not facts. The manager could not possibly know the quality of the employee's "caring" for his job or the condition of his "attitude," but she does know the objective facts—that the employee has been late six times in 2 weeks.

Exploring Stage   Throughout the interview, the counselor focuses on objective facts, being specific about what has been seen, about what behaviors need to be improved, and about the consequences of not changing the behavior. If the complaint is from others, and the supervisor/manager is unable to document the examples from personal observation, discuss the situation with the individual with an emphasis on clarifying the issues and hearing the staff's vantage point.

Resolving Stage   As in nondirective counseling, the counselor should provide adequate opportunity for employees to tell their side of the story, and their remarks should be paraphrased as well. Not only do people not know what they do not know, but they easily fall into traps of seeing, hearing, and selectively perceiving what they expect to see and hear. Giving employees an opportunity to tell their side of the story and then paraphrasing it and empathizing with what the employee is feeling usually leads to collaboration in the conflict-resolution process. There may be extenuating circumstances that no one on the staff is aware of, which account for the dysfunctional behavior of the employee. Having employees explain the problem from their own perspective may add significant insight and understanding.

Concluding Stage After an agreement on a solution has been reached, the counselor should describe as specifically as possible what the consequences will be if the agreed-upon changes in the employee's behavior are not actualized. You might say, for example, "If you are absent without notice again, I am going to file a warning notice with personnel." The manager needs to remember at this point not to exaggerate the consequences or to mention consequences that will not be carried out. If the employee does continue the problematic behavior, the manager must go to the next level of the disciplinary process.

Although verifying understanding is important in nondirective counseling, it is even more important in directive counseling. The tendency for employees to experience physiological stress symptoms from the threat of being called in by the manager heightens the possibility of their misunderstanding some of the communication. Both the manager and the staff member need to paraphrase one another to verify that each has understood the other and that they agree on the final solution. An expression of confidence and support by the manager can help ensure successful implementation of an action plan that both parties have agreed on. Rather than saying, "Well, let's see what will happen," the manager provides more motivation by saying, "I think these are the kinds of ideas that can make a difference." Employees should be reminded that they are an important part of the team, that the manager does indeed care for them personally, and that their contributions to the staff are valued. If the action plan includes a multi-step process for improvement, it would be wise to set follow-up meeting dates. Doing so not only confirms commitment, but adds incentive to begin the performance changes.

As in nondirective counseling, managers must attend to the supporting nonverbal behavior throughout the directive counseling interview. They should select a private place free of interruptions. The spatial dynamics of the location should allow the two people to feel close and intimate, since feelings are being shared and help is being given to solve the problem. The manager needs to act, talk, look, and gesture in a manner that allows the subordinate to infer that the purpose of the counseling session is to change dysfunctional behavior, not to reject or punish. Finally, the manager has to remember to allow adequate time for full expression of thoughts and schedule multiple sessions when appropriate.

Measuring the Outcomes of Counseling

The outcome of successful counseling is attaining the desired goals. These goals may be those of the employer, primary care provider, counselor and, most important, the clients/employees. The measurement may be short-term or long-term. Chapter 5 identifies many nutrition outcomes that can be measured. Beyond individual client/staff outcomes, dietetics practitioners need to systematically assess the results of their counseling to determine effectiveness. Questions such as the number of counseling sessions generally needed to create client change are essential to determine recommendations for care and reimbursement norms. Self- and periodic client evaluation of your counseling skills will assist in your professional counseling skill development.

CASE STUDY 1

Connie, a Registered Dietitian, has worked at Sun Valley Hospital, a 200-bed community hospital for 3 years. Her immediate supervisor, Jill, the clinical manager, is preparing her performance evaluation. While preparing Connie's evaluation, Jill noted that more than 50% of the goals for Connie's performance had not been met. During the evaluation, Connie asked Jill why her merit increase was smaller than the year before. Jill indicated that since 50% of the goals were not met, she was receiving a merit increase based on partial achievement of her goals. Connie left the evaluation session angrily, stating "I don't think this is fair."

1. What could Jill have done to alter the evaluation process?
2. What is the role of Connie in the evaluation process?
3. What steps would you suggest to avoid a similar evaluation next year?

CASE STUDY 2

The dietetic counselor is employed at a WIC (women, infants, and children) clinic. Her client is a 16-year-old who has just learned she is 4 months pregnant with her first child. Her older sister, 18, is accompanying her. Her diet history reveals the following:

Breakfast: None or soda and potato chips
Lunch: French fries, soda, and cookies
Dinner: Meat such as ham, potatoes, bread and butter, and soda
Snacks: Soda, snack foods, crackers, and cookies

Using the motivational interviewing process, respond to the following client's statements reflectively.

1. "My sister says I need to eat differently now that I am pregnant, but I like the foods I eat now."
2. "I'm not hungry in the morning. I have to leave for school at 7:15."
3. "I spend a lot of time with my friends. They can eat whatever they want."

REVIEW AND DISCUSSION QUESTIONS

1. Why is counseling important to both managerial and clinical dietetics practitioners?
2. What are the key outcomes from a counseling or a series of counseling sessions?
3. Differentiate between nondirective and directive counseling.
4. Describe the four characteristics of a quality counselor-client relationship and why they are important.
5. How is motivational interviewing different from the transtheoretical model of counseling?

6. Why is the stage of change important to know when counseling a client?
7. What are the five principles underlying motivational interviewing?
8. Define and give two examples of reflective listening.
9. Why is it better to give the client more than one suggestion when he or she asks for suggestions?
10. Explain the four-stage process of counseling. Provide an example of how this would work with an employee absenteeism issue.

SUGGESTED ACTIVITIES

1. To practice reflective listening statements, form groups of two, one playing the role of a client and one a counselor. Each client should think of two or three things about himself/herself that he or she would like to change (e.g., get more sleep, eat better, lose weight, get more organized and use time better, overcome procrastination, be happier, watch less television, make more friends). This can be stated as: "One thing I would like to change about myself is...." The counselor develops one or two hypotheses of what the person means and puts one of them into a reflective statement rather than a question. A reflection may be started with the following: "You are feeling...." "It sounds like you...." "You are saying that ...." "So you think...."
2. During the next week, practice paraphrasing what others say. What reactions do you get? Does your paraphrasing tend to cause the other to go on talking?
3. Write both a paraphrase and an emphatic comment to the following comments made by a counselee:
   A. I feel awkward discussing my eating habits. I feel I must be disgusting to you.
   B. People tend to think I'm jolly, but I don't believe they take me seriously.
   C. I am at a point now where I don't believe I will ever lose the weight.
4. Form triads consisting of a counselor, counselee, and observer. Each individual should take a turn in each of the roles for 7 minutes. Try three approaches to counseling, the motivational interview, the Rollnick approach, and the four-stage approach. The counselee should play the role of an obese client. After each round, the observer should share reactions to the counselor's approach and encourage feedback from the counselee to the counselor. From the counselee's perspective, what did the counselor do that helped their interaction; what did the counselor do that hindered it? At the end, discuss how each approach helped you.
5. Repeat the activity in number 4. The counselee is a staff member who is not completing his work in a timely manner. Which approach was most helpful here and why?
6. During the next week, make arrangements to view a dietitian's counseling session, noting particularly what occurs during each stage of the process. What behavior on the part of the dietitian facilitates the building of rapport and trust? What techniques did you see that were reflected in the chapter? Discuss which characteristics of a successful counselor were expressed.
7. After each of the statements below, use the FRAME acronym approach to consider the comment.

A. My work situation is impossible. It seems that I'm the scapegoat for everybody. I'm beginning to wonder if I should consider looking for another job.

B. It doesn't seem fair to me that I should have to work weekends when the staff members who have been here only 2 years longer don't have to.

C. It seems easy every morning to promise myself that today I will stick to the program you designed for me. By noon, however, I begin thinking that I'll never be able to comply with the diet for the rest of my life, so why bother?

8. To practice developing understanding and using reflective listening, divide into pairs. Ask each person to prepare to discuss a personal experience that would be difficult for someone else to understand. The counselor can use open-ended questions but primarily reflections. The task is to use verbal and nonverbal skills to seek to understand the experience being described by the other. After 10 to 15 minutes, the pair may switch roles. At the conclusion, the instructor may wish to answer questions and ask for reactions to the activity.

9. Count the F's in the following statement:

> FASCINATING FAIRYTALES ARE THE RESULT
> OF YEARS OF SCIENTIFIC STUDY COMBINED
> WITH THE EXPERIENCE OF CREATIVE MINDS.

Compare answers with several people. Why did you get different answers. How does this relate to issues as a counselor?

10. Explain the relationship between nutrition education and nutrition counseling. How are they similar and different?

REFERENCES

1. Rogers C. Client-centered therapy. Boston: Houghton Mifflin, 1951.
2. Rogers C. On becoming a person. Boston: Houghton Mifflin, 1961.
3. Patterson CH. Theories of counseling and psychotherapy. New York: Harper & Row, 1966.
4. Rogers C. The interpersonal relationship: the core of guidance. Harvard Educ Rev 1962;32:416.
5. Johnson K. How to create trust. Broker World 1989;9:100.
6. Luzaszewski J. How to coach executives. Communication World 1989;6:38.
7. May R. The art of counseling. New York: Gardner Press, 1989.
8. Rollnick S, Mason P, Butler C. Health behavior change—a guide for practitioners. New York: Churchill Livingstone, 1999.
9. Miller WR, Rollnick S. Motivational interviewing: preparing people to change addictive behavior. New York: Guilford Press, 1991.
10. Prochaska JO, DiClemente CC, Norcross JC. In search of how people change: applications to addictive behaviors. Am Psychol 1992;47:1102.
11. Miller WR. Motivational interviewing: research, practice and puzzles. Addictive Behaviors 1996;21(6):835.
12. Berg-Smith SM, Stevens VJ, Brown KM, et al. A brief motivational intervention to improve dietary adherence in adolescents. Health Educ Res 1999;14:399.
13. Newman V. Facilitating health behavior change. Nutrition Educators of Health Professionals. Summer 2001, p. 3.

14. Kinlaw D. Helping skills for human resource development: a facilitator's package. San Diego: University Associates, 1981.
15. Umiker W. Management skills for the new health care supervisor. Gaithersburg, MD: Aspen, 1998.

WEB SITES

www.motivationalinterview.org / information about motivational interviewing
www.oprf.com/Rogers / information about Carl Rogers

5 | Nutrition Counseling

After reading this chapter, you will be able to

1. explain the steps in the nutrition counseling process.
2. explain the stages and processes of change.
3. identify the information needed in a nutrition assessment.
4. explain and practice the steps in goal setting with a client.
5. discuss nutrition intervention and treatment.
6. list ways to evaluate the outcomes of nutrition treatment including how to follow up.
7. explain some of the expanding roles for professionals.

If you don't have time to cook, you can have a regular diet of fast foods or buy entire meals you can microwave at home.

Journal of the American Dietetic Association 2001;101:529

There is no single gold standard method or unifying theory of counseling patients and clients that ensures success in changing food choices and eating behaviors. Instead, dietetics professionals need to be proficient in using a number of different approaches and strategies while adapting them to the people they are counseling.

The previous chapter examined counseling approaches and theories. This chapter explores a basic nutrition counseling process using a model as an outline. It emphasizes assessing the client's stage of change, matching the counseling intervention strategies to the stage, and using the goal-setting process. Later chapters emphasize other counseling approaches, including counseling with behavior modification, counseling for cognitive change since thoughts may influence eating practices, the role of self-efficacy in making lifestyle changes, and preventing or dealing with lapses and relapse.

GOALS OF NUTRITION COUNSELING

Dietetics professionals, whether working in hospitals, medical centers, long-term care, corporate wellness programs, sports nutrition, public health agencies, private practice, or other settings, are responsible for assessing the nutritional status of patients and clients and counseling them about what they are doing successfully and what they may need to change. The goal is to change people's eating behaviors for the improvement of their health and the reduction in the risk of chronic diseases, such as cardiovascular disease, diabetes mellitus, hypertension, and renal disease. The following model depicts this relationship(2):

Nutrition counseling & education	→	Changes in food intake	→	Altered risk factors	→	Desirable health outcomes	→	Economic benefits

(Compliance)

Since changes in eating practices are usually necessary, remember that change is never easy. Changing eating patterns is probably one of the most difficult lifestyle changes a person has to make, since dietary habits are longstanding. Continuing with the current, comfortable lifestyle and avoiding change represent the path of least resistance. The client's resistance to change may occur at an unrecognized, subconscious level and should be expected and probed by the counselor.

Food preferences are determined by many factors, such as cultural, ethnic, socioeconomic, and religious factors. Changing eating patterns is probably a more difficult endeavor than exercising more frequently, stopping cigarette smoking, and taking new medications. Eating provides not only physiological benefits, but also complex psychological benefits. Eating is pleasurable, and food may be associated with reduced stress, boredom, and frustration while providing comfort.

Outcomes are enhanced when a person learns self-management skills, since contact with the counselor is limited. In a person with diabetes, for example, the purpose of nutrition counseling is to change from current eating patterns to nutritional self-management of diabetes. For a pregnant woman, the purpose is to add to her diet foods that meet the nutritional needs of pregnancy while maintaining appropriate caloric levels.

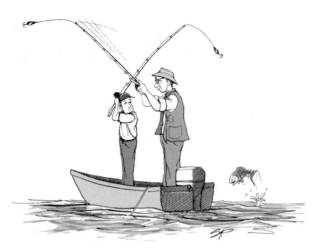

Give a man a fish and you feed him for a day. Teach a man to fish and you feed him for a lifetime.

Eventual client self-management is the goal of all counseling. The counselor must provide the knowledge, skills, and approaches needed by individuals to live independently in their family settings. An old adage states: "Give a man a fish and you feed him for a day. Teach a man to fish and you feed him for a lifetime." The client should take increasing responsibility over time for the dietary change process. Nutrition counseling cannot be a one-time service. Follow-up counseling is necessary until the person is self-sufficient.

MODEL OF THE NUTRITON COUNSELING PROCESS

Several models of the nutrition counseling process may be found in the literature.(3–6) Models help you examine and understand steps in a complex process. A model for medical nutrition therapy includes the following four parts(4):

1. Assessment of the person's metabolic and lifestyle parameters, including dietary, behavioral, physical, social, and cognitive environments as well as stage of change
2. Goal setting based on the assessment
3. Intervention and treatment to achieve the goals
4. Evaluation of outcomes and follow-up

The ideal situation for nutrition counseling consists of a process over a period of time in which clients develop a growing awareness of their food choices and dietary practices and of how these factors influence their health. The process of assisting people in establishing and maintaining good nutrition habits is a complex task, because it requires people to make permanent changes in their eating behaviors.

ASSESSMENT

Nutrition assessment uses a comprehensive approach to evaluating nutritional status by including a number of sources of information: dietary intake, health history including medications taken, laboratory data, anthropometric measurements, lifestyle, and other influences. The assessment assists in identifying the nutritional goals for change, the type of nutrition intervention designed to achieve the goals, and the evaluation of the outcomes.

The first step in nutrition assessment is to gather in advance data or information about the client that may have an impact on treatment. In a hospital or clinic setting, the medical record is the source of data about the patient. Height, weight, pertinent laboratory values, medications, and medical history should be noted. Many factors may make an impact on eating patterns, such as family status, occupation, income, educational level, ethnicity, religion, physical activity, physical disabilities or impairments (seeing, hearing), and place of residence.(5)

Information that is unavailable from the medical record may be obtained during the interview by using a self-administered questionnaire or by collecting anthropometric and dietary data. Nutrition counselors are expected to know their clients physiologically, psychologically, socially, culturally, and economically; that is, they should know what factors influence their clients' eating and lifestyle behaviors. Counselors must view their clients as individuals living and interacting in an environment that influences their motivation for and ability to change.

A second source of data is the dietetics professional's own records kept from previous counseling sessions or previous contact with the client. These records should be reviewed before follow-up counseling. Since the purpose of counseling is to promote change, the dietetics professional needs to collect and assess data that indicate what changes need to be made, what the client wants to discuss, and what personal and lifestyle factors may promote or interfere with changes in eating patterns. After informing the client of the purpose of the interview and after having established good rapport with the client, the counselor may take a nutrition history from the client by using the interviewing skills discussed in Chapter 3.

The dietetics professional may collect data on current eating habits, on the physical, social, and cognitive environments; on previous attempts to make dietary changes.(5) (Behavioral assessment and cognitive assessment are discussed in Chapters 6 and 7.) The physical environment includes where meals are eaten (at home or in restaurants and in which rooms of the home) and events that occur while eating (socializing, watching television, or reading). The social environment, which may or may not be supportive, includes family members, friends, social norms, and trends involved with eating behaviors (e.g., popular food customs of a bridge club, drinking buddies). See Appendix at the end of this chapter for other suggestions.

The cognitive or mental environment involves the client's thoughts and feelings about food and his or her self-image and self-confidence. It concerns what clients say to themselves about their food habits and life, since personal thoughts may or may not promote successful change. Some thoughts may be positive, such as "I love a steak and baked potato," or "My favorite snacks are potato chips and beer." There may be negative and self-defeating thoughts, or thoughts of failure, boredom, stress, and hunger. Examples include: "It's too difficult," "It's not worth it," "I can't do it," "I've been on diets before, always failed, and regained all of the weight I lost," or "I'm happy the way I am and don't want to change." Since behavior is influenced by beliefs and attitudes, you need to explore these in relation to the medical condition, nutrition, food choices, and health. The client's educational level and any language barriers should be noted.

The assessment may have a number of important functions, such as making both parties aware of the current food patterns, problems, knowledge, and misinformation, as well as obtaining the health history. The assessment also provides baseline information from which to gauge progress, alerts both parties to the demands placed on the client so that realistic goals can be identified, provides both parties with ideas for developing the nutrition intervention, provides an opportunity to continue rapport, and enables the counselor and client to work together on a plan for gradual changes that is congruent with the client's lifestyle.(4) Screening for the risk of malnutrition, for example, may require a full nutrition assessment in people with some illnesses such as cancer and AIDS.(7) This assists in determining and prioritizing appropriate nutrition interventions.

Assessing Stages of Change

Prochaska and colleagues have developed a Transtheoretical Model or Stages of Change Model. It is a framework for understanding clients' readiness to change to healthier eating practices. Change is *not* viewed as a single event, such as "I will eat less sodium starting today." People who need to make changes progress through six identified stages: precontemplation (no intention of changing in the next 6 months), contemplation (intending to change but not soon), preparation (intending to change in the next month), action (recent changes in food choices), maintenance (maintained changes for 6 months), and termination (changes maintained for 5 years).(8–10)

People do not change their food choices just because we tell them to or because they know they should. The key to successful nutrition counseling and education is to assess and identify the person's stage or readiness for change and match the intervention to it. Different counseling strategies are needed, for example, for those unaware of a problem, for those resisting efforts to change, and for those intending to change at a future time. This should increase the effectiveness of the intervention, assist the client in progressing to the next stage because of enhanced motivation and readiness, and reduce the likelihood of dropping out of treatment because the intervention was not appropriate. Dietary fat reduction and weight control are the most developed dietary applications of the model.(10–14)

Most health interventions and educational programs are action oriented, assuming that people are making changes or are ready to. However, about 40% to 50% of people are in the precontemplation stage, in denial or resistant to change, 20% are in the preparation stage, whereas only about 20% to 25% are in the action stage.(10,15) Assuming that the client is at the action stage can be counterproductive and lead to failure and dropout. Determining readiness to change is crucial in deciding on the approach to intervention. Practitioners need to provide skills and support change at every stage and help people move to the next stage and eventually to action.

In stage 1, precontemplation, a person is unaware or underaware that a problem exists, denies that there is a problem or is not interested in change, and thus has no plans to change eating practices or start exercising in the near future.(8, 9) The person may have previously tried a change such as weight loss, and failed, and he or she may be resistant to the health professional's efforts to suggest possible changes. Perhaps a visit to the doctor initiated a referral to see the dietitian for weight loss, even if the patient was satisfied with his or her weight. To identify this stage, you may ask: "Are you seriously intending to change (name the problem behavior) in the next 6 months?" For example, for people ignoring the relationship between a high-fat diet and coronary heart disease, you may ask: "Have you thought about eating less fat (or more fruits and vegetables) in the next 6 months?" At this stage, a person with high levels of low-density lipoprotein cholesterol may need to know the benefits of a lower blood level, for example, and the risks of not addressing the problem. An attempt to focus instead on making dietary changes may not be effective in precontemplation. Table 5-1 lists other questions and interventions at each stage.

In stage 2, contemplation, a person is aware that a problem exists and intends to do better eventually, such as eating differently or exercising more. However, he or she has no serious thought or commitment to making a change and keeps putting it off.(8, 9) The person may be mentally struggling with the amount of energy, effort, and cost of overcoming a problem and may be discouraged by previous failures. You may ask:

"What have you been thinking about in terms of making a change?"

"What are the pros and cons of doing it?"

"How can you change your environment?"

"What do you think about eating less fat? What are the barriers or obstacles to doing it?"

The balance between pros and cons can result in ambivalence that keeps people at this stage for long periods of time, even months or years.(11,15)

In stage 3, preparation, a person is more determined to change and intends to take initial action soon, perhaps in about 30 days, but not today.(8,9) He or she may report small changes in the problem behavior, such as reading a few food labels or buying fat-free ice cream.

TABLE 5-1 Stages of Change

Stage	Question for Client	Intervention
Precontemplation	"What can I do to help?"	Consciousness raising
	"Do you ever read articles about...?"	Assess knowledge
	"What do you know about the relationship between..."	Increase self-awareness
		Give information
	"Does anyone in your family have this problem?"	Assess values
		Assess beliefs
	"Are you aware of the consequences?"	Cognitive restructuring
	"How do you feel about making a change?"	Discuss risks and benefits
Contemplation	"What changes have you been thinking about?"	Assess knowledge
	"What are the pros and cons?"	Assess values, beliefs
	"How do you feel about it?"	Assess thoughts, feelings
	"What would make it easier or harder?"	Decrease barriers
	"What would be the results of the change?"	Self-evaluation
	"How can I help?	Cognitive restructuring
Preparation	"Are you intending to act in the next 1–6 months?"	Self-efficacy
		Commitment
	"How will you do it?"	Decision making
	"What changes have you made already?"	Discuss beliefs about ability
	"How will your life be improved?"	Plan goals
Action	"What are you doing differently?"	Stimulus control
	"What problems are you having?"	Self-reinforcement
	"Who can help you?"	Social support
	"How can I help?"	Self-management
	"What do you do instead of (former behavior)?"	Goal setting
		Group sessions
		Self-monitoring
		Relapse prevention
Maintenance	"How do you handle times when you slip up?"	Coping responses
	"What obstacles are you facing?"	Relapse prevention
	"What are your future plans?"	Self-management
	"What issues have you solved?"	Commitment
		Goal setting
		Control environment
Termination		Self-management
		Self-efficacy

In stage 4, action, a person attempts to overcome the problem by actively modifying food choices, behaviors, environments, or experiences.(8,9) Remember that most clients are *not* in the action stage when referred for counseling. Considerable commitment of time and energy is required for the action stage when people are trying to change. You may ask: "What are you doing differently?"

In stage 5, maintenance, a person consolidates and stabilizes gains made over several months to maintain the new, healthier habits and works to prevent relapse.(8,9,15)

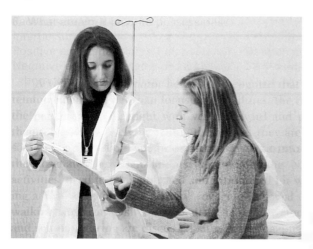

Maintaining weight loss, for example, takes continuing effort. For some people, this stage continues for months, years, or a lifetime, or until the behavior becomes a pattern and is incorporated into their lifestyle. You may ask: "How do you handle small lapses?" (Additional information on counseling about lapses and relapse is in Chapter 7.)

The ultimate goal is the termination stage in which changes have been maintained for 5 years. However, some types of problems, such as weight management, may require a lifetime of mainte-

The dietetic professional needs to assess the patient's stage of change.

nance instead. People, for example, tend to become more sedentary and overweight as they age, thus contributing to continual problems.

SELF ASSESSMENT

"Think of a lifestyle or personal problem you would like to change. Which of the six stages are you in?"

Prochaska proposed that people proceed through the stages in a spiral, rather than a linear, fashion.(8–10) Because lapses and relapse are common problems, recycling to an earlier stage, such as from action to preparation or from preparation to contemplation, may be expected several times as people struggle to modify or cease behaviors. People may avoid high-fat foods, for example, and then start eating them again. Lapse and relapse and the negative emotional reactions (guilt, shame, failure) that may result are discussed in more detail in Chapter 7. It is hoped that people learn from their mistakes with the help of the counselor and continue trying.

A second dimension of the model examines the processes of change or activities people use to progress through the stages of change when there are shifts in behaviors, attitudes, and intentions.(15) The processes of change should be integrated into the stages of change so that the treatment intervention matches the client's stage of change.

In the early stages, focusing on the benefits of making a change and how that change can improve the individual's life or health is suggested. The goal is for the client to think about the problem.(10) However, clients may doubt their ability to change and have decreased self-efficacy at this point. In precontemplation (consciousness raising), providing nutritional information (oral, written, web addresses) about the benefits of healthy choices and about the individual's risk for chronic disease based on dietary habits with the advantages of change is suggested. Self-reevaluation of thoughts, feelings, values, problems, self, and environment is appropriate. The client needs to weigh the pros and cons of change, with the pros ("I'll see my grandchildren grow up.") outweighing the cons ("I can't eat whatever I want."). Cons outweigh the pros at this stage.(10) In the Seattle "5 a Day" worksite intervention to encourage employees to consume more fruits and vegetables, for example, several communication methods were used to move people from precontemplation to contemplation. They included posters, flyers, paycheck inserts, table tents in the cafeteria, and electronic mail.(16)

Cognitive and affective self-reevaluation, in addition to raising awareness, is suggested in the contemplation stage. Self-liberation (a belief that one can change and the actual making of a commitment to it) and behavioral goals (discussed later in this chapter) are important in the preparation stage. In the client's assessment, the benefits or pros must outweigh the cons or costs. In the action and maintenance stages, behavioral techniques (Chapter 6) of stimulus control, reinforcement management, self-monitoring, recipe modification, coping responses during conditions when relapse is likely, and developing a social support system of significant others are useful.(10,11,15,17) Keep in mind that the client may be at an early stage for one change, such as increasing fruit and vegetable intake, while at another stage for a different behavior, such as increasing exercise or decreasing portion size.

The Stages of Change Model was used in defining the energy level of dietary fat in people's diets and was found to be effective in characterizing people by relative fat intake.(18) Those in the stages of precontemplation to preparation may be expected to have higher intakes of fat than those in the action or maintenance stages.(19) One study that assessed stages of change in relation to fat and fiber found that people on a higher fat intake were in the earlier stages (precontemplation, contemplation, and preparation) and those consuming less fat and more fiber were in the later stages (action and maintenance).(20)

Using the stages of change model to achieve Healthy People 2000 objectives of decreasing dietary fat and increasing fruit and vegetable consumption, Campbell and colleagues(21) individually tailored computer messages with the person's current dietary intake and self-reported stage of change. Changes in dietary fat intake were less affected by messages based on dietary guidelines than on those individually tailored to a person's stage of change.

In a study of the 5-a-Day for Better Health initiative, fruit and vegetable consumption, self-efficacy, and knowledge of the 5-a-Day recommendations were positively associated with more advanced stages of change.(22) Among high school students, all were found to be in the earlier stages of change, and none was found to be in action or maintenance related to the 5-a-Day for Better Health program.(23)

After you gather the assessment data, you should analyze and interpret it. Identify influences on eating patterns, and note alternative food choices. Changes may be thought of as problems to be solved by setting goals with the client and should be appropriate to the client's stage of change. This information is baseline data on the client taken before counseling and is recorded later and referred to in future counseling sessions.

GOAL SETTING

The counseling relationship was described in the previous chapter. Counselors should clarify that the responsibility for change rests with the client, but that they are willing to assist in solving problems and helping with goals and new plans. It is recommended that nutrition interventions be based on the self-management approach.(4, 24, 25) This involves clients in their own health care and has them take an active part in their treatment.

Before problems are explored and goals are set, it is advisable to discuss with the client, show approval for, and reinforce those current food choices that do not need changing, that is, what the individual is already doing right according to the diet prescription. Problems—foods that should be limited or foods or cooking practices that should be changed—may be discussed next, perhaps starting with the counselor's estimation of what is most important as well as what the client is willing to consider. Goals should be mutually negotiated based on the nutrition care plan, desired clinical outcomes, or, in the case of normal nutrition, the Dietary Guidelines for Americans (Table 5-2).(26) The conditions and circumstances surrounding food behaviors need to be explored. This stage of counseling requires listening, questioning, accepting, clarifying, and helping clients find solutions to their problems and develop their own plan of action.

Counseling should not be directed solely at the client's knowledge, but also at feelings, attitudes, beliefs, and values, which have strong and powerful influences on dietary behaviors. Several reasonable and appropriate alternatives may be suggested by the counselor, but leaving the final decision to the client on which alternative is pre-

---

TABLE 5-2   **Dietary Guidelines for Americans**

Aim for Fitness . . .
- Aim for a healthy weight.
- Be physically active each day.

Build a Healthy Base . . .
- Let the Pyramid guide your food choices.
- Choose a variety of grains daily, especially whole grains.
- Choose a variety of fruits and vegetables daily.
- Keep food safe to eat.

Choose Sensibly . . .
- Choose a diet that is low in saturated fat and cholesterol and moderate in total fat.
- Choose beverages and foods to moderate your intake of sugars.
- Choose and prepare foods with less salt.
- If you drink alcoholic beverages, do so in moderation

. . . for good health

Source: www.nalusda.gov/fnic/dga.

ferred. Knowledge is a tool only if and when a person is ready to change and is motivated to change. You may ask any of the following questions:

> **EXAMPLE:** *"Which of these alternatives or changes do you think you could try?"*
> *"What would be the easiest?" "The hardest?"*
> *"Is this the right time to make changes?"*
> *"Do you think you can succeed?"*
> *"What foods could you substitute?"*
> *"How will things be better or worse after you make the change?"*
> *"How do you feel about making this change?"*

The client weighs the pros and cons of the options.

Clients (not the counselor) at the preparation, action, and maintenance stages of change should select one or two priorities for change for the next week or so. Clients who are at the precontemplation and contemplation stages of change or who are enthusiastic about making total changes immediately are setting themselves up for frustration and possible failure, which may lead to abandoning the dietary changes altogether. The counselor should guard against this and use other interventions instead. Slow, steady changes that will persist over time are preferable.

The session with a client needing a sodium-restricted diet, for example, may uncover the following problems:

1. Uses salt in cooking and at the table
2. Snacks include crackers and potato chips
3. Uses some high-sodium spices and flavorings
4. Likes bacon, ham, and salami
5. Eats lunch in a restaurant
6. Is only one in the family on a sodium-restricted diet
7. Grocery shopping done by wife, who does not read labels

The problems can be reinterpreted into positive goals for change. A four-step process may be followed in using goal setting with clients: (1) goal identification, (2) goal importance assessment, (3) goal roadblock analysis, and (4) goal attainment.(27–29)

Goal Identification

The first step in goal setting is goal identification. People who have no goals lack a sense of direction in their lives. Personal goals can spur clients to new achievements and changes because they give the person something to strive for as well as a standard against which to judge progress. Because clients are more committed to changes that they select, the counselor may inquire which one or two of the problems does the person want to address first by saying, "Which one or two changes do you think that you can work on this week?" When people play a significant role in selecting goals, they hold themselves responsible for progress. If goals are imposed by the counselor, people do not accept them or feel personally responsible for fulfilling them. If these goals impose severe constraints and burdens, they can render the pursuit aversive and breed dislike rather than nurture interest.(30)

Goals selected by the client should be positively stated as concrete behaviors. Goals should be specific, measurable, reasonable, attainable, and timely. A goal should specify what the person will do or is trying to achieve. Following are examples of goals:

> **EXAMPLE:** *"I will eat fruit instead of baked desserts today."*
> *"I will purchase salt-free pretzels for a snack."*
> *"I will walk for 20 minutes on Monday, Wednesday, and Friday this week."*

The degree to which goals create incentives and guides for action is partly determined by their specificity.(30) Clear, attainable goals produce higher levels of performance than general intentions to do the best one can, which may have little or no effect, such as "I'll look for low-sodium foods the next time I am at the grocery store." When goals are set unrealistically high, performance may prove disappointing. If the client selects problems numbered 1 and 2 from the earlier list, for example, these can be reinterpreted into goals for change as follows:

> **EXAMPLE:** *"I will use low-sodium seasonings in cooking and pepper at the table."*
> *"I will eat fruits and low-sodium crackers for snacks."*

Note that the positive statement of using low-sodium seasonings is preferable to the negative goal of avoiding salt. It is easier to do something positive than to avoid doing something.

Goals should provide a degree of challenge and are standards against which performance attainments are compared.(30) Setting specific goals leads to higher performance when compared with no goals or vague, non-quantifiable goals. "I will walk 15 minutes daily" is better than "I will try to walk daily."(31,32) Having goals can motivate higher performance than having no goals. They should be challenging, yet achievable.

To be realistic and reasonable, goals should be based on the person's past and current behavior. The first challenge should be only a small step away, not a major change, from the current behavior and should be matched with the client's perceived capabilities

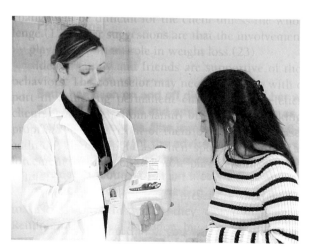

Clients may need an explanation of food labels.

for achieving it. The counselor should guide people toward those goals that they believe they can realistically accomplish.

Goal setting may also be an important part of disease management. Outcomes of interventions may include clinical parameters, such as blood pressure, body weight, lipid levels, and blood glucose levels.(3) However, they may be influenced by factors unrelated to the desired dietary changes.

It is hoped that the client will have a successful experience, not failure, if first changes are not difficult, before returning for follow-up counseling. This is especially important when the individual has negative thoughts or a previous failure at dietary change. Each succeeding subgoal should present new challenges in the mastery of new subskills. Small steps lead to major gains.

A distinction must be made between short-term goals and distal or end goals. The relation between attaining goals and expenditure of effort to attain goals differs.(30) Short-term subgoals that are challenging but attainable with effort are likely to be more motivating and self-satisfying. Self-motivation can be increased by progressively raising subgoals, even though the long-range goals are difficult to realize. For example, people need to commit themselves to the goal of following the dietary changes or goal today, rather than a long-term goal of never eating high-fat foods again. When the distant future is the focus, it is easy to put off the goal and decide to start tomorrow.

Persistence that leads to eventual mastery of an activity is thus ensured through a progression of subgoals, each with a high probability of success. When self-satisfaction is contingent upon attaining challenging goals, more effort is expended than if easy goals are adopted as sufficient.

Goal Importance Assessment

In the second step, after identifying goals, the counselor assesses the goal importance by asking, for example: "On a scale of 1 to 10 with 10 being the highest, how important is that goal to you?" What the counselor thinks is important does not matter. Goals that are not perceived as important by the client are unlikely to be achieved. Other goals should be set instead.

Most of the activities that we now enjoy at one time held little or no interest for us because we were not exposed to them. Certain sports, kinds of music, hobbies, and career choices are examples of activities we learn about and enjoy over time. Subgoals for dietary change, if valued, can cultivate people's intrinsic interest, enlist sustained involvement in activities that will build new skills and competencies, and increase motivation and self-perceptions of efficacy.(30) People who do not set goals for themselves achieve little change in performance.

The strength of a person's goal commitment is affected by several factors. The value the person places on the activity, the perceived attainability of the goals, and binding pledges people make to others concerning their future performance all make a difference.(30) The practitioner needs to inquire about these:

"Do you think you can do it?"

"How important is it to you?"

"Is there someone else with whom you can share your plans?"

In a clinical trial, for example, intense dietary counseling lowered low-density lipoprotein cholesterol.(33) Goal setting that focused on two or three goals was used in the initial counseling session. The second session provided positive feedback on dietary and serum cholesterol changes and continued the goal-setting process. A team approach and counseling over 3 to 4 months enhanced dietary compliance.

Using goal setting, a second intervention with women set 20% of calories from fat as the goal. Twenty dietary behavior change sessions were held. Results showed that 77% met the goal in 6 months, and over two-thirds were maintaining it 2 years later.(34)

Goal Roadblock Analysis

In the third step, obstacles to achieving the goals are examined. You may ask: "What problems do you see in achieving this goal?" "What might interfere?" "How do you feel about this change?" It is important to discuss the problems thoroughly along with the impact of physical, cultural, social, and cognitive environments on the goals selected for change. Roadblocks may be lack of knowledge, such as about the fat content of foods, lack of skills, such as cooking skills or skill in reading food labels, inability to take risks, and lack of social support at home.(27–29)

It is advisable to tell the client to expect some problems, since some things may come up that were not thought of during the counseling session. If the client is aware of the possibility of problems, he or she may avoid abandoning the diet with the first lapse or obstacle. After all, basketball players do not make a basket every time they shoot the ball. But they keep on trying. Supplying a phone number or e-mail address for questions or a website for resources may resolve unexpected problems. However, e-mail should be used cautiously, since there can be issues and potential problems relat-

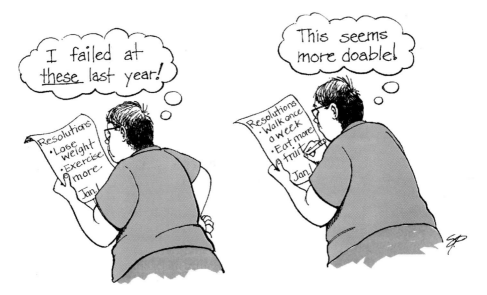

Goals should be specific, measurable, and short-term.

ed to the question asked, possible misinterpretations, legal and ethical implications, and economic reimbursement.(35)

Goal Attainment

In the final step in the goal setting process, if obstacles are overcome, clients can discuss what specific steps they plan to take to achieve the goals. For example, the goal of using low-sodium seasonings may require identifying and purchasing them, acquiring new recipes for using them, and modifying favorite recipes to use them.

By selecting a level of performance, people create their own incentives to persist in their efforts until their efforts match the standards of the goals. Clients compare results against the goals continually so that they know when they are succeeding. The personal standards against which performance attainments are compared affect how much self-satisfaction or self-efficacy is derived for the subgoal. Feedback on progress is provided by mental comparison with the goal and self-evaluation. The counselor should also provide positive feedback. By making self-satisfaction conditional on a selected level of performance, people create their own incentives to persist in their efforts until their performances match their internal standards.(30,36) Clients should reward themselves for their goal accomplishments even if only with self-praise.(30–32,36) Rewards are discussed in Chapter 6.

The attainment of subgoals builds motivation, competencies, interest, and self-perceptions of efficacy. Motivational effects do not derive from the goals themselves, but from the fact that people evaluate their own behavior.(30) They note how well they are doing. When individuals commit themselves to goals, perceived negative discrepancies between what they are doing and what they seek to achieve create self-dissatisfactions that can serve as incentives motivating enhanced effort.

Without standards against which to measure performance, people have little basis for judging how well they are doing nor do they have a basis for judging their capabilities. Subgoal attainments increase self-perceptions of efficacy, and self-satisfaction sustains one's efforts. Attainments falling short of the goals lower perceived self-efficacy and the way one feels about oneself.

SELF ASSESSMENT

"Using the personal or lifestyle problem you selected earlier in the chapter, rephrase it as a specific, measurable, and reasonable goal for change."

"On a scale of 1 to 10 with 10 being the highest, how important is the goal to you?"

INTERVENTION AND TREATMENT

The information from the assessment and goal setting is the basis for the nutrition care plan and nutrition intervention.(4,7) The goals suggest the information, knowledge, and skills the client needs to make dietary changes. The counselor judges what information to provide, how much information can be absorbed at each session, at what educational or literacy level, and what handouts and media to use as supplements. The amount of information to provide and the best method of doing so must be individualized and matched to the client's stage of change and cultural influences.

The intervention may include information, for example, on the following: reading food labels, adapting recipes, menu planning, restaurant or carry out meals, principles of healthful eating, food safety, nutrients in selected foods, nutritional supplements, nutrition misinformation, fat, carbohydrate, sodium or calorie counting, nutrient-drug interactions, managing appetite, and the relationship of nutrition to the health problem. In addition, the client needs to know about exercise, self-monitoring, and self-management. Problem-solving skills for meal planning, food preparation, and food purchasing may be needed. Culturally sensitive interventions are important in meeting the needs, desires, and lifestyles of ethnic clients.

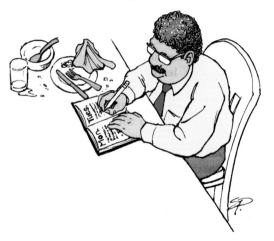

FOOD DIARY ENTRY:

Tues. dinner: skinless chicken breast, rice pilaf, green beans, 1 slice of bread with butter, and a bowl of vegetable soup.

Self-monitoring increases awareness.

Obtain and document the client's commitment to specific action behaviors and at specific times. You may wish to know if there are others with whom the client can discuss the goals, since a public commitment may make it more likely for goals to be accomplished. Practitioners frequently ask their clients to keep self-monitoring records of food intakes and environments, which they should bring to the next appointment as a way for them and the counselor to learn about factors affecting eating behaviors and as a demonstration of their commitment to change. Clients' personal records, observations, and analyses of their environment contribute to their personal awareness and understanding. (Chapter 6, Counseling for Behavior Modification, discusses this matter in more detail.)

By the end of the counseling session, the client should not only know what to do and how to do it, but also be committed to doing it. Clients should be asked to summarize their plans to check for understanding and commitment. The client has to perceive and accept the need for change to succeed. Motivation for change should be explored as well as the dangers in continuing the current dietary patterns. Solely providing information about a dietary regimen is not usually enough to interest or enable people to improve their eating habits. Counseling involves much more than distributing printed diet materials to clients.

In one study, the intervention consisted of eight weekly group sessions, followed by six biweekly sessions, and then monthly sessions for the rest of the year.(37) The goal was to decrease total fat intake to 20% of baseline calories and increase complex carbohydrate consumption to reduce cancer risk. Individual counseling sessions were offered twice. Women were taught fat counting, self-monitoring, reading labels, recipe modification, and other strategies. Those in the intervention group reduced their total fat intake from a mean of 39% to a mean of 22% of total energy.

In the Modification of Diet in Renal Disease (MDRD) study, the intervention emphasized long-term adherence.(38) Dietitians counseled participants about protein intake, weight loss, sodium restriction, and fat modification for managing hypertension and hypercholesterolemia; they met with patients monthly. Dietary and anthropometric data were collected during the nutrition intervention. Instruction included self-monitoring of protein intake, goal setting, and problem solving for meal planning and preparation, food purchasing, and eating out. After 24 months, maintaining motivation, promoting self-efficacy, preventing relapse, and sustaining adherence were emphasized.

EVALUATION OF OUTCOMES AND FOLLOW-UP

An outcome is the measured result of the counseling process. Outcome data identify the benefits of medical nutrition therapy in patient and client care. As systems of quality control, nutrition counselors may wish to evaluate several things: (1) the success of the client in following the goals set and in implementing new eating behaviors; (2) the degree of success of the nutrition intervention including its strengths and weaknesses; and (3) their own personal skills as counselors. A telephone follow-up call to inpatients and outpatients, for example, found positive short-term outcomes of counseling related to understanding, adherence, positive attitudes toward counseling, and improved physical condition.(39)

The counselor should keep records of the client's issues and goals, of the factors influencing them, and of the intervention for future measurement of client change. Examples of outcomes are changes in weight; glycemic, lipid, and other laboratory values; blood pressure control; patient acceptance and progress at self-management; improvements in knowledge, skills, and dietary changes; and lifestyle changes. These indicate the impact of the intervention and can be used to evaluate the effectiveness of the treatment. The counselor and client should engage in evaluation jointly.

A measure of success such as an overweight person eating differently is obvious. Other outcome measures may be indicators of quality of care. The blood pressure and lipid levels of cardiovascular patients can be monitored, although they are more difficult to evaluate since they depend on factors beyond dietary adherence. Monitoring of both glycemic and lipid levels helps to assess results in clients with diabetes mellitus.(40) Despite the client's commitment to dietary change, results may not reflect adherence to the regimen. These outcomes can be used by the health care team working together to adjust the treatment to achieve or maintain treatment goals. Therefore, medical nutrition therapy is an ongoing process. Further information on evaluation is found in Chapter 12.

Frequent follow-up for reassessment, further intervention, coaching, and support is essential until the client is self-sufficient. Discussion at subsequent sessions should focus first on what went well, that is, the successful experiences and subgoals reached—no matter how small. Such positive focus helps clients feel that they can have some control over their eating, health, and life and builds a sense of personal mastery and coping ability. Self-monitoring records kept by the client should be examined jointly and discussed, and difficulties should be resolved. Overlooking the records indicates to clients that they were not considered important. If progress is made, new subgoals for change may be established jointly for the appropriate stage of change. Support and reinforcement to strengthen desirable habits along with gradual, planned changes should continue as long as necessary until the client is successful at self-management.

Enthusiasm for change may decline during the first week and even more during the second week, as obstacles develop. Therefore, frequent follow-up appointments should be scheduled if possible. For long-term follow-up with clients with diabetes mellitus, for example, appointments every 3 to 6 months for children and every 6 to 12 months for adults are recommended.(4) Dietitians in tertiary care settings who do not have the opportunity for follow-up may need to refer patients to dietitians in outpatient clinics or in private practice, since one session with a client is insufficient to promote long-term change in health practices.

DOCUMENTATION

The Joint Commission on Accreditation of Healthcare Organizations (JCAHO) sets standards that are required to address quality-of-care issues in the health care environment. Documentation is essential to quality patient care and reimbursement, and health care professionals need to meet the provision in JCAHO standards. A summary of the medical nutrition therapy should be communicated to the medical team or other referral source in the medical record. The total assessment, the nutrition care plan, the measurable goals set and plans to achieve them, the nutrition intervention, and the evaluation should be documented clearly and concisely in the permanent medical record. All discharge instructions must be documented and provided to the organization or individual responsible for the patient's continuing care.(41)

As the client returns for follow-up appointments, results of health outcomes and goals achieved should be noted. Changes in weight, meal intake, tolerance problems, results of new laboratory values, medications and

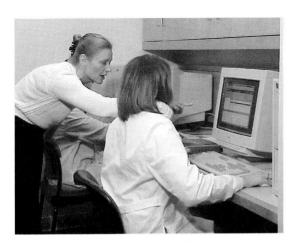

The professional documents in the medical record.

their nutritional significance, and skills in self-management may be assessed. Follow-up reassessment with new goals and interventions should be recorded. Appropriate referrals should be included.

EXPANDING ROLES FOR DIETITIANS

The concept of expanded roles and of the health intervention specialist is a challenge to dietitians who want to expand their counseling in matters other than diet. An intervention specialist is defined as a clinician "who promotes adherence to a variety of prescribed medical and life-style interventions through the health behavior counseling process."(42) Articles in the literature suggest that the dietitian can prepare to counsel clients in other areas.(42–44)

The concept originated in clinical trials, in which dietitians effectively counseled study participants regarding adherence to taking drugs as well as adherence to diet. Many clients, such as those with diabetes mellitus and hypercholesterolemia, are treated with both medication and diet. Counseling in areas of stress management, exercise, and smoking cessation are other examples. Sedentary obese clients may be counseled about exercise principles, such as the speed, frequency, and duration of walking.

Requirements of education and experience for intervention specialists are essentially the same as those for registered dietitians, with added knowledge of the topic area and additional training in interviewing and behavioral counseling.(42) Intervention specialists do require more time with the patient than the usual one or two counseling sessions afforded to some clinical dietitians. The dietitian needs extra time in this counseling approach to achieve long-term health behavior change in cases of adherence problems.

The intervention specialist can coordinate several different prescribed treatments that require behavior changes by the patient. Currently, drug, diet, exercise, stress management, smoking cessation, and physical therapy treatments are often prescribed with no provision for monitoring success of their incorporation into a client's lifestyle. Close cooperation and coordination among the patient, the intervention specialist, and other members of the medical team can help improve the quality of health care.

Some dietitians have expanded into career paths as study coordinators. A study coordinator is responsible for the day-to-day operations of a research study.(43) The registered dietitian can also assume the prominent role of case manager.(44,45) For example, the Diabetes Control and Complications Trial (DCCT) showed that the registered dietitian was an important contributor to health care delivery, research, and case management.(46) In the DCCT, the dietitian's role expanded as the team recognized the relation between adhering to the dietary regimen and achieving targeted blood glucose levels with successful improved diabetes control outcomes.

Dietitians who have credentials as Certified Diabetes Educators (CDE) also have expanded roles in diabetes care, education, and management. Others are certified in nutrition support, pediatric nutrition, health/fitness, and the like.

The term "nutrition therapist" describes dietitians practicing personalized, long-term, client-centered nutrition counseling in which the dietitian and client work as partners in solving problems related to dietary and lifestyle changes.(47) Often the dietitian is part of a multidisciplinary team. For instance, Reiff and Reiff are "nutrition therapists" specializing in behavioral change in clients with eating disorders.(48) The psychotherapy model is used involving the following: (1) long-term care, (2) a relationship that is itself therapeutic, (3) a highly individualized treatment plan evolving over time, and (4) education proceeds from the client's interests and concerns rather than from the counselor.(49) Additional education and training in basic counseling skills through coursework and supervision by a psychotherapist are required for the role of nutrition therapist in eating disorders to have the qualifications to discuss the emotional issues related to weight, food, and body image.(50) Nutrition therapists are a subunit of the Nutrition Entrepreneurs dietetic practice group.

All dietetics professionals need to be knowledgeable in the concepts, processes, and techniques of counseling, although they may apply them in different settings in professional practice. A comprehensive approach to counseling considering lifestyle, environments, culture, and psychological and social factors is needed. Some dietitians, with added training, are expanding their roles dealing with long-term health behavior problems in addition to diet and are counseling to achieve patient adherence. Other chapters discuss the behavior modification approach to counseling and the importance of cognitions to change.

CASE STUDY 1

Len Howard is a 48-year-old male executive in a Fortune 500 company. In a recent physical exam, he was 5'11" tall and 175 pounds. His serum cholesterol was 290 (desirable 200 mg/dL or less) with HDL of 50 (desirable over 40 mg/dL) and LDL 220 (desirable < 100 mg/dL). On the recommendation of his physician, he made an appointment with the dietitian in the corporate wellness program.

Mr. Howard's family history revealed that his father and older brother both died of heart disease. His wife is employed as an attorney, and they have a 15-year-old son.

Dietitian: "You mentioned that the doctor wants you to try modifying your diet before considering medication for your cholesterol level?"

Mr. Howard: "He said to reduce the fat and cholesterol in my diet."

Dietitian: "How much do you know about different foods and their effect on your cholesterol level?"

Mr. Howard: "I've heard of it, but don't know much about it."

Dietitian: "Let's talk about what you are eating now. Then we can identify what you are eating that is ok, and what, if any, changes you may be willing to make."

Mr. Howard' nutrition history revealed the following information:

Breakfast: Orange juice, 2 slices of toast with peanut butter, and black coffee

(continued)

Mid AM snack: Coffee and doughnut

Lunch: Beef sandwich or bacon cheeseburger, French fries, and coke

Mid PM snack: Coffee

Dinner: 6- to 8-oz steak, baked potato with butter and sour cream, green vegetable, salad with blue cheese dressing, cookies, and wine

Evening snack: Beer and pretzels

1. What is Mr. Howard doing that is desirable and that you can encourage him to continue to do (foods low in cholesterol and saturated fatty acids)?
2. Using the goal-setting process described in the chapter, what are possible short-term goals for change for him to consider with you?
3. How would you ask him to assess the importance of the choice of goals?
4. After he selects two goals, how would you discuss any obstacles he sees to reaching the goals?
5. How would you discuss the steps he needs to take to reach the goals, such as discussions with his wife, shopping at the grocery store, or selecting restaurant meals at lunch?
6. What type of follow-up would you like to have with him?

CASE STUDY 2

John Miller, age 48 years, was referred by his physician to Joan Stivers, RD, as a result of a serum cholesterol level of 320 mg/dL. He is 6'0" and weighs 250 pounds.

Mr. Miller has a family history of heart disease. His older brother died of a heart attack. He is married with two children ages 20 and 24 years. His wife is employed full-time and so did not come to the appointment with him.

During the interview Mr. Miller stated: "I know I have a bad family history. I also know that I have put on a few pounds in recent years and should try to lose them. But after a day at work, I enjoy my dinner."

1. What stage of change is Mr. Miller in?
2. How would you match your nutritional intervention to his stage of change? What strategies would you use?

REVIEW AND DISCUSSION QUESTIONS

1. Explain the steps in the nutrition counseling process.
2. List and explain the stages and processes of change.
3. Explain the steps in the process of goal setting.
4. What should be included in the documentation of nutrition counseling?

5. What are some of the newer roles that dietitians are assuming?
6. What is the relationship between nutrition counseling and health promotion?

SUGGESTED ACTIVITIES

1. During the next week, make arrangements to observe a dietitian's counseling session. Afterward, discuss the philosophies of nutrition counseling.
2. Write both a paraphrase and an empathic comment to the following comments made by a counselee:
   A. I feel uncomfortable discussing my eating habits with you. I don't know anything about nutrition.
   B. People tend to think I'm fat and happy, but I don't believe they take me seriously.
   C. I am at a point now where I don't believe I will ever lose the weight.
3. Form triads consisting of a counselor, counselee, and observer. Each person should take a turn in each of the roles for 7 minutes. The counselee should play the role of an obese client, and the counselor should use paraphrasing and empathizing along with open and closed questions to facilitate disclosure and problem solving. After each round, the observer should share reactions to the counselor's approach and encourage feedback from the counselee to the counselor. From the counselee's perspective, what did the counselor do that helped their interaction; what did he or she do that hindered it?
4. Write an open-ended question for each of the statements below:
   A. I never have any fun at a family gathering anymore. Being on this diet has taken the fun our of my life.
   B. Since I developed these health problems, it seems that all I do is think about my diet.
   C. It seems easy every morning to promise myself that today I will stick to the goals we negotiated. By noon, however, I begin thinking that I'll never be able to comply with the diet for the rest of my life, so why bother?
5. In groups of two, take turns discussing a lifestyle problem and restating it as a goal for change.
   A. Think of a lifestyle problem the counselee would like to change, such as eating too much, eating the wrong foods, needing to eat more fruits and vegetables, more fiber, or less fat, exercising too little, not studying enough, needing to budget better, drinking too much, smoking too much, and the like.
   B. Help the person discuss the problem and the conditions and circumstances surrounding it. Then have the counselee restate the problem as a positive goal for change, that is, "I will. . . . "
   C. Assess the importance of the goal on a scale of 1 to 10, with 10 being the highest importance. Revise the goal if necessary.
   D. Ask about and discuss the obstacles and barriers to accomplishing the goal, and try to have the person resolve these.
   E. Have the person list the steps to achieving the goal. What will the person do, and when will it be done?

6. Visit one or more of the internet sites that follow to determine what clients may find and how it may or may not help them change their food choices. Share your results with the class.

7. In groups of two, discuss the following client statements to determine what stage of change the person is in.

   A. "I have made some changes in my food choices within the past 6 months."

   B. "I am intending to change the foods I eat next month."

   C. "I intend to make some changes in the next 6 months."

   D. "I don't eat high-fat foods anymore."

WEB SITES

BOTH PROFESSIONALS AND CLIENTS MAY BENEFIT FROM INFORMATION ON THE INTERNET.

www.nalusda.gov/fnic / Food & Nutrition Information Center, US Department of Agriculture for food guide pyramid, dietary supplements, and much more

www.usda.gov/cnpp / Center for Nutrition Policy Promotion, US Department of Agriculture for dietary guidelines, interactive healthy eating index and more

www.cholesterollowdown.org / cholesterol information

www.americanheart.org / American Heart Association

www.nhlbi.nih.gov / National Heart Lung Blood Institute information on cardio-vascular diseases

www.cancer.org / American Cancer Society

www.fightbac.org / partnership for food safety education

www.foodsafety.gov / government site on food safety

www.diabetes.org / American Diabetes Association

www.healthfinder.gov / consumer health information

www.mayohealth.org / Mayo Clinic health information

www.webmd.com / consumer health information

www.shapeup.org / consumer weight control site

www.cyberdiet.com / nutrition information and self-assessment materials

www.nutrition.gov / nutrition-related material from various government agencies

www.dietitians.ca / site of dietitians from Canada

www.dole5aday.com / educates about fruits and vegetables

www.vrg.org / information about vegetarian diets from the Vegetarian Resource Group

http://vm.cfsan.fda.gov/~lrd/advice.html / Food and Drug Administration Center for Food Safety and Applied Nutrition site on food labeling, supplements, women's health, and more

http://dietary-supplements.info.nih.gov / National Institutes of Health site on dietary supplements

www.merckhomeedition.com / The Merck Manual of Medical Information-Home edition

REFERENCES

1. Johnson DB, Eaton DL, Wahl PW, et al. Public health nutrition practice in the United States. J Am Diet Assoc 2001;101:529.
2. Olendzki MC, Tolpin HG, Buckley EL. Evaluating nutrition intervention in atherosclerosis. J Am Diet Assoc 1981;79:9.
3. Pastors JG, Barrier P, Rich M, et al. Facilitating lifestyle change: a resource manual. Alexandria, VA: American Diabetes Association. and Chicago: American Dietetic Association, l996.
4. Tinker LF, Heins JM, Holler H.J. Commentary and translation: 1994 nutrition recommendations for diabetes. J Am Diet Assoc 1994;94;507.
5. Curry KR, Himburg SP. Establishing an effective nutrition education/counseling program: skills for the RD. Study Kit 11. Chicago: American Dietetic Association, 1988.
6. Rosal MC, Ebbeling CB, Lofgren I, et al. Facilitating dietary change: the patient-centered counseling model. J Am Diet Assoc 2001;101:332.
7. Position of the American Dietetic Association and Dietitians of Canada: nutrition intervention in the care of persons with human immunodeficiency virus infection. J Am Diet Assoc 2000;100:708.
8. Prochaska JO, DiClemente CC, Norcross JC. In search of how people change: Applications to addictive behaviors. Am Psychol 1992;47:1102.
9. Prochaska, JO, Norcross, JC, DiClemente CC. Changing for good. New York: Avon Books, 1994.
10. Greene GW, Rossi SR, Rossi JS, et al. Dietary applications of the Stages of Change Model. J Am Diet Assoc 1999;99:673.
11. Summerfield LM. Nutrition, exercise, and behavior: an integrated approach to weight management. Belmont, CA: Wadsworth, 2001.
12. Finckenor M, Byrd-Bredbenner C. Nutrition intervention group program based on preaction-stage-oriented change processes of the Transtheoretical Model promotes long-term reduction in dietary fat intake. J Am Diet Assoc 2000;100:335.
13. Hargreaves SMK, Schlundt DG, Buchowski MS, et al. Stages of change and the intake of dietary fat in African-American women: improving stage assignment using the Eating Styles Questionnaire. J Am Diet Assoc 1999;99:1392.
14. Nitzke S, Auld G, McNulty J, et al. Stages of change for reducing fat and increasing fiber among dietitians and adults with diet-related chronic disease. J Am Diet Assoc 1999;99:728.
15. Prochaska JO, Velicer WF. The transtheoretical model of health behavior change. Am J Health Promot 1997;12:38.
16. Thompson, B, Shannon, J, Beresford, SA, et al. Implementation aspects of the Seattle "5 a Day" intervention project: strategies to help employees make dietary changes. Top Clin Nutr 1995;11:58.
17. Greene GW, Rossi SR, Reed GR, et al. Stages of change for reducing dietary fat to 30% of energy or less. J Am Diet Assoc 1994;94:1105.
18. Sandoval WM, Heller K, Wiese WH, et al. Stages of change: a model for nutrition counseling. Top Clin Nutr 1994;9:64.
19. Sigman-Grant M. Stages of change: a framework for nutrition interventions. Nutr Today 1996;31:162.
20. Glanz K, Patterson RE, Kristal AR, et al. Stages of change in adopting healthy diets: fat, fiber and correlates of nutrient intake. Health Educ Q 1994;21:499.
21. Campbell MK, DeVellis BM, Strecher VJ, et al. Improving dietary behavior: the effectiveness of tailored messages in primary care settings. Am J Public Health 1994;84:783.

22. Campbell MK, Reynolds KD, Havas S, et al. Stages of change for increasing fruit and vegetable consumption among adults and young adults participating in the national 5-a-Day for better health community studies. Health Educ Behav 1999;26:513.

23. Brinley C, Barrar C, Cotugna, N. Stages of change tools to increase fruit and vegetable consumption in high school students. J Nutr Ed 2001;33:57.

24. National standards for diabetes self-management education programs. Diabetes Educ 1995;21:189.

25. Gillis BP, Caggiula AW, Chiavacci AT, et al. Nutrition intervention program of the Modification of Diet in Renal Disease Study: a self-management approach. J Am Diet Assoc 1995;95:1288.

26. Diabetes Care and Education Dietetic Practice Group. Scope of practice for qualified dietetics professionals in diabetes care and education. J Am Diet Assoc 2000;100:1205.

27. Laquatra I, Danish SJ. A primer for nutritional counseling. In: Frankle, RT, Yang, MU, eds. Obesity and weight control: the health professional's guide to understanding and treatment. Rockville, MD: Aspen Publications, 1988.

28. D'Augelli AR, D'Augelli JF, Danish SJ. Helping others. Monterey, CA: Brooks/Cole Publishing, 1981.

29. Laquatra I, D'Augelli AR, Danish SJ. Helping Skills II: life development intervention leader's manual. New York: Human Sciences Press, 1983.

30. Bandura A. Social foundations of thought and action: a social cognitive theory. Englewood Cliffs, NJ: Prentice-Hall, 1986.

31. Strecher VJ, Seijts GH, Kok GJ, et al. Goal setting as a strategy for health behavior change. Health Educ Q 1995;22:190.

32. Cullen KW, Baranowski T, Smith SP. Using goal setting as a strategy for dietary behavior change. J Am Diet Assoc 2001;101:562.

33. Shenberger DM, Helgren RJ, Peters JR, et al. Intense dietary counseling lowers LDL cholesterol in the recruitment phase of a clinical trial of men who had coronary artery bypass grafts. J Am Diet Assoc 1992;92:441.

34. Burrows ER, Henry HJ, Bowen DJ, et al. Nutritional applications of a clinical low fat dietary intervention to public health change. J Nutr Ed 1993;25:167.

35. Rodriguez JC. Legal, ethical, and professional issues to consider when communicating via the internet: a suggested response model and policy. J Am Diet Assoc 1999;99:1428.

36. Bandura A, Cervone D. Self-evaluative and self-efficacy mechanisms governing the motivational effects of goal systems. J Personality Soc Psych 1983;45:1017.

37. Gorbach SL, Morrill-LaBrode A, Woods MN, et al. Changes in food patterns during a low-fat dietary intervention in women. J Am Diet Assoc 1990;90:802.

38. Dolecek TA, Olson MB, Caggiula AW, et al. Registered dietitian time requirements in the Modification of Diet in Renal Disease Study. J Am Diet Assoc 1995;95:1307.

39. Schiller MR, Miller M, Moore C, et al. Patients report positive nutrition counseling outcomes. J Am Diet Assoc 1998;98:977.

40. Franz MJ, Horton ES, Bantle JP, et al. Nutrition principles for the management of diabetes and related complications. Diabetes Care 1994;17:490.

41. Krasker GD, Balogun LB. 1995 JCAHO standards: development and relevance to dietetics practice. J Am Diet Assoc 1995;95:240.

42. Insull W. Dietitians as interventions specialists: a continuing challenge for the 1990s. J Am Diet Assoc 1992;92:551.

43. Schmidt L. A new career path for dietitians: study coordinators. J Am Diet Assoc 1993;93:749.

44. Mackey CS. New roles for RDs: diabetes case manager. J Am Diet Assoc 1993;93:401.

45. Position of the American Dietetic Association: weight management. J Am Diet Assoc 1997;97:71.

46. Powers MA, Wheeler ML. Model for dietetics practice and research: the challenge is here, but the journey was not easy. J Am Diet Assoc 1993;93:755.

47. Licavoli L. Dietetics goes into therapy. J Am Diet Assoc 1995;95:751.

48. Reiff DW, Reiff KKL. Eating disorders: nutrition therapy in the recovery process. Gaithersburg, MD: Aspen Publishers, 1992.

49. Kiy AM. The philosophy of nutrition therapy. Top Clin Nutr 1998;13:51.

50. Position of the American Dietetic Association: nutrition intervention in the treatment of anorexia nervosa, bulimia nervosa, and binge eating. J Am Diet Assoc 1994;94:902.

APPENDIX A Counseling Guidelines—Initial Session

Step	Topic	Questions To Ask	Questions To Avoid
1	Candidly review the problems of dietary change. 1. Review overall rationale and objectives for recommended diet. 2. Acknowledge difficult nature of dietary change. 3. Listen to patient's concerns about the recommended diet.	 What are your thoughts and feelings about changing your food intake?	 Do you have any opinion about about this diet?
2	Build some commitment to solve problems. 1. Indicate your willingness to work with the patient. 2. Clarify to patient that he must assume primary responsibility for making dietary changes. 3. Propose program of frequent meetings for next 3 months, close observation of diet, phone contact. 4. Emphasize slow but steady approach to change. 5. Obtain patient's verbal commitment to meet any of your proposals.	 What aspects of this program are you willing to try now?	 Do you want to try anything now?
3	Plan some specific changes in diet during coming month. 1. Emphasize good points of 3-day record.[a] 2. Look on record for ideas on dietary changes. 3. Probe patient for more ideas. 4. Pinpoint *one aspect* of diet pattern to change. 5. Acknowledge patient's desire for radical and fast changes in diet, but reemphasize that the most successful approach is slow and steady. 6. Help patient set realistic dietary change goals (e.g., one meatless evening meal per week, substitution of a salad bowl for usual main entree at one lunch per week.)	 What do you see that could be changed or improved? What are realistic goals for you?	 Do you see anything to change? Is this a realistic goal?

4 Plan how to make a change successful.		
1. Identify obstacles that are likely to interfere with achieving goal. Consider problems in the following areas:	What obstacles are likely to interfere with your plans?	Are any problems going to interfere with plans?
a. Physical environment (e.g., what foods are available in house, snacking in front of TV in evening, absence of reminders on refrigerator or dining table.)	What can you change in your home, office, or car that will help you achieve your goals?	Do you need any reminders?
b. Social environment (e.g., influential people, such as spouse, children, business associates, whose approval and support or criticism can affect achievement of dietary change goal.)	Who can help, what can they do, and what can I do to help during the next few weeks?	Do you need any help?
c. Cognitive or private environment (e.g., what patient says to himself when confronted with personal thoughts such as the following: What others will say about his planned behavior; thoughts of failure or disappointment when he is not perfect in his behavior.)	What encouraging things can you say to yourself when confronted with these inevitable thoughts?	Will you give yourself encouragement?
5 Plan how to keep track of progress. Devise an unobtrusive and convenient way for patient to keep a record of the desired or target behavior (e.g., count egg cartons, measure side of vegetable oil container, attach pencil *and* paper to refrigerator, table, wallet.) Plan counseling continuity and support.	How are you going to keep track of (target behavior)?	Can you keep track of (target behavior)?
6	When is it convenient for us to discuss your progress? Let's schedule our next appointment. What would you like to discuss next time?	Do you want me to contact you sometime?
7. Make certain that spouse, if present, is involved in answering questions, providing ideas, and discussing potential problems and solutions.	Would it be possible for someone to come with you at our next visit?	

ᵃ Before initial counseling session, patient should be given materials and instructions for completing a 3-day food diary. Adapted from and reprinted with permission from Wilbur CS. Nutrition counseling skills. Audiocassette series 5. Chicago: American Dietetic Association, 1980.

6 Counseling for Behavior Modification

CHAPTER

DIANE RIGASSIO RADLER, MS, RD, CDE

After reading this chapter, you will be able to

1. define and distinguish learning styles of classical conditioning, operant or instrumental conditioning, and observational learning or modeling.
2. apply learning styles to behavior change and specifically in clinical situations, such as obesity, eating disorders, diabetes mellitus, and cardiovascular disease, and in human resource management.
3. analyze eating behaviors according to the ABC framework.
4. apply behavior modification to case study examples.

ose weight! Quit smoking! Control your blood sugar! This advice is easily uttered but requires a process to implement and maintain. This process is referred to as behavior modification. Changing behaviors is one of the most difficult tasks for people because human behavior is quite complex. Complex behaviors usually are based on a combination of inherited and acquired characteristics. The inherited characteristics cannot be changed, just as it is impossible to alter any genetic attribute. However, the acquired characteristics, those shaped by a person's environment and experience, are possible to change. Behaviors that are learned or acquired can be changed or modified.

This chapter reviews the principles of learning and the process of behavior modification that have evolved from research studies. Included are classical conditioning, operant or instrumental conditioning based on positive reinforcement or rewards, and observational learning or modeling after others. The role of cognition, the individual's mental perceptions of events, and their effect on behavior, a newer area of research, is covered in more detail in the next chapter.

In behavior modification, the therapist attempts to alter previously learned behavior or to encourage the development of new behavior. Wilson and O'Leary in *Principles of Behavior Therapy*(1) point out that most abnormal behavior is acquired and maintained by the principles as normal behavior. As obvious as this seems, it is difficult to influence patients who may not see the health danger in their current habits. Food preferences and eating behaviors have deep roots within the individual and may be highly resistant to change. In addition, behaviors may define individuals in terms of what they think and feel and how they react to certain situations.(2) Reluctance to making changes may occur when a good rationale and a stepwise process to change are not identified.

Furnishing information concerning what to eat is frequently insufficient to promote alterations in eating behaviors or adherence to modified diets. Israel and Moore differentiate between diet instruction and behavior modification.(3) Contrary to traditional diet instructions, nutrition counseling for behavior modification steers the client into assuming responsibility for change. The transfer of decision-making power from the professional to the client reduces the risk of relapse and failure. Over time, even an individual in the best-designed, short-term intervention can relapse after the formal program ends. If the decisions are transferred to the hands of the clients, they are much more likely to modify eating choices. As challenging as this seems, it is more challenging to effectively implement this in acute care nutrition intervention settings. Along with information on nutrition, behavior modification principles may be used because they offer the dietetics professional an additional dimension to counseling—that of combining the sciences of psychology and physiology with the art of therapy.(4)

Behavior modification principles are applied in the treatment of various nutritional problems. One of the earliest and the most frequently used applications was in the treatment of obesity. Therapy for eating disorders, such as anorexia nervosa and bulimia, and inappropriate eating behaviors related to diabetes mellitus and cardiovascular diseases are other potential uses of behavior modification. In prevention, behavior modification can be applied in wellness and disease risk reduction. If unhealthy eating behaviors are modified in favor of healthy alternatives, the incidence of nutrition-related diseases could decrease.

Also, in human resource management, supervisors may be interested in altering the behavior of subordinates and encouraging the development of new behaviors. More

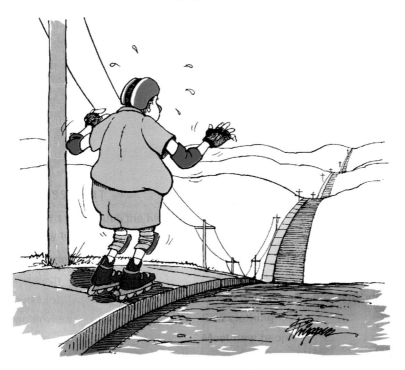

The road to long-term behavioral change is not easy.

effective interaction between peers and superiors may also be a goal. Although the term *behavior modification* in the context of human resource management may sound manipulative, an honest and understanding supervisor may use the principles by sharing with employees the goals of the process. These learning principles are the basis for the advice in the book, *The One Minute Manager*.(5) Modeling is a technique that is used frequently in employee training programs.

CLASSICAL CONDITIONING

The methods of behavior modification are based on principles of learning that have been discovered mostly in the experimental laboratory. According to Hill, the best-known animals in the history of psychology were the dogs housed in the laboratory of Ivan Pavlov, the Russian physiologist, who was conducting research on digestive processes.(6) Serendipitously, Pavlov noted that his laboratory animals salivated not only when food was presented, but also when the laboratory assistant who regularly fed them came into the room; at times, they even salivated at the sound of the laboratory door opening. Pavlov spent the rest of his life investigating a type of learning based on association, now known as classical conditioning.

Pavlov realized immediately that the response of salivation to laboratory assistants and noisy doors was not a part of the physiological makeup of the dog. The dogs were salivating when events occurred that had regularly and repeatedly come before the presentation of their food. An association was apparently formed between some event and the future appearance of food.

Pavlov noted that certain environmental events or stimuli would reliably trigger or elicit a particular behavioral response. For example, food in a dog's mouth would reliably produce saliva. The triggering event (food in the mouth) became known as the *unconditioned stimulus* (US), whereas the response that was triggered (salivation) was called the *unconditioned response* (UR). This relationship was built into the organism and hence unconditioned.

Conditioning occurs when a stimulus (a neutral stimulus) that originally does not trigger the particular response (salivation) eventually comes to produce that response. This occurs by pairing the originally neutral stimulus with the unconditioned stimulus. When conditioning has occurred, the conditioned stimulus (CS), which was originally neutral, produces the same, or very similar, response as does the US. In the example, the CS was the presence of the laboratory assistant. Pavlov showed that bells, tones, lights, and many other stimuli could serve as the CS and could come to elicit the response of salivation, which is labeled a conditioned response (CR) after it is triggered by or produced by a CS.

Many types of responses have been found to be responsive to classical conditioning principles. Not only reflexive responses, such as salivation and eye blink, but complex emotional responses can be classically conditioned. The heart pounds and beads of perspiration appear on the forehead as one hears the siren of an ambulance approaching a neighbor's home. The same phenomenon may occur when the teacher passes out examination questions. Try to construct a scenario to account for this response in terms of classical conditioning principles, or think of other situations in which classical conditioning might play a part in human behavior or emotional responses.

OPERANT CONDITIONING

At about the same time that Pavlov was delineating the principles of classical conditioning, a young American scientist, Edward Thorndike, was pursuing the investigation of learning principles from another perspective. Thorndike used many types of animals in his research and designed and constructed "puzzle boxes" for cats. A hungry cat was placed inside the box with food located outside. To have access to the food, the cat had to solve the puzzle of how to escape from the box. Thorndike observed that the cats made trial-and-error responses until escape was achieved and the food consumed. Gradually, the time required to complete the puzzle decreased, and the behavior that achieved success in solving the puzzle became dominant, and unsuccessful behaviors were eliminated.

Thorndike proposed an explanation for this phenomenon based on a principle he called the Law of Effect. This law stated that behaviors could be changed by their consequences. Responses that were followed by satisfying consequences would be strengthened. Behaviors not followed by satisfying consequences, or behaviors followed by annoying consequences, would be weakened and less likely to occur in the future. Thorndike's Law of Effect led to much research in principles of learning and formed the foundation for the study of operant or instrumental conditioning, which is learning based on reinforcement or reward.

The focal point of research on the Law of Effect is the relationship between responses, or behaviors, and the consequences of those behaviors. Schwartz described four types of response-consequence outcomes.(7) First, responses or behaviors may produce positive outcomes; a consequence known as *positive reinforcement*. An example would be the lavish praise and attention a person may receive after achieving a svelte new figure. Second, responses may produce negative outcomes; this consequence is known as *punishment*. Punishment decreases the future likelihood of a response. Examples of punishment include the receipt of a traffic ticket for an improper left turn and the inability to fit into a favorite outfit after gaining weight. Third, responses may result in the removal of adverse stimuli that are already present. This consequence is known as *negative reinforcement* or escape and is similar to positive reinforcement in that it increases the future likelihood or probability of a response. Examples include escaping devastating cold by going into a heated building, escaping a poor television show by changing channels, or eliminating or reducing hypoglycemic agents in type II diabetes by losing weight and following a sound meal plan. Finally, responses may prevent an unpleasant event from occurring. Examples include avoiding the cold by staying indoors and avoiding unfavorable comparisons with others by maintaining a trim figure. The avoidance of adverse events increases the likelihood of the response, as does positive reinforcement. Behaviors that are not positively or negatively reinforced should decrease in strength.

Later behaviorists continued where Thorndike concluded. B.F. Skinner is best known for his championing of a set of methods and terms to explain behavior on the basis of the principles of operant conditioning. Skinner developed a situation in which behavior could be observed in discrete units and subsequently recorded. This situation was an operant chamber, which has been dubbed a "Skinner box." The lever presses of rats and key pecks of pigeons have been the most frequently studied responses. Skinner's enthusiasm for the behavioristic approach was not limited to lower animals, however, since he proposed wide application for the principles that were established.

In recent years, the behavioristic approach has become an increasingly important practical technique in many settings, such as classrooms, mental hospitals, prisons, clinics, the workplace, and self-management situations.(1)

MODELING

In addition to classical and operant conditioning as modes of behavior change, a third form of learning is known as observational learning, or modeling. Learning by modeling involves the observation of some behavior or pattern of behaving, which is followed by the performance of either the same or a similar behavior. Albert Bandura is associated with this method of learning by modeling.(8) In obesity behavior modification, for example, a person could "eat like a thin person" to model after the appropriate food choices, portion sizes, and duration of meals of someone who demonstrates the skill.

The effectiveness of learning by modeling appears to be directly related to certain characteristics of the model. The two characteristics found to be most relevant are the observer's similarity to the model and the status of the model. The more similar the characteristics of the model are to those of the observer, the higher is the probability that learning by modeling will occur. Movie and television stars and other well-known persons capitalize on

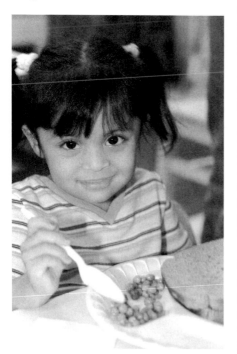

Parents and caregivers shape children's eating habits.

modeling by producing books and videotapes of their fitness/nutrition programs. Many people model after the behavior of a person with "status," even though equally effective or superior programs could be developed by relatively unknown but professionally trained nutritionists and exercise physiologists.

Shaping behavior begins at an early age. Parents and caregivers of children serve as role models in forming good eating habits and healthy behaviors. Long-term food choices of children can stem from the dietary patterns of parental figures. Nutrition counseling may be geared toward parents for their benefit and for the health of the children.(9,10)

To take advantage of modeling, dietetics professionals may try sharing success stories of people who have made permanent dietary modifications for the benefit of their health. In group therapy, clients who have succeeded in changing eating practices may serve as models for others. Keep in mind that the client often views the counselor as a model, and, to this end, dietetics professionals should be following the healthy nutrition recommendations given to others.

Behavior modeling is used in employee training programs to teach basic supervisory techniques, selling skills, and a variety of other verbal skills through observation of films and videotapes. New employees may be assigned to work with current employees who serve as models of desirable behaviors. Managers should make sure that their own behaviors are exemplary of what they expect of subordinates.(11) If the supervisor adds an extra 10 minutes to the allowed time for a coffee break, for example, employees may model after the example set.

A great deal of human learning and behavior undoubtedly is a result of modeling, even though traditionally, emphasis has been placed on the stimulus-response (or behavior-consequence) approach to explaining changes in behavior, or the acquisition and extinction of responses.(6) These three approaches—conditioning, operant conditioning, and modeling—form the basis of behavior modification. The behavioristic position is that many behaviors are learned or alterable through use of these three learning principles.

Note, however, that behaviors might be more or less resistant to change depending on where the individual is on the continuum of Stages of Change (see Chapter 5 for in-depth discussion of Stages of Change). One barrier to effective communication is that perhaps a counseling approach is implemented erroneously in a particular stage, but may be effective in a different stage. Miller suggests the use of various approaches to counsel at particular stages.(4)

CHANGING EATING BEHAVIORS

As the principles that govern behavior and behavior change became more clearly defined, it became increasingly apparent that nutritionists and behavioral scientists should work together to provide methods of using these principles in applied settings where changes in dietary habits are the primary goal. The National Heart, Lung, and Blood Institute (NHLBI) has been one of the leaders in encouraging this type of collaboration.(12) The most common application has been the behavioral management of obesity, but cooperative programs have led to application in such diverse areas of concern as cardiovascular diseases, eating disorders, and diabetes mellitus.

Dietary behaviors should be studied in terms of the client's total environment, which includes physical, social, cultural, psychological, physiological, and environmental factors compounded by all conditions and events that precede and follow eating. Behavioral scientists have referred to this framework as the ABCs, derived from analysis of the Antecedents (stimuli or cues), the Behavior (response itself or eating), and the Consequences (reinforcement or reward) of the behavior.(13)

$$A \longrightarrow B \longrightarrow C$$

For example, seeing a package of cookies left on the kitchen counter may be the antecedent or cue. The behavior is eating some or all cookies in the kitchen. The consequences may be pleasure from the taste of the cookies and reduced feelings of hunger or frustration, with increased feelings of happiness and satisfaction, which reinforce the behavior. The dietetics professional and the client must find ways to decrease undesirable eating behaviors and increase new desirable ones.

Antecedents

Behavior modification techniques work by regulating the antecedents, the behavior of eating itself, and the consequences or rewards. Analysis of antecedents of behavior

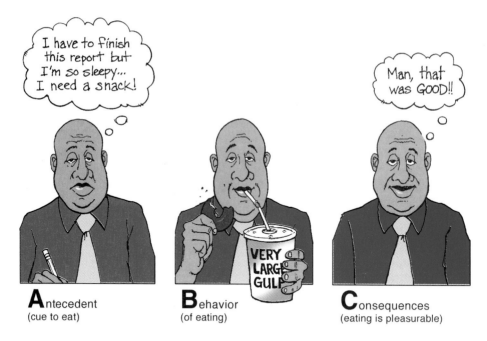

Antecedent
(cue to eat)

Behavior
(of eating)

Consequences
(eating is pleasurable)

Counselors need to examine the As, Bs, and Cs.

seeks to control or limit the stimuli or cues to eating. For example, a cue may be seeing or smelling food, watching television, arriving home from work or school, attending a social event, or noticing the presence of extra food on the table at mealtime. Behavior may be influenced by both internal and external factors. There may be internal cues, such as physiological feelings of hunger or psychological feelings of loneliness or boredom. A number of external variables may cue eating, such as noting the time of day or passing an ice cream shop in the street. Both internal and external factors may be mediated by cognitive factors, such as not caring about current weight levels or not wishing to dull one's appetite for the next meal.(14)

The behavior-modifying strategy involves decreasing the exposures to situations in which food is used as a reward or as a focal point of an activity. A list of suggestions for changing behavior that have been recommended by various authors for persons desiring to lose weight is found in Table 6-1.(14–16) To modify antecedents, the dietetics professional may suggest removing negative cues (not buying inappropriate foods), introducing new, more positive cues (exercising instead of eating), restricting behavior to one set of cues (eating only at designated times), cognitive restructuring discussed in the following chapter, and role-playing new responses to old antecedents (telling a friend you would rather go to a movie than out for pizza). Breaking response chains and preplanning behavior are other strategies.(17)

Preplanning meals and snacks and having only appropriate foods in the house are preferable to expecting self-control when hungry. Preplanning social occasions and exercise are also helpful. Small portions of favorite foods may need to be included in the diet to avoid feelings of total deprivation and potential abandonment of dietary changes. Doing the right thing is enhanced by stimulus control. The goal of preplanning to con-

TABLE 6-1 Techniques for Behavior Modification

I. Provide Incentives to Aid Patients In Maintaining Commitment
  A. Determine ways to focus attention on successful experiences. A positive comment by the counselor is helpful, and you can always find something positive to say.
  B. Encourage people to tell others about dietary goals. This public commitment often will aid in maintaining a course of action.
  C. Have the person anticipate problems that might come up and consider possible solutions before a problem arises. Having a plan ready will make focusing on the goal easier.
  D. Concentrate on allowed foods and portions rather than the disallowed. Be positive.
  E. Keep reminding the person that dietary change is a gradual process. Dietary habits were not developed in a brief period of time and probably will not be significantly changed in a short time. Set realistic goals for immediate and long-term change. Encourage successive approximations to the desired behavior.

II. Learn Eating Habits (and Exercise Habits) by Record Keeping

  A person cannot change a habit until he or she knows what it is. Self-monitoring with accurate records of the foods consumed is necessary for behavioral control of eating. Information to consider recording would be:

  A. What food was eaten.
  B. Quantity of each food.
  C. What the person was doing just before eating (to help identify cues)
  D. Place of eating (cue providing)
  E. With whom eating occurs, or alone (cue providing)
  F. How the person felt (cue providing)
  G. Time of eating (cue providing)

  This record keeping exercise can identify the person's patterns of food intake and those cues that are associated with food consumption as well as the emotional outcome of eating. The person will become more aware of the environmental stimuli that are associated with eating behavior.

III. Control the Stimuli (Cues) and Restructure the Environment
  A. Physical environment
    1. Based on the records kept, have the person identify physical stimuli in the environment that are associated with, and therefore are cues to, inappropriate eating behaviors. Different stimuli become associated with the act of eating and can become signals for appropriate or inappropriate food consumption.
    2. Ask the person to identify physical stimuli that could remind him or her to eat properly. Examples of these would be charts or graphs, cartoons, signs, and the like. The presence of appropriate foods in the home is probably the best cue to appropriate eating, supplemented by the elimination of inappropriate foods.

(continued)

TABLE 6-1 Techniques for Behavior Modification (*Continued*)

3. Have the person specify a special place where food should be consumed, such as at the dining table, and not in front of the television set or kitchen sink.
4. Make those foods that are acceptable in the nutrition plan as attractive as possible. Use good dishes, crystal, and so forth to make dining a pleasant event.
5. Set up shopping trips based on the following suggestions:
   a. Shop for food only after eating.
   b. Use a shopping list.
   c. Avoid ready-to-eat foods.
   d. Do not carry more money than needed for shopping list.
6. Set up specific plans and activities:
   a. Substitute exercise for snacking.
   b. Eat meals and snacks at scheduled times.
   c. Do not accept food offered by others.
   d. Store food out of sight.
   e. Remove food from inappropriate storage areas in the house.
   f. Use smaller dishes.
   g. Avoid being the food server.
   h. Leave the table immediately after eating.
   i. Discard leftovers.
7. Regarding special events and holidays:
   a. Drink fewer alcoholic beverages.
   b. Plan eating before parties.
   c. Eat a low-calorie snack before parties.
   d. Practice polite ways to decline food.
   e. Do not get discouraged by occasional setbacks.
B. Social environment
   1. Have the person identify the types of social situations that contribute to poor eating habits. Examples of stimuli in the social environment that might contribute to difficulty for the person would be negative statements from family members or friends, social situations in which there are expectations for eating inappropriate or disallowed foods.
   2. Have the person identify the kind of social interactions that would be supportive of good eating habits and following the nutrition plan. Role playing can be useful with the person practicing how he or she will ask others to help change his or her eating habits.
C. Cognitive or mental environment
   1. Have the person identify what thoughts and feelings are likely to make attempts to change eating habits unsuccessful.
   2. After the person has identified possible negative thoughts that could lead to discouragement, help him or her develop some positive thoughts that can be used to counteract the negative ones.
   3. Avoid setting unreasonable goals.

TABLE 6-1   Techniques for Behavior Modification (*Continued*)

IV. Change Actual Eating Behavior
    A. Slow down.
        1. Take one small bite at a time.
        2. Put the fork down between mouthfuls.
        3. Chew thoroughly before swallowing.
        4. Take a break during the meal. Stop eating completely for a short period.
    B. Leave some food on the plate.
    C. Make eating of inappropriate foods as difficult as possible.
    D. Control snacks.
        1. Save allowable foods from meals for snacks.
        2. Establish behaviors incompatible with eating.
        3. Prepare snacks the way one prepares meals—on a plate
        4. Keep on hand a quantity of low-calorie foods such as raw vegetables. Have them ready to eat and easy to get.
    E. Instruct the person that when eating, he or she should not be performing any other act. The cues associated with eating should be restricted to that act, so the person should not eat while reading, sewing, watching television, and so on.
    F. Have the person continue self-monitoring.
V. Change Exercise Behavior
    A. Routine activity
        1. Increase routine activity.
        2. Increase use of stairs.
        3. Keep records of distance walked daily.
    B. Exercise
        1. Begin supervised exercise program under specialist's direction.
        2. Keep records of daily exercise.
        3. Increase exercise gradually.
VI. Set Up A Reward-and-Reinforcement System
    A. Have family and friends provide this help in the form of praise and material rewards.
    B. Clearly define behaviors to be reinforced.
    C. Use self-monitoring records as a basis for rewards.
    D. Plan specific rewards for specific behaviors. Use written contracts.
    E. Gradually make rewards more difficult to earn.
    F. Use creative reinforcers, such as dropping quarters in a bank, putting money away for each goal reached and earmarked for something desirable. Take money back as a punishment if the goal is not reached.

Adapted from Stunkard A, Berthold H. What is behavior therapy? Am J Clin Nutr 1985;41:821; Rabb C, Tillotson JL, eds. Heart to heart. Washington, DC, US Dept of Health and Human Services, 1983; and Fensterheim H, Baer J. Don't say yes when you want to say no. New York: Dell Pub Co, 1975.

trol antecedents is to decrease the number of times the person is exposed to tempting situations so that the client's behavior is tested as rarely as possible.(18) Think about how you could suggest modifying the behavior of snacking on cookies in the prior example.

In some instances, responses occur in chains in which each response produces the stimulus for the next response. An example of a chain is watching television, going to the kitchen at commercial breaks, getting a snack, eating the snack, feeling satisfied or less bored (reinforcer). The components of the chain should be identified, and then a break in the chain should be planned, such as doing stretching exercises or laundry at commercials.

Behavior

After identifying antecedents, explore the eating behavior itself by investigating the speed of eating, the reasons for eating, the presence of others, and activities carried on during meals or snacks, such as watching television. Breaking a chain of eating too rapidly, for example, is accomplished by introducing delays in eating, such as resting the utensils after a bite of food or pausing for conversation. Also, eating behaviors can be modified by eating only as a single event in which a person can concentrate on the act of eating and enjoying the flavors of the foods.

Consequences

Consequences of eating are described as reinforcements or rewards. Because behavior may be maintained by its consequences, efforts are made to arrange consequences that will maintain desirable behaviors. The consequences of eating may be positive, negative, or neutral. In general, positive consequences are more effective in promoting change than negative or punishing consequences. Alternatives to eating may be included, such as walking or exercising, writing a letter, cleaning a part of the house, working on a hobby, and so on. One recommendation related to sodium restriction was for the client to set aside a quarter (or dollar) as a reward for using a spice or flavoring in place of salt.(15)

If the client's current eating habits are pleasurable and if food is considered its own reward, then new and different rewards must be established. Eating is a powerfully motivated behavior, the occurrence of which is necessary to maintain life, a positive reinforcement. The dietetics professional needs to identify new reinforcers with clients and introduce healthier food choices. Acquired taste can be developed for a broader selection of foods and can steer choices to healthier selections. In some cases, a client may be aware of foods prepared only one way, which were not pleasing to eat. If a new preparation method is described, the client may be receptive to trying the food. For example, a client may dislike asparagus because he or she knows it only as the long skinny vegetable that is boiled and covered with Hollandaise sauce. If the client is told that asparagus can be grilled for a delicious flavor, he or she may be open-minded enough to try it again and perhaps develop a taste for this low-fat vegetable. Changes in eating patterns should be pleasurable to be self-reinforcing. If new patterns are a chore and are disliked, they will fail to provide self-reinforcement.

The counselor can work with the client to establish reinforcers. Asking, "What do you like to do with your leisure time," may identify activity reinforcers. Reinforcers may be walking, attending movies, plays, or sporting events, taking a bath, gardening, doing hobbies, playing cards, reading, or doing whatever the person prefers. Social reinforcers may be found by asking, "Whom do you like to be with?" Reinforcers may include visiting family or friends or phoning. Other questions are, "What do you find enjoyable?" and "What do you like to buy when you have extra money?" (other than inappropriate foods, of course).(18) Table 6-2 summarizes the identification of reinforcers.

TABLE 6-2 Identifying Reinforcers

1. Make a list of leisure time activities and hobbies that you enjoy.
2. Make a list of people you like to be with.
3. Make a list of things you would like to purchase with small amounts of extra money.
4. What do you find relaxing?
5. What do you do for fun?
6. What are your favorite possessions?

A very important point here is to recognize that the counselor is also part of the reinforcement. Rather than focusing on failures, the counselor should emphasize what the person has done right with verbal reward and praise. Remind clients to reward themselves cognitively by telling themselves they are making progress and have done something right. For the obese, the ability to fit into smaller-sized clothes hanging in the closet and the weight loss itself are reinforcing. New reinforcers, such as enjoyable activities, need to be established and introduced for weight maintenance, such as joining a YMCA for physical activity, engaging in social events not centered on eating, or walking laps around shopping malls. The reinforcement provided by significant others and self-monitoring are discussed later in this chapter.

After one or two eating changes or goals are identified, a schedule of reinforcement needs to be discussed and established. The schedule specifies which behaviors, if any, will be reinforced and how frequently reinforcement will be provided. Continual reinforcement is the simplest method, but this may lose its effectiveness if the reinforcer is used excessively. An alternative is intermittent reinforcement, such as reinforcement three times a day, or once a day. Eventually, the time may be lengthened between reinforcements. The schedule should be appropriate to the behavior one is trying to strengthen, convenient for the person to apply, and applied immediately for the greatest effect. Never reinforcing a behavior leads to its extinction.(19)

In some cases, contracts may be desirable. Contracts are clear statements of target behaviors of the individual; they specify the type of reinforcers to be used, the person who will deliver the reinforcers, and the frequency of reinforcement. They are signed and dated by the counselor and the client. Contracts ensure that all parties agree on the goals and procedures and provide a measurement of how close the client is to reaching the goals. The signatures help to ensure that the contract will be followed, since signing is a commitment and may provide added motivation to change.(15) Figure 6-1 is an example of a contract.

An alternative to a formal contract is encouraging the client to write out a list of behaviors to change and a few strategies to implement the change. Also, a simple list of pros and cons of modifying food choices can become a key eye-opener to some.

Completion of behavioral assessment, including a consideration of the Stage of Change, is needed before counseling begins. Examination of the ABCs (antecedents, behaviors, and consequences) by the dietetics professional and the client assists both parties in understanding current eating behaviors and allows discussion of what can be changed. Maintaining new behaviors when under pressure or stress is especially diffi-

Patient/Client Name_____

Date _____

Goals:

    Example: Increase physical activity 3 times a week.

    1.

    2.

Strategy to Modify Goal:

Time Frame:

    Example: Get up a half-hour earlier than usual for a brisk walk in the neighborhood Tuesdays, Thursdays, and Saturdays.

    Use the stairs instead of the elevator, especially if only one floor.

    1.

    2.

_____   _____
Patient/Client Signature   Dietitian's Signature

Figure 6-1 EXAMPLE OF A BEHAVIORAL CONTRACT FOR CHANGE.

cult. The counselor may consider assessing client self-confidence and ability to cope with stress or anxiety. This may help identify those clients who will need additional support at particularly stressful times.

    The role of the counselor is to provide an integrated plan for the total nutrition program of each client. The nutrition counselor serves as a guide or facilitator of change rather than a director or controller of change by suggesting behavioral techniques appropriate to the situation. The counselor should assist the client in learning to analyze the eating problems and should suggest possible goals, strategies, and techniques to deal with them.(20) Ultimately, the client must determine which suggestions seem manageable at that time and must be willing to implement them. It is also a good idea to ask the client to give an example of the specific behavior change rather than the concept by stating, for example, "the next time I am out of milk I will buy low-fat milk instead of whole milk." This is a concrete action plan compared with merely stating the concept "I'll try to follow a low-fat diet."

Goal setting is one of the critical steps of behavior modification. Goals must be set realistically yet high enough to provide significant change. Cullen and colleagues suggest using a multiple-step goal-setting process. The four-step process is (1) recognizing the need for change, (2) establishing a goal, (3) monitoring goal-related activity, and (4) rewarding yourself for goal attainment. These components can be easily adapted to nutrition interventions.(21)

Since clients are not routinely in daily contact with the counselor, they must be ready to assume personal responsibility for sound dietary changes and eventually become independent. They must learn to analyze and solve their own eating behavior problems. Have the client start with small, easy changes, which are most likely to be successful, and progress incrementally to more difficult ones in later sessions. To be self-reinforcing, the eating changes should be pleasurable ones. If clients enjoy potato chips, ice cream, pizza, and beer, they have to find substitutes they enjoy, such as baked chips, fresh grapes, unbuttered popcorn, and dietetic beverages or light beer. It may be sufficient to start by reducing the quantity of favorite foods consumed. However some people may elect to avoid a food item entirely to reduce the temptation of having more. Needless to say, strategies must be highly individualized, and what is appropriate for one client may be inappropriate for another.

Nutrition therapists have the opportunity to share the experiences of others. By having counseled patients and clients on various issues and using customized approaches, counselors learn to assist patients at every point of change. A great analogy applied to counseling is comparing it with making bread, as described by Miller.(4) Just as every baker knows that there are essential ingredients, kneading, and rising time to make a loaf of bread, every baker also introduces artistic expression and ingredient variation to make a unique loaf of bread to meet the distinct tastes of his loyal customers. When learning to bake, Miller states, "it may be helpful to see pictures of the finished product, and when baking at different altitudes, adjust the recipe."(4) Similarly as counselors, we need to be cognizant of the right things to convey at the right time and customize along the way.

The client should be told to expect problems and some inappropriate eating episodes, especially when under physical or emotional stress. Expecting immediate total control over change is unrealistic and may lead to diminished self-esteem in clients who have problems following diets, with eventual abandonment of the dietary changes. Learning any new skill requires practice over a period of time. Repetition of the same new behaviors gradually becomes reinforcing and habitual. Support and forgiveness should be provided during any lapses. (Analyzing high-risk situations and dealing with lapses is dealt with in the next chapter.) Enthusiasm for change may be expected to drop rapidly after the initial period, especially if frustration and disappointments arise. Weekly appointments with the counselor may be needed and are desirable in the beginning, tapering to bi-monthly and monthly.

SELF-MONITORING

Self-monitoring, or keeping records of eating behaviors to be controlled, was intended originally as a means of supplying the counselor and client with data for analysis. Clients record what, where, when, and how much they eat; the circumstances (e.g.,

TABLE 6-3	Self-Monitoring Food Record				
Time	Food/ Amount/ Method Prep	Room Place	Others Present	How You Felt Before Eating	Activities Same Time
Example:					
9:30 PM	8 cookies, 10 oz milk	Family room	Husband	Bored, tired	Watching TV

eating while watching television or while feeling bored); and the persons present (Table 6-3). The exercise of keeping records has additional value of its own; it increases client awareness and understanding of current eating behaviors and the influences on them and leads to such realizations as "I'm eating too much during evening hours while I read." Data provide a basis for setting goals for change ("I'll eat a low calorie snack instead") and finding ways to reinforce new behaviors ("I'll tell myself how well I'm doing"). Keeping records serves as a measure of the person's commitment to change. In addition, by having to write down the foods and beverages consumed, the client may think twice about actually consuming the item rather than eating it out of habit or with distraction. Weight loss graphs for the obese and records of physical exercise, blood sugar, and blood pressure are other self-monitoring techniques. However, knowledge of the relation between muscle mass and weight and the concepts of weight plateaus are essential to avoid misinterpretation regarding total health.

SELF-MANAGEMENT

In most behavior modification programs for weight control, the client and counselor are together only for a brief duration at specified intervals. Consequently, the counselor cannot be continually in control of dispensing rewards and punishments or withholding them for appropriate and inappropriate behavior, which is the basis of behavior modification. Therefore, self-regulation or self-management techniques are taught to clients so that they can regulate and control their own behavior. In this way, progress may be achieved in the interval between meetings of the client and counselor.

Research has shown the importance of developing behavioral self-management techniques. Skinner explained that self-management or "self-control" occurs when the individual manipulates the variables on which the behavior rests.(22) Self-management programs have been designed to help persons become aware of and modify antecedents of eating and to self-administer rewarding consequences for eating differently. As self-management programs have evolved, more emphasis has been placed on cognitive change. People have been helped to modify thoughts and beliefs that interfered with adherence to specific dietary regimens and to make use of self-reinforcing thoughts when appropriate behaviors occur. Becoming aware of one's inner state can assist in achieving the desired self-management. For example, referring to a diet has connotations of an ephemeral event, whereas adapting a lifestyle change leads to a more permanent behavior modification.

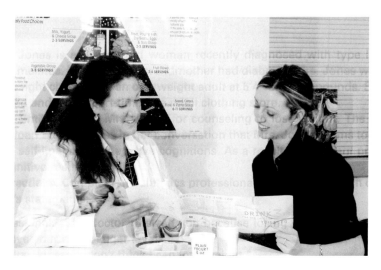

The goal of counseling is self-management.

SOCIAL SUPPORT

A client's social environment consists of people contacted daily. It is important to include the person's family and significant others when planning lifestyle and dietary changes. The dietetics professional should include family members in counseling for change whenever possible, since the changes in food plans at home may affect them as well. Cultural and social factors may be contributing factors to obesity. If the family system supports an obese lifestyle with high-calorie foods and little physical activity, change will be difficult for the client unless the whole family participates in the challenge.(15) Other suggestions are that the involvement and support of spouse and family play an important role in weight loss.(23)

Ideally, family and friends are supportive of the client's efforts to change eating behaviors. The counselor may need to discuss with clients the important role of support in achieving permanent change. The dietetics professional may suggest that clients request help from family or friends by seeking their agreement not to eat inappropriate foods in front of them or not to purchase or prepare the wrong foods. In addition, clients might ask their spouses, families, and friends to offer positive reinforcement for their efforts. Role-playing some of these situations with clients may be helpful.

When family members are present at the counseling session, they should be asked to discuss ways in which they can contribute to the client's lifestyle change. Reinforcing proper behavior by the use of praise is an example. Controlling antecedents by having proper foods available is of great assistance. Family and friends should avoid acting the role of judge. "You shouldn't eat that," "It's bad for you," and "I told you so" are not helpful remarks. Jealous and envious reactions may also be expected. "You've lost enough weight," "Just this once won't hurt your diet," and "Your skin is getting to look awful" are remarks that the client may need to tolerate or confront.

APPLICATIONS

Obesity

The most common application of behavioral principles and methods to the treatment of nutritional problems has been in the management of obesity. Although there has been much success using behavior modification in weight loss regimens, weight regain is common and is a result of the failure to impose weight maintenance behaviors.(24) James Hill, PhD, an expert in weight maintenance, states, "People mistakenly assign most of their effort to losing weight instead of maintaining weight loss . . . weight maintenance should be the focus."(25)

Opinions differ regarding the efficacy of behavior modification techniques developed for use in treating overweight clients. Brownell reports that behavior therapy is an essential part of any weight reduction program.(26) Obesity is a complex state and is not treated easily. The obese may be overweight for a variety of reasons, only one of which may be related to improper eating behaviors.(27) This does not mean, however, that it is futile to attempt to control one's weight.

The American Dietetic Association's position on weight management states that a successful approach "requires a life-long commitment to healthful lifestyle behaviors emphasizing eating practices and daily physical activity that are sustainable and enjoyable."(28) The American College of Sports Medicine, in a position statement, stressed that lifelong weight control requires commitment, an understanding of your eating habits, and a willingness to change them.(29) Realistic goal setting, combined with a reduction of caloric intake plus a sound exercise program is recommended. Behavioral methods have been used successfully in diet planning, nutrition education, and a strenuous physical education program in a residential summer camp for obese boys. This combined approach resulted in significant improvement in body weight for the group.(30) Caban, and colleagues(31) detail a model for individualizing treatment for specific patient needs, particularly for patients who have or are at risk for developing diabetes. Tailoring practical applications to a client's lifestyle achieves the greatest success.

A study designed to include a 2-year follow-up to assess the effectiveness of a behavioral weight control program revealed that after 2 years, 65.3% of the subjects were still below their baseline weights.(32) The researchers indicated that the behavioral weight control program had an important and long-term impact on the weight status of a large sample of obese men and women.

However, long-term weight loss remains a difficult task. Clearly, improved methods to facilitate a higher level and longer duration of success are needed. Four common behaviors among dieters who have been successful in weight maintenance according to James Hill and research from the National Weight Control Registry are (1) eating a low-fat, high-carbohydrate breakfast, (2) eating breakfast almost every day, (3) self-monitoring (weighing, food journals), and (4) engaging in high levels of physical activity (approximately 1 hour a day).(25)

Motivation and readiness must be present for behavior change. This is particularly true of eating behaviors. Several factors are relevant to the prediction of success in weight control, one of which is motivation to reduce weight. A free download from Shape Up America may be used in motivating by revealing barriers to change.(33)

Explaining realistic weight loss achievements is also critical. Clients should consider weight loss successful with an initial reduction of about 10% of their body weight over a 6- to 12-month period.(34, 35) To expect more than that initially would be a set-up for disappointment; however, weight goals can be reevaluated after successful weight loss. Requiring a fee for treatment is another approach; a deposit-refund system may also be used.(36) In the latter system, patients are asked to deposit money, which is later returned if the patient attends meetings faithfully and/or achieves a previously determined weight loss. This system appears to be effective in reducing the dropout rate.

An added benefit of significant weight reduction based on cognitive-behavioral treatment in a long-term therapeutic setting has been the reduction in psychosomatic symptoms, anxiety, and depression in treated clients. More adaptive behavioral alternatives in longer goal-oriented programs seem effective in promoting continued weight loss.(37,38) Research results, therefore, emphasize the fact that there is no quick-fix in weight reduction and that the outlook must be long-term.(39)

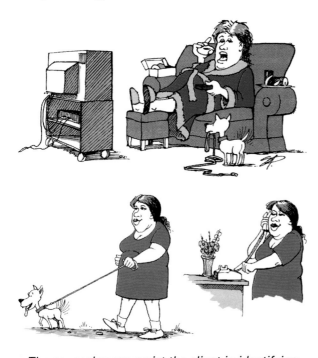

The counselor can assist the client in identifying new behaviors. (top) Old behavior. (bottom) New behaviors.

Eating Disorders

Anorexia nervosa, bulimia, and binge eating are estimated to occur in up to 5% of females and 1% of males, with approximately 85% developing in adolescent years.(40) Therapist errors in treating eating disorders have apparently contributed to patient resistance, treatment ineffectiveness, and premature treatment termination. Various medical and psychological approaches have been used in treatment. It is most important for the therapist to be aware of the alternatives for treatment. The behavior modification approach is one of these alternatives.(41–43)

A now classic report detailed the use of behavior modification techniques for the nutritional disorder, anorexia nervosa, a chronic failure to eat.(44) A female who was 5 feet, 4 inches tall weighed only 47 pounds at the start of her behavior therapy. Before therapy, the hospital environment provided many amenities and privileges. Because she appeared to enjoy them, these privileges and amenities were removed so that they could be used to reinforce appropriate behaviors, in this case, eating. All the attention and sympathy that the hospital staff had used to coax the patient to eat were withdrawn. The therapist ate one meal a day with the patient, and the staff was allowed only to greet the patient on entering the room.

The social reinforcement that had helped to maintain non-eating behavior was withheld so that it could be used later to strengthen eating behaviors. The therapist talked to the patient to reinforce her behavior when she picked up her fork, lifted food toward her mouth, chewed food, or performed any other eating behavior. She was then allowed the use of radio or television, but only after meals at which she increased her food intake over previous meals. As she gained strength and weight, other reinforcers were introduced, such as the privilege of choosing her own menu or inviting other patients to dine with her. Later reinforcers included walks, visitors, and mail.

The treatment was successful, and after 8 weeks of therapy, the patient was discharged weighing 64 pounds to a program of outpatient follow-up. Five years later, she had maintained her weight between 78 and 80 pounds and was successfully employed.(45) Locating potential reinforcers or behavior strengtheners is an essential first step in any treatment program. What reinforces behavior for one person may not function as a reinforcer for another.

A more recent study reported on the use of contracts in behavior modification therapy for anorexia nervosa.(46) On admission, patients with anorexia nervosa signed a contract specifying the weight gain necessary to earn privileges such as phone use and visitors. The report supported the use of behavior contracting in this type of eating disorder.

Other earlier studies have noted the importance of self-monitoring and daily logging of intake, weight, and details of binge-purge episodes on progress and successful treatment of anorexia and bulimia.(47–49) These reported successes of behavioral treatment of anorexia and bulimia have involved inpatient therapy and outpatient follow-up.

Another finding from the research on anorexia nervosa concerned the effect of size of food portions on eating behavior. The serving of larger portions was associated with increased food intake. Apparently, the subjects ate a relatively fixed proportion of the amount of food presented, whether the portion was large or small. This pattern of eating has been noted to occur in obese people as well, but not in normal adults or in young children.(50)

Behavior modification has also been used successfully in the treatment of chronic food refusal in handicapped children. Records of conditions before treatment began indicated that all patients accepted little food, expelled food frequently, and engaged in disruptive behavior. Treatment methods used were social praise, access to preferred foods, brief periods of play with toys, and forced feeding. Marked behavioral improvement was noted for each patient as well as an increase in the amount of food consumed. Further improvements were noted at 7- to 30-month follow-up.(51)

Participation in a behavioral treatment program proved useful when multiple problems were dealt with in the case of a 29-year-old married woman, hospitalized with anorexia after a diagnosis of multiple sclerosis at 21 years of age.(52)

Many drug and hormonal therapies have been tried as treatments for anorexia nervosa. The most common treatment is behavior modification, combined with individual and family counseling.(53)

A position paper by the American Dietetic Association on eating disorders recognizes the role of the registered dietitian in therapy for disordered eating, but also emphasizes the importance of interdisciplinary collaboration with this population.(54)

Diabetes Mellitus

Behavior modification methods have proved to be a useful component in the management of diabetes mellitus. Historically, poor patient adherence to dietary regimens has been a problem. Behavioral interventions such as cueing, self-monitoring, and reinforcement for appropriate behavior can be successfully implemented to improve glycemic control and reduce risks of complications in patients with diabetes.(55) As previously noted, though, the problem of control of obesity from the standpoint of any particular treatment is complex.

Behavioral management techniques may be used to reduce the burden of diabetes complications.(56) Proactive management by care providers and patients is warranted and has demonstrated positive outcomes.(57–59) Implementation of internet technology to increase therapist and social support may be on the rise as care providers continue to seek better ways to achieve optimal behaviors.(60)

The National Diabetes Education Program (NDEP) supports the work of the other organizations in diabetes management and sets forth initiatives for comprehensive care. The initiatives and additional resources can be viewed from their website at http://ndep.nih.org.

Behavioral interventions, when used in the management of diabetes mellitus, should be geared to the developmental stage of the individual in treatment.(58) An understanding of life-span changes (i.e., preadolescence, adolescence, and adulthood) in relation to life role, peer conformity pressure, eating disorders, and hormonal changes needs to be taken into account. The strategy that is effective with a diabetic adolescent struggling with peer conformity pressures may well be markedly different from that which will be of assistance to a pregnant woman with diabetes. There is a definite need to individualize interventions directed toward behavior change.(61)

Cardiovascular Diseases

In the Multiple Risk Factor Intervention Trial (MRFIT), behavioral scientists and nutritionists worked cooperatively with the aim of changing behaviors related to diet and smoking on a long-term basis to reduce the risk of cardiovascular disease. A self-evaluation system for monitoring food intake was developed so that the counselor could estimate the subject's progress in making appropriate dietary changes. A scoring system was used for classifying foods according to their fat and cholesterol content as well as their predicted effect on blood cholesterol. Subjects could use the system and select alternative food choices to meet appropriate eating goals. The self-monitoring records were used as a method of measuring compliance and also served to reinforce change and provide positive feedback for appropriate behavior.(62)

The research on the DASH (Dietary Approaches to Stop Hypertension) diet, which is rich in fruits, vegetables, and low-fat dairy foods, concluded that food selection lowered blood pressure. Follow-up studies have further demonstrated that "the DASH diet affects coronary heart disease (CHD) risk favorably."(63)

Studies of healthy populations, of those at increased risk, and of patients with cardiovascular disease have shown that risk-related behavior can be altered and, in some cases, the incidence of cardiovascular disease can be reduced.(64–66) Since it is generally recognized that cardiovascular disease may result from self-selected behaviors such as smoking, inappropriate eating behaviors, and the pursuit of stress-prone lifestyles, it is most encouraging that we can emphasize the initiation of the behavior is by choice and that modification of these self-defeating behaviors is possible. Because the risk factors are behavioral in nature, it is particularly appropriate to attempt to alter them using psychological methods based on behavior modification. The degree of difficulty with such behavior modification partially depends on how long the undesirable behavior has been in place.

Human Resource Management

The behavior of employees is of major concern to supervisors interested in productivity and good human relations. Blanchard and Johnson's book, *The One Minute Manager*, provides examples of behavioral modification strategies.(5) Goals begin new behaviors and in the "one minute goal," the manager uses observable, measurable behavioral terms to describe the discrepancy between the actual and desired performance. Supervisors need to convert ambiguous affective goal statements into a format that is useful for producing improved performance. For example, it is useless to encourage employees to do better, if "better" is not defined and stated in behavioral terms.(67) Because behaviors are believed to be maintained by their consequences, the "one-minute praise" and the "one-minute reprimand"—examples of rewards and punishments—are recommended. Although most supervisors attempt to catch subordinates doing things wrong, Blanchard and Johnson suggest that they notice employees doing something right or approximately right and then gradually move them toward the desired behavior. The one-minute praise is used immediately to reinforce proper behavior. Eventually, some employees begin to praise themselves for the proper behavior, which provides additional reinforcement. Table 6-4 lists positive reinforcers for employees. The one-minute reprimand is also used immediately and concentrates on the improper behavior, not on the person.

An important aspect of job satisfaction and performance is the employee's sense of personal control; so it is imperative that supervisors do not use behavior modification in ways that are seen as manipulative and degrading to employees.(68) Intrinsic motivation should be encouraged to emphasize the importance of a self-reinforcing loop.

TABLE 6-4   **Positive Reinforcers**

Praise	Social events
Positive feedback	Knowledge of results
Recognition (employee of the week, month)	Thank you letter
Added responsibility	Salary increase
Compliments	Bonus
Special assignments	Promotion

CASE STUDY 1

Gail is a 23-year-old single woman who has landed her first professional job as a lawyer in a large New York City law firm. She is 5'4" and weighs 105 pounds. She lives alone in a small apartment and spends most of her time at work or out with friends. Typically, she consumes three cups of black coffee in the morning at work before 9:00 AM. Gail usually works through lunch and may eat a light yogurt or a banana while doing other things. After work she meets with clients or friends for dinner, where she will pick at a tossed salad but rarely finishes the meal. She accompanies the meal with several martinis and a half-pack of cigarettes.

1. What are the health risk factors for Gail?
2. What tool(s) for behavioral change could be implemented in Gail's lifestyle?

CASE STUDY 2

Steve is a 45-year-old banker at a small local bank. He has recently been found to have high cholesterol. He is 6'1" tall and weighs 255 pounds. His wife Susan is employed full-time in the same bank and is also overweight. They have no children.

The dietetics professional discovers that Steve enjoys eating and looks forward to his meals. He skips breakfast, but has coffee with cream and sugar and one or two doughnuts or rolls at his desk at work. He usually eats at a local restaurant for lunch. One of his most common meals at lunch is a cheeseburger with French fries, a large cola, and an ice cream sandwich for dessert. If time permits, he may have an afternoon snack of another large cola and some cookies. He looks forward to arriving home after work and relaxes with one or two glasses of wine. A typical dinner includes fried chicken, baked potato with sour cream, corn, a roll and butter, and apple pie for dessert. Steve and Susan watch television in the evening and snack on popcorn and potato chips with cola or beer.

1. Identify Steve's antecedents or cues to eating.
2. Eating is enjoyable and a reward for Steve. What could the dietetics professional do to help Steve identify new rewards?

IMPLICATIONS FOR THERAPY

Brownell and Cohen(14) have pointed out major advantages of behavior therapy. Programs integrating behavioral approaches appear to hold the most promise. A comprehensive program, however, considering psychological, cultural, environmental, and behavioral factors, is more apt to be successful.

Eating patterns are not altered easily, but behavior modification therapy offers promising techniques that may be helpful to both the client and the counselor. Analysis of the ABCs—the antecedents of eating, the eating behavior itself, and the consequences of eating—by the counselor and client leads to understanding of the problems, the setting of goals, and the development of strategies for change. Efforts should be made to arrange consequences that reinforce and maintain desirable changes, with an ultimate goal being independent client self-management. Behavior modification may be used in conjunction with other counseling and education strategies.

REVIEW AND DISCUSSION QUESTIONS

1. Describe the similarities and differences in learning styles of classical conditioning, operant conditioning, and modeling. Are there situations or cases in which you would prefer using one style over another?
2. Give two examples of a chain of events using the ABC framework.
3. Describe two methods of self-control discussed in the chapter, and discuss how each aids in successful behavior modification.
4. List one of the most important behavior modification strategies for each of the applications discussed: eating disorders, obesity, diabetes, cardiovascular disease, and human resource management.

SUGGESTED ACTIVITIES

1. Complete a food diary for 3 days. Identify your cues for eating. Identify your reinforcers. Set one goal for change with identified reinforcers.
2. Record and identify your own ABCs related to an activity other than eating, such as studying, exercising, smoking, and the like. How can these behaviors be made to occur more or less often by rearranging the antecedents and/or consequences?
3. Role play and tape-record a counseling session. How often did you reinforce positive behaviors?
4. Arrange to watch an adult interact with a child or children for half an hour. Tally the number of times the adult attends to desirable behaviors, which reinforces them, versus the number of times desirable behaviors are ignored, which may lead to their extinction. Note whether the adult responds to undesirable behaviors, which reinforces them.
5. Identify your own reinforcers by making a list of leisure time activities that you enjoy, people you like to be with, and things you would purchase with extra money. Select an appropriate reinforcer for yourself for the next time you have a book to read or a paper to write. Identify a time schedule for dispensing the reinforcer.
6. Select an undesirable behavior of your own that you would like to diminish. Record the situations in which the stimulus or the behavior occurs for 3 days. Identify the controlling stimulus conditions just before the behavior and the reinforcement.
7. Identify three situations in which modeling occurs.
8. In a social situation with friends, tally the number of times in a half-hour that you dispense social approval (smiles, nods, appreciative words) compared with disapproval (frowns, disparaging words).
9. List 10 phrases of social approval that you are comfortable using with others.

10. Discuss your personal experiences at work and compare them with those of others. Does your supervisor praise or punish? What are the consequences of the supervisor's actions on your behavior and that of other employees?

WEB SITES

http://www.diabetes.org / American Diabetes Association
http://www.cyberdiet.com / Cyberdiet
http://www.renfrew.org / Renfrew Center for eating disorders
http://www.freeweightloss.com/article3.html / behavior modification article
http://www.nationaleatingdisorders.org / National Eating Disorders Association

REFERENCES

1. Wilson G, O'Leary K. Principles of behavior therapy. Englewood Cliffs, NJ: Prentice Hall, 1980.
2. Brownell KD. The central role of lifestyle change in long-term weight management. Clin Cornerstone 1999;2(3):43.
3. Israel D, Moore S, eds. Beyond nutrition counseling: achieving positive outcomes through nutrition therapy. Chicago: American Dietetic Association, 1996.
4. Miller WR, Rollnick S. Motivational interviewing: preparing people to change addictive behavior. New York: The Guilford Press, 1991.
5. Blanchard K, Johnson S. The one minute manager. New York: Berkley Books, 1981.
6. Hill WF. Principles of learning. Palo Alto, CA: Mayfield Pub Co, 1981.
7. Schwartz B, Lacey H. Behaviorism, science and human nature. New York: WW Norton, 1982.
8. Bandura A. Self-efficacy: the exercise of control. New York: WH Freeman Company, 1997.
9. Tibbs T, Haire-Joshu D, Schechtman KB, et al. The relationship between parental modeling, eating patterns, and dietary intake among African-American parents. J Am Diet Assoc 2001;101:535.
10. Nicklas TA, Baranowski T, Baranowski JC, et al. Family and child-care provider influences on preschool children's fruit, juice, and vegetable consumption. Nutr Rev 2001;59(7):224.
11. Sims HP, Manz CC. Modeling influences on employee behavior. Personnel J 1982;61:58.
12. National Heart, Lung, and Blood Institute (NHLBI) mission statement available at http://www.nhlbi.nih.gov/about/org/mission.htm. Accessed 11/6/01.
13. Mahoney MJ, Caggiula AW. Applying behavioral methods to nutritional counseling. J Am Diet Assoc 1978;72:372.
14. Brownell KD, Cohen LR. Adherence to dietary regimens 2: components of effective interventions. Behav Med 1995;20:155.
15. Rabb C, Tillotson JL, eds. Heart to heart. Washington, DC: US Department of Health and Human Services, 1983.
16. Fensterheim H, Baer J. Don't say yes when you want to say no. New York: Dell, 1975.
17. Building nutrition counseling skills, vol. II. Washington, DC: US Department of Health and Human Services, 1984.
18. Storlie J, Jordan HA. Behavioral management of obesity. New York: Spectrum Pub, 1984.
19. Martin G, Pear J. Behavior modification. Englewood Cliffs, NJ: Prentice-Hall, 1978.
20. Holli BB. Using behavior modification in nutrition counseling. J Am Diet Assoc 1988;88:1530.
21. Cullen KW, Baranowski T, Smith SP. Using goal setting as a strategy for dietary behavior change. J Am Diet Assoc 2001;101:562.
22. Skinner BF. Science and human behavior. New York: Macmillan, 1953.

23. Poston WS II, Foreyt JP. Successful management of the obese patient. Am Fam Physician 2000;61(12):3615.

24. Latner JD, Stunkard AJ, Wilson GT, et al. Effective long-term treatment of obesity: a continuing care model. Int J Obes Relat Metab Disord 2000;24(7):893.

25. American Medical Association Media Briefing July 12, 2001. Four behaviors that can spell success in maintaining weight loss. Available at http://www.ama-assn.org/ama/pub/article/4197-5159.html. Accessed 12/27/01.

26. Brownell KD. Diet, exercise and behavioural intervention: the nonpharmacological approach. Eur J Clin Invest 1998;28 S2:19.

27. Stunkard AJ. Current views on obesity. Am J Med 1996;100(2):230.

28. Cummings SM, Goodrick GK, Foreyt JP. ADA position paper: weight management. J Am Diet Assoc 2002;102:1145. Available at http://www.eatright.org/positions.html. Accessed 1/15/03.

29. American College of Sports Medicine: Position statement: appropriate intervention strategies for weight loss and prevention of weight regain for adults. Med Sci Sports Exerc 2001. Available at http://www.acsm-msse.org/. Accessed 12/27/01.

30. McKenzie TL. A behaviorally oriented residential camping program for obese children and adolescents. Educ Treatment Children 1986;9:67.

31. Caban A, Johnson P, Marseille D, Wylie-Rosett J. Tailoring a lifestyle change approach and resources to the patient. Diabetes Spectrum 1999;12(1):33.

32. Lavery MA, Loewy JW, Kapadia AS, et al. Long-term follow-up of weight status of subjects in a behavioral weight control program. J Am Diet Assoc 1989;89:1259.

33. Shape Up America. Patient education materials available at http://www.shapeup.org/profcenter/education/index.asp. Accessed 12/01/01.

34. NIH First Federal Obesity Clinical Guidelines. Available at http://www.nih.gov/news/pr/jun98/nhlbi-17.htm. Accessed 11/06/01.

35. Collazo-Clavell ML. Safe and effective management of the obese patient. Mayo Clinic Proc 1999;74(12):1255.

36. Helm K, Klawitter B. Nutrition therapy: advanced counseling skills. Lake Dallas, TX: Helm Seminars, 1995.

37. Anonymous. Dieting and the development of eating disorders in overweight and obese adults. Arch Intern Med 2000;160(17):2581.

38. Williamson DA, Perrin LA. Behavioral therapy for obesity. Endocrinol Metab Clin North Am 1996;25(4):943.

39. Jeffery RW, Drewnowski A, Epstein LH, et al. Long-term maintenance of weight loss: current status. Health Psychol 2000;19(1 Suppl):5.

40. Anonymous. Adolescent Medicine Committee, Canadian Paediatric Society. Eating disorders in adolescents: principles of diagnosis and treatment. Paediatrics and Child Health 1998;3(3):189.

41. Yager J. The treatment of eating disorders. J Clin Psychiatry 1988;49:18.

42. Thompson RA, Sherman RT. Therapist errors in treating eating disorders: relationship and process. Psychother 1989;26:62.

43. Cox GL, Merkel WT. A qualitative review of psychosocial treatments for bulimia. J Nerv Ment Dis 1989;177:77.

44. Bachrach A, Erwin W, Mohr J. The control of eating behavior in an anorexic by operant conditioning techniques. In: Ullman L, Krasner LP, eds. Case studies in behavior modification. New York: Holt, Rinehart, & Winston, 1965.

45. Reese E. The analysis of human operant behavior. Dubuque, IA: William C. Brown Co, 1966.

46. Solanto MV, Jacobson MS, Heller L, et al. Rate of weight gain of inpatients with anorexia nervosa under two behavioral contracts. Pediatrics 1994;93(6):989.

47. Leitenberg H, Gross J, Peterson J, Rosen J. Analysis of an anxiety model and the process of change during exposure plus response prevention treatment of bulimia nervosa. Behav Therapy 1984;15:3.

48. Cullari S, Redmon W. Treatment of bulimorexia through behavior therapy and diet modification. Behav Therapist 1983;6:165.
49. Smith G, Medlik L. Modification of binge eating in anorexia nervosa. Behav Psychotherapy 1983;11:249.
50. Barlow DH, Tillotson JL. Behavioral science and nutrition: a new perspective. J Am Diet Assoc 1978;72:368.
51. Riordan MM, et al. Behavioral assessment and treatment of chronic food refusal in handicapped children. J Appl Behav Anal 1984;17:327.
52. Touyz SW, Gertler R, Brigham S, Somerville B. Anorexia nervosa in a patient with multiple sclerosis: a case report. Int J Eating Disord 1989;8:231.
53. Hsu LKG. The treatment of anorexia nervosa. Am J Psychiatry 1986;143:573.
54. Spear BA, Myers ES. American Dietetic Association position paper: Nutrition intervention in the treatment of anorexia nervosa, bulimia nervosa, and eating disorder not otherwise specified (EDNOS). Available at: http://www.eatright.org/adap0701.html. Accessed 11/06/01.
55. Wing R, Goldstein MG, Acton KJ, et al. Behavioral science research in diabetes: lifestyle changes related to obesity, eating behavior, and physical activity. Diabetes Care 2001;24(1):117.
56. Clark CM Jr, Fradkin JE, Hiss RG, et al. The National Diabetes Education Program, changing the way diabetes is treated: comprehensive diabetes care. Diabetes Care 2001;24(4):617.
57. Meyer-Davis E, D'Antonio A, Martin M, et al. Pilot study of strategies for effective weight management in type 2 diabetes: pounds off with empowerment. Fam Community Health 2001;24(2):27.
58. Clark CM Jr, Snyder JW, Meek RL, et al. A systematic approach to risk stratification and intervention within a managed care environment improved diabetes outcomes and patient satisfaction. Diabetes Care 2001;24(6):1079.
59. Ridgeway NA, Harvill DR, Harvill LM, et al. Improved control of type 2 diabetes mellitus: a practical education/behavior modification program in a primary care clinic. South Med J 1999;92(7):667.
60. Wing R, Tate DF. Lifestyle changes to reduce obesity. Curr Opin Endocrinol Diabetes 2000;7(5):240.
61. Glasgow RE, Fisher EB, Anderson BJ, et al. Behavioral science in diabetes: contributions and opportunities. Diabetes Care 1999;22(5):832.
62. Remmell PS, Gorder DD, Hall Y, Tillotson JL. Assessing dietary adherence in the Multiple Risk Factor Intervention Trial (MRFIT). J Am Diet Assoc 1980;76:351.
63. DASH Hypertension Diet Also Lowers Cholesterol, Finds New NHLBI-Funded Study. Available at: http://www.nhlbi.nih.gov/new/press/01-06-21.htm. Accessed 11/06/01.
64. Blair SN, Horton E, Leon AS, et al. Physical activity, nutrition, and chronic disease. Med Sci Sports Exerc 1996;28(3):335.
65. Henritze J, Brammell HL, McGloin J. LIFECHECK: a successful, low touch, low tech, in-plant cardiovascular disease risk identification and modification program. Am J Health Promot 1992;7(2):129.
66. Johnston DW. Prevention of cardiovascular disease by psychological methods. Br J Psychiatry 1989;154:183.
67. Stuart JA, Wallace SG. Analyzing "affective" goal statements. Performance and Instruction 1988;27:10.
68. Greenberger DB, Strasser S, Cummings LL, Dunham RB. The impact of personal control on performance and satisfaction. Organ Behav Human Decision Processes 1989;43:29.

Counseling for Cognitive Change

CHAPTER 7

After reading this chapter, you will be able to

1. identify the types of cognitions a person may have and their effect on behavioral change.

2. discuss the types of cognitive distortions and the effects they have on people's behaviors.

3. explain the phases of cognitive restructuring.

4. discuss self-efficacy's role in the initiation and maintenance of health behavior changes and the person's choice of activities.

5. list the advantages and disadvantages of the sources of efficacy information.

6. explain how people appraise information cognitively.

7. define relapse prevention and the difference between a lapse and a relapse.

8. explain high-risk situations and the cognitive-behavioral model of the relapse process.

9. list determinants and predictors of lapse and relapse and how to assess them.

10. identify treatment strategies to prevent lapses and relapses.

Behavior modification, based on learning principles, examines the influence of external environmental factors on an individual's behaviors. A person's eating responses are linked to stimuli or cues in the environment, and food choices are shaped by their immediate consequences (positive reinforcement) without requiring conscious thought. A second approach by psychologists, which can be classified as internal rather than external, is exploring the relation between cognitive processes and eating behaviors. Cognitions may be defined as one's thoughts or perceptions at a particular moment in time. Thinking patterns can profoundly influence how people behave and the way they feel.(1) Strategies for dealing with a client's cognitions are frequently incorporated into behavioral programs, known as cognitive-behavioral therapy.

Since behavior is molded and changed through the interaction of a person's external environmental influences as well as internal cognitive processes, there is a role that thoughts can and do play in explaining a person's behaviors. In addition to examining external environmental cues and reinforcement, the dietetics professional needs to assess the client's internal thoughts when teaching them to implement coping strategies

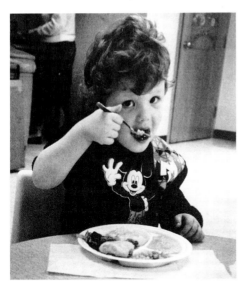

"This tastes good" is a positive cognition.

for promoting better dietary adherence. Combining several approaches to treatment holds the promise of better results. Weight control programs, for example, may include treatment components of behavior modification, cognitive change, exercise, social support, and nutrition.(2–4)

This chapter explores three interrelated areas: cognitions and cognitive restructuring, self-efficacy, and relapse prevention. Assessing a client's cognitions can provide valuable information about the maintenance of adaptive and maladaptive behaviors, since negative thoughts inhibit behavioral change. The dietary counselor can help clients identify distorted thoughts, their effect on behavior, and ways to modify them into more positive coping cognitions.

Self-efficacy, another cognitive process, deals with people's judgments about their competence to perform specific behaviors. These perceptions, not necessarily a person's true capabilities, influence the initiation and maintenance of health and other behavior changes.

Relapse prevention is a self-management program with both cognitive and behavioral components. To prevent relapse from a dietary change, the counselor works with the client to anticipate and prevent dietary lapses that may occur during high-risk situations and to help the person recover from minor slips before they become a full relapse or total breakdown in self-control.

Negative cognitions and low self-efficacy ratings are of concern to counselors because they are predictive of relapse. Individuals with positive cognitions and perceived self-efficacy tend to call on their coping skills and regulate their behavior better. Albert Bandura does not believe that appropriate behavior, such as eating what one should, is achieved by a feat of willpower.(5,6) When people do not behave optimally, even though they know what they should do, thoughts or cognitions may be mediating the relationship between what they know and what they do.

COGNITIONS

Cognitive events are conscious thoughts that occur in a person's stream of consciousness. Beck refers to them as "automatic thoughts," since they run through the mind automatically, whereas Meichenbaum, calls them ongoing "internal dialogue."(7) A person's thoughts, also referred to as self-talk, can influence how he or she behaves, feels, and appraises the outcomes of a behavior. Although our actions are not governed solely by thought, thought does enter into the determination of many actions. An example of an internal dialogue is: "Shall I cook supper or eat out? I guess I'll cook in. I wonder what's in the freezer that won't take too long to cook. I'll check as soon as I get home."

Although people do not engage in self-talk all the time, there are times in which they are more likely to do so. These instances include when they are integrating new thoughts and actions, such as making lifestyle and dietary changes or performing a new job; exercising choices and judgments as in novel situations; and anticipating and/or experiencing intense emotions.(7) According to Bandura, cognitive processes play a major role in the acquisition and retention of new behavior patterns.(6) See Table 7-1 for examples of self-talk.

SELF-ASSESSMENT

Add some of your own examples of self-talk to Table 7-1. What are you thinking right now?

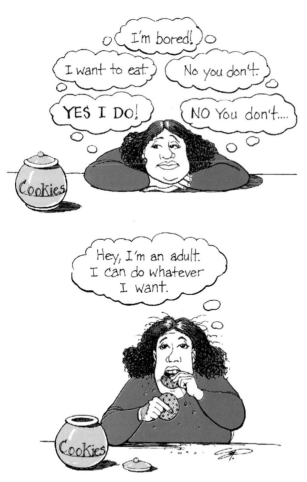

The counselor needs to have the client keep a record of cognitions.

The client's internal dialogue is viewed as a learned response. This self-talk may be positive and supportive, negative and upsetting, or neutral. Positive cognitions support behaviors, such as, "These dietary changes are not so bad." Negative cognitions inhibit people's ability to change behaviors, such as, "This dietary regimen looks difficult to follow." Cognitive variables are important in modifying dietary habits and in maintaining eating disorders, such as anorexia nervosa and bulimia. Dysfunctional thoughts and beliefs about "fattening" foods, fear of weight gain, and body image require identification, challenging, and restructuring.(8) In managing subordinates, an employee may be thinking: "I like my job," or "this job is boring."

Since cognitions are learned responses, the counselor may view the client's cognitions as behaviors to be modified or changed. Counselors need to assist

TABLE 7-1	Examples of Self-Talk

"I'm going to get a college degree so I'll have a successful career."
"I need to get up earlier tomorrow so I'll arrive on time."
"It's the holidays so I'm going to eat whatever I want."
"My New Year's resolution is to get more exercise."
"I'd be in better health if I lost some weight."
"I look fat."
"I hate to exercise because it makes me sweat."
"I have no will power."

clients in altering thought patterns, beliefs, attitudes, and opinions. Many people cannot improve their eating habits until they change their thoughts about food, eating, and drinking. Overeating and drinking can be a person's way of coping with stress, depression, and other emotions. The cognitive approach is to help the client by getting rid of unproductive, debilitating thoughts or beliefs and adopting more positive, constructive ones.

Cognitive Distortions

Since negative thoughts inhibit behavioral change, it is necessary for people to first become aware of distortions in their thought patterns. Faulty thinking almost always contains gross distortions, often has little to do with actual reality, and may be self-defeating and destructive. Burns identified 10 common cognitive distortions.(1)

1. **All-or-nothing thinking.** This refers to the tendency to evaluate personal qualities in black and white, good or bad, and it is the basis of perfectionism. Either a person has high goals or standards and performance is perfect, or that person is a failure. For example: "I ate this piece of pie, and I shouldn't have. I'm a weak person and a failure."
2. **Overgeneralization.** A person concludes that if one negative event happens, it will happen over and over again. For example: "I shouldn't have eaten that. It's no use. I will never be able to follow the diet." Or, "I tried to lose weight before and was unsuccessful, so I will never be able to lose."
3. **Mental filter**. A person dwells on a negative detail in a situation, and the whole situation is perceived as negative. For example: "If I can't eat whatever I want at the party, the party won't be any fun."
4. **Disqualifying the positive.** Some individuals transform neutral and even positive experiences into negative ones. For example: "I am following the diet now, but this is a fluke. I probably won't be able to do it tomorrow."
5. **Jumping to conclusions.** A person makes a negative interpretation even though there are no facts to support it. There are two types of jumping to conclusions: mind reading and fortune teller error. In mind reading, people assume that others are looking down on them. For example: "People don't want to be my friend because I am so fat." In fortune teller error, a person predicts that things will turn out badly and assumes that this is a fact. For example: "I don't think I can follow

the diet." A positive prediction is "I'll feel less lonely if I eat this bag of cookies." This is not entirely true, and later the person may feel guilty and have less self-respect. These negative feelings may lead to more binge eating. "I'll only eat one chocolate candy" is another prediction.

6. **Magnification and minimization**. A person either blows things up out of proportion, called *catastrophizing* or shrinks them into the small and unimportant. For example: "I goofed up. Everyone will hear about it. I'm ruined." Or, "I did it this time, but that is such a small gain that it doesn't amount to anything." The anorexic client, for example, overinterprets small increases in weight and has dysfunctional beliefs about shape, body weight, and eating.(9)

7. **Emotional reasoning**. Negative emotions are taken as evidence of the truth. For example: "I feel inadequate. Therefore, I must be inadequate." Or, "I'm so bored that I deserve a hot fudge sundae."

8. **"Should" statements**. People try to motivate themselves with "should," "must," and "shouldn't" statements. For example: "I should eat fruit," and "I shouldn't eat cake." When behavior falls short of one's personal standards, guilt results. To assert their independence when others tell people what they "should" or "shouldn't" do, some people feel rebellious and do just the opposite.

9. **Labeling and mislabeling**. Instead of describing an error, individuals attach a label to themselves. Instead of thinking that a lapse occurred on the diet, for example, the person thinks, "I'm a pig" or "I'm an idiot."

10. **Personalization**. A person sees him- or herself as the cause of some negative external event when this is not true. For example: "What happened was my fault because I am inadequate."

Cognitive distortions are thinking traps that have been learned. These negative thoughts create feelings that may lead to a negative self-image or sense of worthlessness. In addition, they can become a self-fulfilling prophecy. Because they have been learned, they can be changed or relearned with practice. However, since some people have had these thoughts for years, change may require extended effort and counseling.

To improve dietary adherence and outcomes, the dietetics practitioner can ask clients to keep self-monitoring records of their thoughts. Then counselors should reinforce any positive and coping thoughts and help clients recognize and restructure the negative ones. Cognitive assessment allows a person to examine the role of thoughts and thinking processes in the development of adaptive and maladaptive behaviors. Table 7-2 is an example of a client log of cognitions.

TABLE 7-2   Log of Cognitions

Date	Time	Place	Food Eaten	Thoughts About Eating Before/ During Eating	Thoughts About Eating After Eating
1/10	2:15	Home	6 cookies, coke	"I feel hungry and tired. The cookies taste great."	"I'm not hungry any more. I feel better."

Cognitive Restructuring

Cognitive restructuring techniques refer to a variety of approaches involved with modifying the client's thinking and the assumptions and attitudes underlying these cognitions.(7) The focus is on the false thoughts, inferences, and premises. Thus, the counselor attempts to become familiar with the client's thought content, feelings, and behaviors and to understand their interrelationships. As a dietetics professional, you need to help the client identify specific misconceptions and distortions and to test their validity and reasonableness.(7)

Phases of Cognitive Behavior Modification

Cognitive behavior modification consists of three phases, not necessarily in progression. The first phase is concerned with helping the client understand the nature of the problem.(7) A basic principle is that people cannot change a behavior without increasing their awareness, raising their consciousness, or noticing a pattern in how they think, feel, and behave and the impact of their behavior in various situations. The client's recognition is a necessary first step, although not a sufficient condition to bring about change.

Rarely does a client recognize that thinking processes are a source of the eating problems. The counselor should enlist clients in a collaborative, investigative effort to understand. The client needs to keep a written log of self-observations to heighten the awareness of the relation between dysfunctional thoughts, feelings, and maladaptive eating behaviors.

Burns suggests having the client keep written, self-monitoring records with three columns, including, first, the false thought or self-criticism, then the type of cognitive distortion or thinking error it represents, and, finally, a self-defense response or the substitution of a more objective, coping thought.(1) Table 7-3 shows examples.

In addition to written records, the counselor can discuss in an interview the range of eating situations, past and present, during which the client has false thoughts, such as hopeless thoughts about previous attempts to lose weight or follow specific dietary changes. The dietetics professional should ask clients to verbalize their thoughts and feelings concerning food, eating, and the dietary goal or change during the counseling session

TABLE 7-3   Assessing and Altering False Thoughts

Daily Record		Date
False Thought or Belief	**Type of Distortion**	**Self-defense, Coping Thought**
"I shouldn't have eaten those cookies. I'm a failure."	All-or-none thinking	"Eating 3 cookies does not make me a failure. I can improve."
"I ate the pie. I'm a pig."	Mislabeling	"Pigs are animals and I am human. I don't have to be perfect."
"I don't have time to eat right."	Fortune teller error	"I have just as much time as anyone else."

by asking: "How do you feel about...?" and "What do you think about...?" to determine what their clients are thinking to themselves about the eating behavior to be changed, about their ability to change it, and, at follow-up appointments, about their progress.

> **EXAMPLE:** *"How do you feel about eating more fruits and vegetables?"*
> *"How do you feel about cutting down on the amount of fried foods you eat?"*
> *"What do you think about your ability to make these changes starting tomor-row?"*
> *"On a scale of 1 to 10 with 10 being the highest, how important is this to you?"*

In group counseling, cognitions can be discussed, such as the negative self-talk of obese people. Clients need to realize the false, self-defeating, and self-fulfilling aspects of their self-statements.

During the second phase, the counselor helps the client to explore and consolidate the cognitive problem. As the client reports negative, self-defeating, and self-fulfilling prophecy aspects of thoughts, the counselor can ask how these affect actual behavior. For example: "What happens when you are thinking you are bored and want to eat something?" "What happens when you think you are too tired after working all day to do any cooking?" "What happens when you think the food isn't as good tasting or sat-isfying as before?" The client needs to interrupt the automatic nature of negative self-talk and appraise the situation. The negative cognitions are viewed as hypotheses wor-thy of testing rather than as facts. The client should be encouraged to ask the follow-ing questions:(1)

> What good does it do to focus on negative thoughts? Is there another way to view the situation?
>
> What is the worst that could happen compared with the likeliest?
>
> What is the factual evidence for thinking this thought? Is it really true?
>
> What can I say about myself in self-defense?
>
> Am I exaggerating a negative situation?
>
> Is it as bad as it seems?

Asking clients questions about their thoughts, rather than providing answers, pro-motes self-discovery, thus helping clients solve their own problems.(10) The client needs to recognize that negative thoughts sabotage dietary change and decrease motivation.

In the third phase, actual change takes place. The counselor helps clients to mod-ify internal dialogue or self-statements and accompanying feelings and to produce new more adaptive thoughts and behaviors. Clients are encouraged to control negative self-destructive statements, to offer positive self-statements as a coping strategy, and to rein-force themselves for having coped. An obese woman who is eating differently, for exam-ple, can tell herself how well she is doing and to keep it up. The "power of positive thinking" enhances motivation and results greatly.

Besides these techniques, it may be necessary to teach the person other coping skills, such as problem-solving skills, mental rehearsal, and "thought stopping." Problem-solving approaches help to teach a client to stand back and systematically ana-lyze a problem situation. A problem-solving method called STOP requires the person to: (1) Specify the problem; (2) Think of options; (3) Opt for the best solution; and (4) Put the solution into practice.(11) Cognitive rehearsal with visual imagery permits attention to the important details of a future desired behavior. A client may rehearse, for example, his or her food order at a restaurant or the amount of food and beverages to consume at a party. If people think about or imagine themselves overcoming barriers and performing adequately, actual performance is likely to improve.

Another behavior therapy procedure is "thought-stopping." Clients are trained to self-instruct themselves by saying "STOP!" whenever they are having false thoughts or negative self-talk and focus on a positive thought instead. In addition, some of the same behavioral techniques to modify overt behaviors, such as modeling and operant conditioning, can be used for covert thoughts. More suggestions are offered in a cognitive behavioral therapy package for obesity including six lesson plans.(12)

Besides the role of cognitions in acquiring and regulating behaviors, motivation is partly rooted in cognition. The ability to represent future consequences or outcomes in positive thoughts provides a source of motivation.(6) For example, having positive thoughts that one will feel better, look better, or be in better health may contribute to motivation.

SELF-EFFICACY

The concept of self-efficacy is a useful part of social cognitive theory in predicting and promoting behavior change. In addition to correcting faulty ways of thinking, the dietetics counselor should focus on increasing the client's self-efficacy. Self-efficacy is a person's belief or confidence in his or her ability to perform specific tasks, such as eating differently or exercising more, under a variety of conditions. A client on a weight reduction or diabetic regimen, for example, may have a strong degree of self-efficacy when eating at home, but a weaker degree when eating in a restaurant. Feelings of self-efficacy can be a powerful influence on problem solving and coping skills.

Bandura recognized that learning and behavior change are influenced not only by external cues, rewards, and environmental influences (discussed in the previous chapter), but also by the interaction of demands on a person's coping capabilities. In his view, successful therapies work by increasing a person's confidence in his or her ability to engage in or practice a specific behavior.(6) This, in turn, allows people to exercise greater control over their own behavior, motivation, and environment.

SELF-ASSESSMENT

On a scale of 1 to 5 with 5 the highest, rate your level of confidence (self-efficacy) in your ability to do the following:

Exercise 3 times a week	Ski
Give a speech	Control your weight
Make wise food choices	Give a dinner party for 10 people
Arrange flowers	Sew clothing
Lift weights	Meet new people

What effect does a high or low rating have on your choice of activities?

Although it has not been studied extensively in the literature of health education research and practice, self-efficacy appears to play a critical role in the initiation and maintenance of nutrition and health behavior change.(13,14) There is overwhelming evidence that there is a close association between perceived self-efficacy and nutrition and health behavior change and that self-efficacy is a powerful predictor of change.(13,14)

Self-efficacy is a cognitive process dealing with people's judgments about their capabilities to perform a behavior or set of behaviors adequately in specific situations and the influence of their perceptions on motivation and actual performance.(6) An individual's competent functioning requires both a set of skills to organize and execute actions and self-beliefs of efficacy to use them effectively.

Bandura distinguishes between "outcome" expectancies and "efficacy" expectancies.(15,16) An outcome expectancy is a person's estimate or belief that a given change will or will not lead to a valued outcome. For example, the behavior of reducing dietary sodium will lead to an outcome of lower blood pressure and better health; following a dietary regimen will lead to an outcome of weight loss; reducing dietary fat will lead to a lower cholesterol level in the blood; or successfully completing a project for one's superior will lead to a salary increase or promotion.

A self-efficacy expectation is a person's belief that he or she is or is not capable of performing the change in behavior required to lead to the desired outcome. A male client may or may not believe, for example, that he can reduce his dietary sodium intake sufficiently to attain the outcome of lower blood pressure. With staff, an employee may believe that performing work optimally will lead to the desired outcome of a promotion, but may or may not believe that he is capable (self-efficacy) of optimum performance on a continuing basis.

Self-efficacy and outcomes are differentiated because people may believe that certain actions can produce the outcomes, but they may have serious doubts about whether or not they can cope with the necessary changes to reach the outcome. One study defined self-efficacy toward nutrition behaviors as the ability to follow the dietary regimen, to follow general nutrition principles and practices, to select healthy foods, and to change food purchasing and preparation practices.(17)

Choice of Behaviors

Self-percepts of efficacy can affect people's choices of activities, how much effort they expend, and how long they persist in the face of difficulties. The line, "I think I can" from the children's story, *The Little Engine that Could*, for example, provides a vision of succeeding in performing a difficult task through sustained effort.

A person's self-efficacy is generally a good predictor of how that person is likely to behave on specific tasks.(6) Survey studies of self-efficacy by Strecher suggest a strong association between self-efficacy and progress in health behavior change and maintenance.(13) Where the health practice is believed to lead to desired outcomes, but the change is difficult to make, self-efficacy considerations are probably paramount.

In addition, goal setting appears to enhance a person's self-efficacy and satisfaction with performance.(18) It can improve motivation to perform a task in part through cognitive self-evaluation of performance compared with the adopted goal or standard. A person with strong self-efficacy increases effort and persistence in achieving subgoals, which results in higher performance. The dietetics counselor should break down tasks into easily mastered steps within the person's capabilities with some degree of effort required.(16)

People commonly have a higher sense of confidence about one type of activity than they have about another. For example, a woman may feel confident in increasing daily walks, but may doubt that she can sustain the effort to reduce her fat intake in the face of family food preferences. In evaluating osteoporosis, for example, different levels of self-efficacy were found for physical activity and for calcium intake.(19) A male employee may feel confident in his ability in one job, such as using a computer, but not in another, such as giving a 30-minute oral presentation.

Efficacy expectations are a major determinant of people's choice of activities.(6) The client involved in a change of behavior, such as eating or exercise, must make decisions about whether or not to attempt different food choices, how long to continue, how much effort to make, and, in the face of difficulties or aversive experiences, whether or not to persist. Bandura believes that these decisions are partly governed by judgments of self-efficacy.(6) People tend to avoid situations that they believe exceed their coping abilities, but they are willing to undertake activities they judge themselves capable of executing. The stronger the perceived self-efficacy, or sense of personal mastery, the more persistent are the efforts, even in the presence of obstacles. When difficulties arise, those with lower perceptions of self-efficacy make less effort or may give up entirely.

Dimensions of Efficacy Expectations

The dietetics practitioner needs to assess their clients' thoughts about their abilities to make changes in eating and exercise behaviors or employees' thoughts about work behaviors. Different dimensions of thoughts may be examined, such as the level of difficulty of the task, strength of self-efficacy, and generality. When tasks have different levels of difficulty, efficacy expectations may limit some people to the simple tasks, whereas other people may feel comfortable with the moderately difficult or difficult ones. Self-efficacy differs also in strength or confidence for regulating eating behaviors. Weak self-beliefs are easily extinguished by disconfirming experiences, whereas those with strong efficacy expectations persevere in their coping efforts even through difficulties. Perceived efficacy may or may not be generalized to other activities or behaviors requiring similar skills.(14,16)

A two-step approach to measuring self-efficacy is suggested. First, given a group of tasks of varying levels of difficulty, ask clients which dietary goals or changes they can undertake. It is preferable to start off with the simpler ones to guarantee success; this increases self-efficacy. Then, you can work up slowly to more difficult ones. Second, for each designated task in the behavior change, ask clients to rate the strength of their expectancy of success. The dietetics professional can ask the client to rate his or her confidence in making a specific change on a 5-point scale, with 5 being very confident to 1 being not at all confident.

Self-appraisals are reasonably accurate, and the individual's verbalized intentions are useful in predicting a client's behavior. People successfully execute tasks within their perceived capabilities, but shun those that exceed their perceived coping abilities. In relation to adherence to a diabetes self-care regimen by patients who did not view self-care as a high priority, self-efficacy appeared to be an important variable in relation to dietary adherence, although it was unstable over different time frames.(20)

According to Bandura: "Unless people believe they can master and adhere to health-promoting habits, they are unlikely to devote the effort necessary to succeed."(5) One study found that those with high initial self-efficacy had better outcomes in an intervention to lower serum cholesterol levels.(21) Another study reported that self-efficacy was a powerful correlate for vigorous activity in overweight people.(22) Other studies have also found self-efficacy to be a key cognitive variable in behavior change.(23,24)

Efficacy expectations and performance should be assessed periodically during the dietary change process, since the stronger the perceived efficacy, the more likely people are to persist in their efforts until they succeed. Self-efficacy scores have generally been found to increase from precontemplation to maintenance in the Stages of Change Model. It is low in precontemplation and contemplation, but higher in action.(25)

Sources of Efficacy Information

When planning interventions with clients, it is important to consider the four major sources of efficacy information. Expectations of personal efficacy are based on four major sources of information: (1) actual performance accomplishments, (2) vicarious experiences (modeling) by observing the performance of others, (3) verbal persuasion, and (4) physiological and emotional states.(6,16) Although verbal persuasion is used commonly by counselors, it is among the least effective approaches in influencing another's capability for coping with change.

Actual Performance

The most influential source of efficacy information is based on the experience of successfully performing the behavior in question.(16) "Nothing succeeds like success" reinforces this idea. Personal successes raise mastery expectations, but failures lower them, especially early in the course of a change. Repeated successes in overcoming obstacles through perseverance strengthen self-efficacy. People also perfect their coping skills and reduce their vulnerability to stress. Success begets success; failure begets failure.

Vicarious Experiences

A second source of efficacy information comes from modeling followed by guided performance. Clients can learn how to handle situations by observing a model demonstrating the appropriate behavior, such as ordering the proper food from a restaurant menu. The vicarious experience of seeing another perform, which relies on inferences from social comparison, can generate expectations of "if another can do it, so can I." To enhance self-efficacy, the model should be perceived as similar to oneself or possessing competencies to which one aspires. Clients should then be given an opportunity to perform the modeled behavior successfully. Employees also learn by observing and modeling after other employees. Stronger efficacy expectations, however, are produced by personal performance accomplishments than by only observing a model.

Verbal Persuasion

A third approach, verbal persuasion, is widely used by counselors in attempts to influence behavior. Telling people what to do and that they possess the ability to do it, and informing them of the benefits, is not as effective, however, especially if an individual has had a previous disconfirming experience, such as a failure to follow dietary changes or perform a task at work. The impact of verbal persuasion, the encouragement of the counselor or support from others, may vary greatly depending on the perceived credibility of the persuaders, their prestige, trustworthiness, and other factors.

Physiological and Emotional States

Finally, people partly judge their capabilities from physiological states or emotional arousal. Situations in which the individual has to cope with lifestyle changes may produce anxiety, stress, hunger, fatigue, and tension. Whether or not a person can perform in the face of negative signals varies with the individual. People who diet and regain the weight, for example, may express negative physiological effects and lowered self-esteem.(26) Those susceptible to anxiety may become self-preoccupied with their perceived inadequacies in the face of difficulties rather than with the task at hand. Stress-reducing exercises and discussion of correct interpretation of body signals may be of help when these problems arise.

An effective intervention program should increase self-efficacy as well as increase the value of the outcome.(27) The dietetics practitioner may use one or more of the four sources of efficacy information to raise or strengthen self-perceptions of clients and employees. Personal mastery of a dietary change or accomplishment of a goal is compelling. Small "wins" build confidence for additional changes. Models, such as former clients, may be enlisted to explain how they overcame difficulties by determined effort. Persuasive information is given by informing people that they are capable. The meaning of physiological information, such as anxiety, hunger, and stress, should be explained to make sure that the individual does not misread body signals and abandon efforts.

With employees, personal accomplishments give better efficacy information than telling people that they are capable of performing a job. Modeling after the performance of others, such as seeing that hard work leads to a promotion, is another source of efficacy information. Behaviors are adopted from seeing what others are doing.

Cognitive Appraisal of Efficacy Information

Many factors affect successful performance. The extent to which success raises self-efficacy depends in part on the amount of effort expended. Laborious effort suggests less self-efficacy than success achieved through minimal effort. A person's performance suggests a higher self-efficacy attained through continuous progress than through discouraging reversals and plateaus.

In addition, many factors enter into personal appraisals. Some individuals underestimate their capabilities. If people are not fully convinced of their personal efficacy, they abandon the skills they have been taught when they fail to get quick results or when they experience obstacles to success. People with high self-efficacy attribute failure to lack of effort, whereas those with low self-efficacy may attribute it to low ability. Those with negative self-beliefs do not discard them readily. Even when actual performance attainments are beyond their previous expectations, they may discount their importance through faulty cognitive evaluation or credit their achievements to factors other than their own capabilities.

The counselor can guide clients to increased self-efficacy through small manageable steps or goals that gradually lead them to do more than they ever thought they could. Attainment of subgoals indicates personal mastery, which can enhance self-efficacy and motivation, whereas distant future goals are not as good, because they are too far removed to have an effect.(6) For example, attaining the subgoal of following the dietary change today is an immediate commitment rather than a future goal of never eating desserts again. With employees, a goal of improving performance today is better than a more distant goal of improving during the month.

In a study of dropouts from obesity treatment, at the beginning of treatment self-efficacy was an important predictor of the decision to drop out.(28) Dropouts had lower expectations of success and were more likely to have doubts about whether they would ever reach their goal weights, whereas stayers felt confident that they would.

In the obesity study, perceptions of success proved more important than actual success in predicting who would drop out. Although it might seem that actual success in weight loss would have an important relationship to dropout, little relationship was found. Success results in greater increases in self-efficacy only when the subjects' successful experience is appropriately evaluated. People are influenced more by how they read their performance successes than by the successes per se, and this determines the course of cognitive and health behavioral change. Thus, efficacy expectations reflect a person's perceived rather than actual capabilities, and it is these perceptions and not a person's true abilities that often influence behavior.(13)

If a person ascribes success to his or her ability or effort, self-efficacy is reinforced. Cognitive appraisal of the difficulty of the task accomplished further affects self-efficacy. Even in the face of a setback, if relative progress is perceived, efficacy may be raised.

Thus, in their daily lives, people approach, explore, and try to deal with situations within their self-perceived capabilities, but avoid situations they perceive as exceeding their ability. People weigh and integrate various sources of information about their capabilities. They regulate their choices of behaviors, how much effort they put forth, and how long they will persist in the face of difficulties.(6,16) Efficacy expectations are presumed to influence the level of performance by enhancing intensity and persistence of effort. Thus, the dietetics professional needs to discuss with clients and employees their judgments of their capabilities to perform a variety of tasks and the strength of the belief.

RELAPSE PREVENTION

The problem of relapse, or giving in to temptation, is a challenge for clients engaging in dietary changes and for the practitioners who counsel them. Most people making dietary changes experience temporary setbacks. When people are not prepared, they may give up all efforts to change. Relapse rates on dietary regimens are high, varying from 50% to 100%. In the Stages of Change model, recycling to a previous stage is expected as people go through the five stages of precomtemplation to contemplation, preparation, action, and maintenance. The likelihood of relapse may be increased by social or psychological events or situations, emotional reactions to initial slips, and problems in reestablishing control.

Marlatt and Gordon define relapse prevention as a cognitive-behavioral self-management program designed to help individuals anticipate and cope with relapse during the "habit-change process."(29,30) The change process is one in which old eating habits are unlearned or modified, and new healthier behaviors are gradually learned and acquired to replace previous eating practices. Errors may occur, but each mistake is viewed as an opportunity for new learning, not a personal failure. The goal is to teach the individual involved in a behavior change program how to identify situations with a high risk for lapse and relapse, to use problem-solving and coping strategies when confronted with these situations, and to deal with the negative thoughts that accompany a lapse.

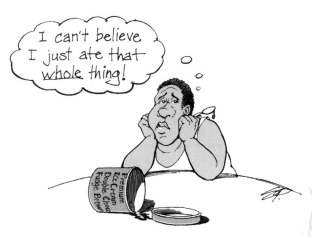

Unless one's thoughts are redirected positively, a lapse can turn into a full-blown relapse.

Marlatt does not view relapse as an all-or-none phenomenon in which there is either absolute control and total restraint or, in the other extreme, loss of control and total indulgence. He makes a useful distinction between a lapse and a relapse.(29) A lapse, such as making poor food choices at dinner, overeating, or skipping exercise, is a single act, a slight error, a temporary fall, a reemergence of a previous habit or behavior, or a slip, not a total failure. Control is not lost and corrective action can be taken. A lapse may provide a learning experience if the person examines the immediate precipitating circumstances and ways to correct them in the future. After a lapse, a person may continue with positive change or proceed to total relapse. A relapse may be defined as the individual's response to a series of lapses or a loss of control. A lapse does not necessarily become a relapse.

Relapse prevention is based on the principles of social learning theory and includes both behavioral and cognitive components.(29) In the social learning view, behaviors may be viewed as overlearned, maladaptive habits which can be analyzed and modified. The eating behavior of people with anorexia nervosa, bulimia, and obesity, for example, may be viewed as overlearned, maladaptive habit patterns with maladaptive coping mechanisms.(8) These maladaptive behaviors are generally followed by some sort of immediate gratification, such as feelings of pleasure or the reduction of anxiety, tension, boredom, or loneliness. When eating takes place during or before stressful or unpleasant situations, it represents a maladaptive coping mechanism.

Food habits or eating behaviors are assumed to be shaped by prior learning experiences. Changing these habits involves the active participation and responsibility of the client, who eventually becomes the agent of change. In a self-management program, the person acquires new skills and cognitive strategies so that behaviors are under the regulation of higher mental processes and responsible decision making. As applied to a program to prevent relapse, the goals are (1) "to anticipate and prevent the occurrence of a relapse after the initiation of a habit change" and (2) "to help the individual recover from a 'slip' or lapse before it escalates into a full-blown relapse."(29)

Dietetics counselors need to advise clients of the possibility of lapses and relapse and how to handle them. Failure to do so deprives the client of the opportunity for developing skills to cope with these situations and/or minimizing damage if one occurs. Using the term "lapse" avoids the value judgment associated with a term like "cheating" on the diet.

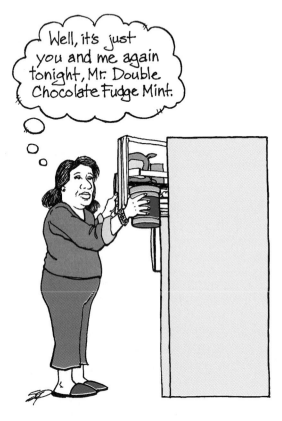

The individual is in a high-risk situation related to the time of day (arriving home from work) and the cognition.

A Relapse Model

Marlatt and Gordon have defined a Cognitive-Behavioral Model of relapse based on the coping response process in high-risk situations. They believe that an individual's control continues until the person encounters a high-risk situation, defined as "any situation that poses a threat to the individual's sense of control and increases the risk of potential relapse."(29,30) Examples of high-risk situations for a person on a dietary regimen are attendance at a social gathering, interpersonal conflicts, feelings of anxiety, boredom, fatigue, or hunger, and the like. When high-risk situations, temptations, and urges occur, relapse prevention techniques are designed to enhance self-efficacy in coping.(31)

There are two possibilities when a person is in a high-risk situation—a coping response or lack of a coping response (Fig 7-1). If the individual copes, self-efficacy is increased, and there is less probability of a lapse or relapse. For example, the client thinks: "I'm not hungry so I won't eat" or "I'll take a walk instead of eating" or "I'll phone my friend instead of eating."

If there is no coping response and the person feels unable to exert control, he or she experiences a decrease in self-efficacy, sometimes combined with a sense of helplessness and passive "giving in" to the situation. ("It's no use. I can't stop myself.") In this all-or-nothing perspective, a single lapse leads to giving up. If the person has positive outcome expectancies of immediate gratification from eating ("It will taste

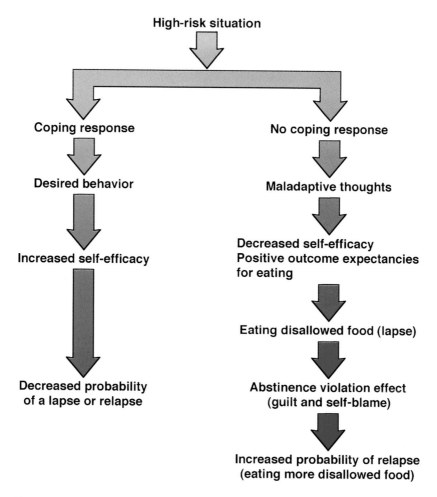

Figure 7-1 COGNITIVE-BEHAVIORAL MODEL OF THE RELAPSE PROCESS. (MODIFIED FROM MARLATT GA, GORDON JR, EDS. RELAPSE PREVENTION. NEW YORK: GUILFORD PRESS, 1985.)

delicious." "I will feel better if I eat this.") and ignores the negative health consequences, the probability of lapse or relapse is enhanced. The individual experiences a conflict of motives between a desire to maintain control and the temptation to give in.(32,33) The person consumes less desirable foods and a slip or lapse has occurred.

Abstinence from less preferable foods is frequently viewed by individuals from an all-or-nothing perspective. Marlatt postulates a cognitive "abstinence violation effect" when a person violates the commitment to change food choices and consumes a food that he should not eat.(29) This brings elements of guilt, lowered self-esteem, and blaming oneself for the loss of control or indulgence in food ("I shouldn't have eaten it, but I did. I'm guilty."). An obese person may continue to eat to relieve the guilt ("I ate one cookie and I blew it. I might as well eat the whole bag.")

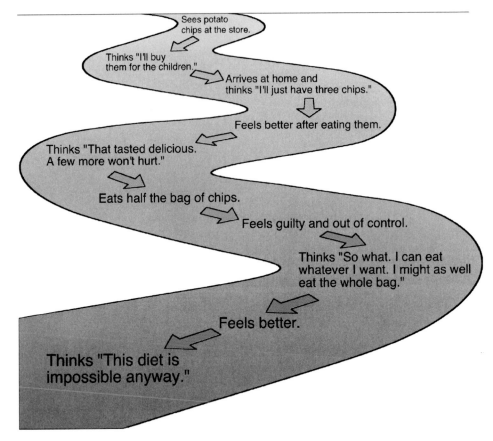

Figure 7-2 IN FAILING TO COPE, ONE'S THOUGHTS AFFECT EATING.

or alter his cognition from being a restrainer to an indulger ("I never could follow the diet anyway."). The reward of instant gratification may far outweigh negative health effects in a distant future.

People may even justify backsliding by rationalizing, "I deserve a break today. I owe myself this food," or change their commitment to save face, as "I changed my mind about following this dietary regimen and decided to eat whatever I want."(32) Thus, a single lapse, or series of lapses, may snowball into a full-blown relapse from which it is more difficult to recover. Figure 7-2 is an example of failing to cope at the grocery store and at home in the presence of the external cue of potato chips. The loss of control and dysfunctional self-talk result in binge eating and relapse.

A multidimensional paradigm for the prevention, treatment, and management of weight-related problems recommends counseling to prevent relapse and inappropriate reactions to lapses. The program recommends client awareness of high-risk situations and the possibility of lapse and the identification and management of these situations. High-risk situations include negative emotional states, stressful events, inadequate problem-solving skills, inability to cope with different eating situations, thinking errors, and the like.(34)

TABLE 7-4 Examples of High-Risk Situations

Physiological feelings of hunger, fatigue, food cravings, tension
Attending social affairs, parties, eating in restaurants
Holidays
Low self-efficacy or inadequate motivation
Stress
Negative self-talk
Lack of social support
Interpersonal conflicts
Positive emotional states, i.e., fun and celebration of an event
Negative emotional states or moods, i.e., depression, anxiety, frustration, anger,
   boredom, lonely, feeling deprived, upset, sad, worried

Determinants and Predictors of Lapse and Relapse

High-risk situations are of several types. Individual factors occur within the individual or are reactions to environmental events. They include negative or unpleasant as well as positive emotional states, moods or feelings, inadequate motivation, social situations or pressures, interpersonal conflicts, responses to treatment, and coping skills. Table 7-4 lists examples.

SELF-ASSESSMENT

Using the examples of high-risk situations in Table **7-4**, identify those that are high-risk situations for your own eating.

Negative emotional moods and states such as depression, anxiety, stress, frustration, anger, boredom, loneliness, feelings of deprivation, and the like before or at the time of the lapse are related to relapse. Uncontrolled eating is a common response when a person is alone. The emotional reactions increase the chance that a dietary slip will occur and become a relapse.

Positive emotional states in which one desires to increase feelings of pleasure and/or celebrate an event are also a problem. A study of dieters found that negative emotional states occurring when the person was alone and positive emotional states involving other people, such as at social gatherings, were both difficult high-risk situations to handle, suggesting that emphasis on managing these situations should be incorporated into counseling programs.(35)

Clients initiate dietary changes with varying degrees of motivation. In addition, some who appear to be highly motivated initially may discover that long-term change is more difficult than first imagined. Initial response to treatment may predict later success. Patients on weight reduction diets who lose some weight, for example, and those who struggle but adhere to their dietary regimens, may be able to cope with temporary setbacks. Coping skills include cognitive responses, such as positive self-talk ("I can do it."), behavioral responses, such as calling a friend instead of eating less preferable foods, and beliefs about self-efficacy or judgments concerning whether or not one can respond effectively in a situation.

Besides individual factors, situational or environmental factors also play a role in relapse. These include social support and environmental cues. The support of family, friends, and self-help groups is associated with better success in several studies. However, the opposite situation, interpersonal conflicts in relationships, namely disagreements or hassles with family, friends, or employer, are a sign for relapse.(22,23,36) In addition, events in the environment may provoke a relapse. Eating cues in the environment, for example, may include holidays, restaurants, and parties where overeating is socially acceptable. Social pressures from others occur when people tempt or coax ("Eat it. Just this once won't hurt you.") and when a person sees others consuming foods not on the person's dietary regimen ("Everyone else is eating it. Why shouldn't I?").

Finally, negative physiological factors may contribute to relapse. Urges and cravings for foods, feelings of hunger, fatigue, or headache, changes in metabolic rate during weight loss, and metabolic tendencies toward weight regain when lapsing from a diet may increase the likelihood of relapse.

Identification and Assessment of High-Risk Situations

Assessment of high-risk situations may be viewed as a two-stage process.(37) In the first stage, an attempt is made to identify specific situations that may pose a problem for a client in terms of lapse or relapse. The use of self-monitoring records is helpful in identifying high-risk situations as well as in raising the individual's level of awareness of food choices made. Eating may be an automatic response that cannot be dealt with until there is a conscious awareness that one is eating without any conscious decision to do so. Self-efficacy ratings in which the client is given a series of descriptions of specific situations and asked to rate how difficult it would be to cope, autobiographical statements about the history and development of the dietary problem, and descriptions of past relapses are other techniques that may be used.(37)

Problem situations creating obstacles to dietary adherence in adults with diabetes were studied. Twelve types of situations were identified: negative emotions and stress tempted people to overeat; food, food cues, or cravings made it difficult to resist temptation; eating in restaurants was another problem situation as well as feeling deprived, having time pressures, being tempted to give up, lacking time for advance planning of what and when to eat, having competing priorities, attending social events, lacking family support, being unable to refuse inappropriate food offered, and lacking the support of friends. An individual's ability to cope in these high-risk situations should be assessed so that problem-solving strategies can be a part of counseling.(38)

In adolescents with diabetes mellitus, 10 obstacles were found: being tempted to stop trying; having negative emotional eating; seeing forbidden foods; having interpersonal conflicts with peers; having competing priorities; eating at school; attending social events and holidays; having food cravings; snacking when home alone or bored;

and experiencing social pressures to eat. The counselor can assist clients in dealing with these situations.(39)

After identifying high-risk situations, the second stage is an assessment of the client's coping skills or capacity to respond. Coping responses should involve both thoughts and actions. One can evaluate these in simulated situations with role playing or in written form. The individual can role play responses to high-risk situations with the counselor or fellow group members. Videotapes of these sessions may be helpful if they are available.

Treatment Strategies

Lapses are inevitable. The counselor needs to prepare the client for the possibility of a lapse and a relapse. Everyone on occasion overeats or eats tempting foods. Marlatt and Gordon use the metaphor of a fire drill.(29) A person practices to escape a fire even though fires are rare.

Relapse prevention strategies are important both in initial treatment or in action and maintenance phases of change. The cornerstone of the relapse prevention approach is to teach the client to recognize high-risk situations and develop coping strategies with skill training.(37) Skill training implies the actual acquisition of a new behavior through overt practice and rehearsal. One does not acquire a new skill, such as playing tennis, by verbal instruction alone. Actual practice of coping skills is essential.(37) Both cognitive and action coping strategies may be needed. "Practice makes perfect," as the saying goes. Baseball players do not hit a home run every time they are at bat. In fact, they may not even get a hit. If they strike out once, they just try again the next time.

Modeling, behavioral rehearsal, positive self-talk, direct instruction, and coaching and feedback from the counselor are useful. Role reversal with the client teaching the dietary counselor how to cope with a high-risk situation and how to handle a lapse gives the client more convincing arguments than any counselor could provide. Increasing self-efficacy through successful performance and modeling of positive self-statements are recommended, such as "I can handle it."(37)

Mental rehearsal through imagined scenarios in which the client engages in coping responses when temptations are present and feels good about it, called *covert modeling*, may be used to cope with reactions to a slip or lapse.(37) Marlatt uses a strategy called "urge surfing."(40) When confronted with an urge to binge, the clients are asked to imagine their urge is an ocean wave building to a crest. The challenge is to surf the wave and remain in balance without being wiped out. The person continues until the urge has passed.

Relaxation training, positive self-talk, meditation, exercise instead of eating, visualization of relaxing, imagining pleasant scenes or carrying out coping behaviors when tempted, and stress management procedures may be needed as antidotes to stress. In visualization, clients can be asked to think ahead about a situation in which they might find themselves. With their eyes closed and with the counselor's help, they can learn to create a mental image of the situation by asking questions that create a visual picture of the situation and the accompanying emotions. If imagining a party, for example, the counselor may ask: "What do the surroundings look like?" "What are you doing?" "What are other people doing?" "Where are the foods and beverages?"

"What will you choose?" "Who can you turn to for support?" "What will you say?' "How do you feel?"

Adopting a problem-solving orientation to stressful situations or modeling problem solving by thinking out loud with clients can be helpful. When lapses are discussed, it is preferable to discuss how the person might have succeeded in preference to focusing on the failures.

Cognitive restructuring teaches people to interpret events, attitudes, and feelings rationally and to respond in high-risk situations. Cognitive restructuring may be used also to counter the cognitive and affective components of the "abstinence violation effect."(39) Instead of seeing the first lapse as a sign of failure characterized by conflict, guilt, and personal attribution, the client is taught to see it as a single event or small mistake rather than a total disaster and that it is possible to resume the dietary regimen right away and learn from mistakes.

When the person's high-risk situations are identified, you can teach the person to look for cues, such as an upcoming party, vacation, or stressful time at work. The client can take preventive action and make advance decisions about how to cope.

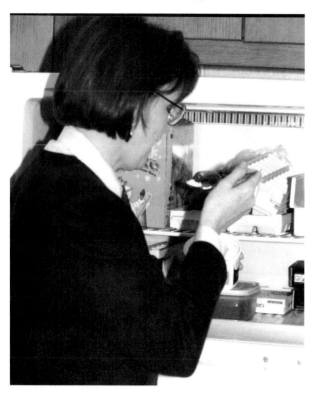

When you are hungry or upset, the availability of high-calorie foods presents a high-risk situation.

Long-term or chronic problems may require long-term treatment even in the maintenance stage of change.(41) Just as Rome was not built in a day, neither is successful dietary change established in a short period of time. It may not be sufficient to teach new ways of eating and turn people loose and unaccountable on a maintenance program. They need to learn strategies to cope with the normal urge to lapse into old habits. Self-monitoring and self-management skills are needed. They should be more successful when they keep in contact with a counselor, at least by phone, for a year or more. The model of lifelong treatment is used by several groups, such as Alcoholics Anonymous, Overeaters Anonymous, and the lifetime membership offered in Weight Watchers.

CASE STUDY 1

Carol Jones is a 50-year-old woman recently diagnosed with type II diabetes mellitus. Her maternal grandmother had diabetes. Mrs. Jones was an overweight child and is an overweight adult at 5'4" and 180 pounds. She is married and works part-time at a retail clothing store.

Dr. Smith referred Mrs. Jones for counseling to lose weight. The dietitian, Joan Stivers, notes in her conversation that Mrs. Jones seems to have a low self-image with negative cognitions. As a result, her current priority is cognitive restructuring.

Directions: Complete the dietetics professional's response to each of the client's statements:

Professional: "The doctor referred you because losing weight will help to improve your blood sugar levels."
  1. Mrs. Jones: "I don't think I can lose weight."
Professional:
  2. Mrs. Jones: "My husband likes me the way I am. He does not think I am overweight."
Professional:
  3. Mrs. Jones: "I lost 10 pounds once before. But it was just a fluke. I couldn't do it again."
Professional:
  4. Mrs. Jones: "When I go out to eat at a restaurant, I won't get my money's worth if I don't eat the food they serve."
Professional:
  5. Mrs. Jones: "When the holidays come, my friends bring me candy and other goodies. So my husband and I eat them. We can't waste food."
Professional:

CASE STUDY 2

Betty has been on and off diets to control her weight for the past 10 years. She is 35 years old and employed full-time as a librarian. She is 5'5" and weighs 200 pounds. She is married with one 6-year-old son.

Betty has sought the advice of Joan Stivers, RD, in private practice, to lose weight. The dietitian is concerned with Betty's yo-yo dieting and has decided to counsel her on lifestyle modification, emphasizing counseling her about relapse prevention so that she can maintain any weight she loses.

  1. Identify the things you would teach her about preventing lapses and relapse as she loses weight with lifestyle modification.

Counselors should give clients a summary or overview of the relapse prevention model. Together, they should identify the individual's high-risk situations and coping skills. If clients have a level of awareness in high-risk situations, they are better prepared to use their coping skills and take remedial action. People need to see themselves as capable agents of control rather than as helpless victims in situations beyond their control.

REVIEW AND DISCUSSION QUESTIONS

1. What effect do negative cognitions have on behavioral change?
2. What types of cognitive distortions do people have?
3. Explain the three phases of cognitive restructuring.
4. What are examples of coping skills the counselor may teach to the client?
5. What is the relationship between an outcome expectancy and an efficacy expectancy?
6. How do self-percepts of efficacy affect people's choice of activities?
7. Explain an individual's sources of efficacy information.
8. What is the difference between a lapse and a relapse?
9. Explain the relapse model.
10. What are examples of high-risk situations?
11. What strategies can help to prevent relapse?

SUGGESTED ACTIVITIES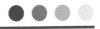

1. Keep a log of what you eat during one day, noting your thoughts about food before eating, during eating, and after eating. Are the thoughts positive or negative? What percent are positive? Negative? This will increase your awareness.
2. Identify you own high-risk situations for eating and how you respond. What happens if you cope with the situation? What happens if you are unable to cope with the situation? How do you feel?
3. For each of the following client cognitions, forecast how the client will behave. Then develop a more positive, coping thought.
    A. "I've never been able to stick to any low-calorie diet for more than a week."
    B. "The food doesn't taste any good without salt."
    C. "There are chocolate chip cookies in the cupboard, and I sure could use a few after the day I've had. I deserve a treat."
    D. "This television show is boring. Here is a commercial break—a good time to see what's interesting in the kitchen."
    E. "That leftover pie looks good, but I don't need it."
    F. "I've blown my whole diet eating that apple pie with ice cream. What's the use?"
    G. "I don't have time to prepare all of that special food today."
4. For 2 days, keep a tally of the number of times people use the terms "should," "shouldn't," "must," "have to," or "ought to" in statements about themselves. Or, keep a tally of the number of times you use these terms.

5. For 2 or more days, consume a modified diet (low fat, low calorie, restricted sodium, high fiber, etc). Keep a log of your thoughts. Identify any high-risk situations.

6. Each evening for 2 days, make a written list of all your successes or things you accomplished. Give yourself a verbal pat on the back with a positive cognition.

WEB SITES

www.mirror-mirror.org/relprev.htm / relapse prevention, eating disorders
www.mirror-mirror.org/relplan.htm / relapse prevention plan
http://nationalpsychologist.com/articles/art_v9n5_3.htm / article on relapse prevention from *National Psychologist*
www.nacbt.org/whatiscbt.htm / National Association of Cognitive-Behavioral Therapists
www.emory.edu/EDUCATION/mfp/effpage.html / information on self-efficacy
www.emory.edu/EDUCATION/mfp/bandurabio.html / biographical sketch of Albert Bandura

REFERENCES

1. Burns DD. The feeling good handbook. New York: Plume, 1999.
2. Dornelas EA, Wylie-Rosett J, Swencionis C. The DIET study: long-term outcomes of a cognitive-behavioral weight-control intervention in independent-living elders. J Am Diet Assoc 1998;98:1276.
3. Foreyt JP, Poston WSC. The role of the behavioral counselor in obesity treatment. J Am Diet Assoc 1998;98:S27.
4. Foreyt JP, Goodrich GK. Evidence of success of behavior modification in weight loss and control. Ann Intern Med 1993;119:698.
5. Bandura A. Social foundations of thought and action: a social cognitive theory. Englewood Cliffs, NJ: Prentice-Hall, 1986.
6. Bandura A. Exercise of personal and collective efficacy in changing societies. In: Bandura A, ed. Self-efficacy in changing societies. New York: Cambridge University Press, 1995.
7. Meichenbaum D. Cognitive-behavior modification. In: Kanfer FH, Goldstein AP, eds. Helping people change, 3rd ed. New York: Pergamon Press, 1986.
8. Williamson DA, Muller SL, Reas DL, Thaw JM. Cognitive bias in eating disorders: implications for theory and treatment. Behav Mod 1999;23:556.
9. Spangler DL. Cognitive-behavioral therapy for bulimia nervosa: an illustration. J Clin Psychol 1999;55:699.
10. Holli BB. Using behavior modification in nutrition counseling. J Am Diet Assoc 1988;88:1530.
11. Glasgow RE, Tooberi DJ, Mitchell DL, et al. Nutrition education and social learning interventions for type II diabetes. Diabetes Care 1989;12:150.
12. Fremouw WJ, Heyneman NE. Obesity. In: Hersen M. Outpatient behavior therapy. New York: Grune & Stratton, 1983.
13. Strecher VJ, DeVellis BM, Becker MH, Rosenstock IM. The role of self-efficacy in achieving health behavior change. Health Educ Q 1986;13:73.

14. AbuSahba R, Achterberg C. Review of self-efficacy and locus of control for nutrition- and health-related behavior. J Am Diet Assoc 1997;97:1122.
15. Schwarzer R, Fuchs R. Changing risk behaviors and adopting health behaviors: the role of self-efficacy beliefs. In: Bandura A, ed. Self-efficacy in changing societies. New York: Cambridge University Press, 1995.
16. Bandura A. Self-efficacy: the exercise of control. New York: WH Freeman, 1997.
17. Matheson DM, Woolcott DM, Matthews AM, Roth V. Evaluation of a theoretical model predicting self-efficacy toward nutrition behaviors in the elderly. J Nutr Educ 1991;23:3.
18. Strecher VJ, Seijts GH, Kok GJ, et al. Goal setting as a strategy for health behavior change. Health Educ Q 1995;22:190.
19. Horan ML, Kim KK, Gendler P, et al. Development and evaluation of the Osteoporosis Self-Efficacy Scale. Res Nurs Health 1998;21:396.
20. Skelly H, Marshall JR, Haughey BP, et al. Self-efficacy and confidence in outcomes as determinants of self-care practices in inner-city, African-American women with non-insulin-dependent diabetes. Diabetes Educator 1995;21:38.
21. Van Beuren E, James R, Christian J, Church, D. Dietary self-efficacy in a community-based intervention: implications for effective dietary counseling. Aust J Nutr Diet 1991;48:64.
22. Hovell MF, Barrington E, Hofstetter R, et al. Correlates of physical activity in overweight and not overweight persons: an assessment. J Am Diet Assoc 1990;90:1260.
23. DeWolfe JA., Shannon BM. Factors affecting fat consumption of university students: testing a model to predict eating behaviour. J Can Diet Assoc 1993;54:132.
24. Littlefield CH, Craven JL, Rodin GM, et al. Relationship of self-efficacy and bingeing to adherence to diabetes regimen among adolescents. Diabetes Care 1992;15:90.
25. Herrick HB, Stone WJ, Mettler MM. Stages of change, decisional balance, and self-efficacy across four health behaviors in a worksite environment. Am J Health Promot 1997;12:49.
26. Turner LW, Wang MQ, Westerfield RC. Preventing relapse in weight control: a discussion of cognitive and behavioral strategies. Psychol Rep 1995;77:651.
27. Hinton PS, Olson CM. Postpartum exercise and food intake: the importance of behavior-specific self-efficacy. J Am Diet Assoc 2001;101:1430.
28. Mitchell C, Stuart RB. Effect of self-efficacy on dropout from obesity treatment. J Consult Clin Psychol 1984;52:1100.
29. Marlatt GA. Relapse prevention: theoretical rationale and overview of the model. In: Marlatt GA., Gordon JR, eds. Relapse prevention. New York: Guilford Press, 1985.
30. Marlatt GA, George WH. Relapse prevention and the maintenance of optimum health. In: Shumaker SA, Schron EB, Ockene JK, McBee WL, eds. The handbook of health behavior change, 2nd ed. New York: Springer, 1998.
31. Marlatt GA, Baer JS, Quigley LA. Self-efficacy and addictive behavior. In: Bandura A, ed. Self-efficacy in changing societies. New York: Cambridge University Press, 1995.
32. Marlatt GA. Cognitive factors in the relapse process. In: Marlatt GA, Gordon JR, eds. Relapse prevention. New York: Guilford Press, 1985.
33. Marlatt GA. Cognitive assessment and intervention procedures in relapse prevention. In: Marlatt GA, Gordon JR, eds. Relapse prevention, New York: Guilford Press, 1985.
34. Senekal M, Albertse EC, Momberg DJ, et al. A multidimensional weight-management program for women. J Am Diet Assoc 1999;99:1257.
35. Sternberg B. Relapse in weight control: definitions, processes, and prevention strategies. In: Marlatt GA, Gordon JR, eds. Relapse prevention. New York: Guilford Press, 1985.
36. McCann BS, Retzlaff BM, Dowdy AA, et al. Promoting adherence to low-fat, low-cholesterol diets: review and recommendations. J Am Diet Assoc 1990;90:408.
37. Marlatt GA. Situational determinants of relapse and skill-training interventions. In: Marlatt GA, Gordon JR, eds. Relapse prevention. New York: Guilford Press, 1985.

38. Schlundt DG, Rea MR, Kline SS, Pichert JW. Situational obstacles to dietary adherence for adults with diabetes. J Am Diet Assoc 1994;94:874.
39. Schlundt DG, Pichert JW, Rea MR, et al. Situational obstacles to adherence for adolescents with diabetes. Diabetes Educator 1994;20:207.
40. Mindfulness and metaphor in relapse prevention: an interview with G Alan Marlatt. J Am Diet Assoc 1994;94:846.
41. Marlatt GA. Lifestyle modification. In: Marlatt GA, Gordon JR, eds. Relapse prevention. New York: Guilford Press, 1985.

8 Cross-Cultural and Life-Span Counseling

CHAPTER

After reading this chapter, you will be able to

1. discuss the problem of diversity.
2. discuss the management of diverse employees.
3. identify the stages of cultural competence in nutrition counseling.
4. list the problems that may appear in counseling culturally diverse clients and how to handle them.
5. explain ways to learn about different cultures.
6. describe potential problems in cross-cultural communication.
7. describe the nutritional problems to be aware of when counseling at different ages in the life span.
8. explain the strategies for working with individuals throughout the life span and for those with limited literacy.

EXAMPLE: *In the United States, the population is 12.9% African American, 12.4% Hispanic or Latino, and 4.2% Asian.[1] The Hispanic population increased by more than 50% since 1990.[2]*

The issue of diversity is not new. After all, we are a nation of immigrants. The United States population is increasingly heterogeneous and is projected to continue to change until minorities outnumber the current majority. The government health objectives for the nation published in Healthy People 2010 reflect the health needs of a diverse population.[3] Dietetics professionals encounter diverse clients and employees and must be competent in communicating with them.

What is diversity? Diversity consists of the many ways in which individuals are unique or different while at the same time being similar in other ways.[4] There are many individuals and families, for example, with different cultures and languages. In addition, there are different ethnic groups, races, religions, genders, sexual orientations, body sizes, physical abilities, levels of health, educational levels, ages from infancy to old age, previous work experiences, lifestyles, values, marital status, socioeconomic status, and others. It is important to value all types of diversity.

This chapter examines the dietetics professional's role in communicating with culturally diverse clients and workplace employees. In addition, the challenges of counseling individuals and families at various stages in the life span are included. Finally, there is information on communicating with those of limited literacy.

WORKPLACE DIVERSITY

Although there has always been diversity in the workforce, federal legislation covering equal employment opportunities, affirmative action, and disabilities increased its significance in the 1970s and beyond. The annual influx of new immigrants creates a challenge in integrating them into the workforce. Food service attracts and employs a large proportion of immigrant and ethnic groups, thus making bilingual kitchens a challenge. The pool of available employees continues to change, and our organizations become more culturally diverse. By 2010, almost half of the nation's new workers will be people traditionally classified as "minorities."(5)

The goal is to provide an environment in which everyone is a member contributing a variety of talents and abilities.(6) All employees must work together toward achieving the goals and objectives of the organization while prospering individually. Everyone in the organization, including those of the dominant culture, must not only accept diversity, but also make a commitment to it and value it. This requires an undertaking at all levels in the organization.

There are many benefits to a diverse organization. Employees contribute a broader variety of ideas, backgrounds, experiences, interests, and viewpoints.(4,6) This can be critical in companies that want to serve diverse consumer or customer groups. Dealing with someone from one's own group helps the consumer identify with the service provider. Thus, it is good for business and the bottom line. The company may need to understand a certain segment of the market that they are targeting for a product or service. If the organization reflects the community it serves, there is an increased chance that it will provide the goods and services needed, wanted, or willing to be purchased. To create this environment requires considering diversity in job interviews, supervising employees, staff development, and a harassment-free work environment. Management professionals need to develop and support effective teams in a culturally diverse workforce.(7)

In diversity-driven environments, individuality is nurtured. Differences in ideas and experiences can lead to more creative solutions to problems and better decisions.(4) Collaboration, consensus, and shared power make everyone feel more equal. The workforce is more productive, and the company is more competitive in achieving it objectives.

All workers must be viewed as assets. Everyone must be respected, respectful of others, and treated fairly and equally. Sensitivity to others may not come naturally, however. People must be aware of and examine their own prejudices, suppress them, and try to overcome them. It is important not to just accept diversity, but also to value it. A permanent change in how employees work together may take time.

Younger workers in their 20s and 30s may seem to have more opportunities for advancement than older workers. The former may have a greater interest in balancing work and career with family responsibilities and outside interests. They may be seeking jobs that are more fulfilling and may be willing to seek other employment if job satisfaction falls or fails to satisfy. Their values and ethics may differ.

In earlier years, most immigrants came from Europe and Canada.(4) Recently, they come from Asia, Mexico, Latin America, and Central America. Intent on making the United States their home, many immigrants have to deal with the issues of assimilation. The first generation has the most difficulty adapting to American culture, and many have problems with language. Literacy can be a bigger problem than culture for people who cannot read or write in their native language, making training difficult. Training materials need to be translated and graphically illustrated or color-coded.

In some environments, race and ethnicity have been used to identify nonwhite workers. Are we, for example, still referring to the African-American supervisor, Mexican cook, Japanese hostess, or the Puerto Rican dishwasher?

Following are some questions to consider when evaluating workplace diversity:(4)

- Are all employees viewed as assets?
- Are there lower expectations of any group?
- Is there an overall atmosphere of acceptance and encouragement for all workers?
- Do diverse workers have levels of responsibility comparable to the dominant group?
- Are managers' expectations lower for certain groups or individuals?
- Are certain groups overrepresented or underrepresented in some departments or areas?
- Are hiring and promotion opportunities open to all? What percent of management positions are filled with women and minorities? Are they tokens, or are they respected? Are they resented?
- Are everyone's ideas, proposals, and suggestions taken seriously?
- Do all groups participate in the normal socialization and networking during work hours?
- Are native-born employees impatient with those who speak English slowly or poorly?
- Are cultural mannerisms and body language accepted or misunderstood and ridiculed?
- Are all people treated with patience, tolerance, and understanding?

CULTURAL COMPETENCE IN COUNSELING

Besides dealing with the diversity of workplace employees, dietetics professionals communicate with diverse clients and patients. This section includes ways to develop cultural competence in counseling, counseling throughout the life span, and communicating with persons with limited literacy.

As the United States becomes increasingly heterogeneous, the need to be cross-culturally competent is critical. Health care professionals continue to see patients and clients from many cultures; each group has its own traditional foods and food practices. Food choices and practices are probably best understood in the context of a person's culture. Effective communication with these groups requires that the differences or variations be recognized, respected, understood, and acknowledged. Otherwise, nutrition counseling and education will be ineffective.

What is culture? Culture is broadly defined as "the values, beliefs, attitudes, and practices accepted by a community of individuals."(8) It is a "framework that guides and bounds life's practices."(9) Culture is helpful. It allows people to share beliefs, values, and practices while living together harmoniously. On the other hand, it can create disharmony because of ethnocentrism when people consider that their values and practices are the true ones and they judge all others based on these beliefs.(10) Culture is deeply ingrained, affecting and guiding the group's activities and behavior of daily life. Dietetics professionals need to understand themselves and their cultural and world view and realize that it is not inherently "right."(9)

Culture is learned, not inherited. It is passed from generation to generation in the home by a process called *enculturation*. Yet, within each culture there are differences. In the countries of the world, there may be one major group as well as other subgroups that differ. India, for example, has several groups, and not all Indians are Hindus. Not all Arabs are Muslims. It is a mistake to stereotype people just because you know they are from Italy, Mexico, or India. The Latino population includes Mexican Americans, Puerto Ricans, Cubans, Central and South Americans, and others. There are probably similarities, but also definite differences.(10) First-generation immigrants cling most closely to their cultural ways. Second and third generations change over time and accept some American ways while keeping some of their cultural practices and food choices. Children, for example, adapt to new cultural patterns more easily than adults, and this may lead to conflict in the family.

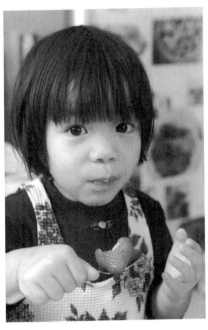

The professional counseling ethnic groups needs a knowledge of their food practices.

Cultural practices evolve gradually and people may or may not adhere to their cultural norms and practices. Individuals are unique in the degree to which they adhere to cultural patterns, some identifying with the group more strongly than others.(9) The process by which groups adopt the practices of a new country is termed *acculturation*, and the degree of acculturation to American eating practices needs to be assessed. Assumptions about food practices based on the person's cultural group or on a stereotype may result in inaccurate or inappropriate generalizations and counseling. Those who are more acculturated need help selecting healthful American foods, whereas those less acculturated need help modifying traditional recipes. The clients are our teachers and guides in learning about their cultures, so we need to listen to them carefully.(11)

"Cultural pluralism" has tended to replace the "melting pot" concept. "Tossed salad," in which different cultures combine to make a whole is sometimes used as well as rejected.(10,12) The "smorgasbord" or the "flower garden" in which each culture maintains its own identify may be better choices of metaphors. Although dietetics professionals cannot be culturally competent in every culture they see, they *must* be culturally competent with the few cultures that they encounter often.

Culture determines how a person defines health, recognizes illness, and seeks treatment.(8) Each culture holds values, beliefs, and practices about good health and disease prevention, the care and treatment of the sick, whom to consult when ill, and the social roles and relationships between patient and health care provider. The United States, for example, believes in scientific medicine, individual decision through informed consent, the health care provider as the manager of care, and the separation of body, mind, and spirit in treatment programs. The health care orientation of other cultures, however, may differ. A family member or community may have decision-making responsibility, for example, rather than the individual alone; science may be less important than emotional and psychological support; and body, mind, and spirit may be seen not as separate, but as joined.(10) Folk remedies including teas, herbs, and powders may need to be assessed.

In Mexico, for example, health is believed to be a matter of chance or God's will. Illnesses are influenced by "hot" and "cold" imbalances with food choices determined accordingly.(10) Pregnancy is a hot condition during which hot foods (garlic, grains, expensive meats, alcohol) are avoided. Cold foods are vegetables, dairy, inexpensive meats, and tropical fruits. Note that the concept does not refer to the food temperature or spiciness.(13) Family interdependence takes precedence with the male family member dominant, consulted, and included in decisions. Folk healers may be consulted.

In India, in contrast, diseases are believed to be caused by an upset in body balance. The husband's ownership of his wife is quite pervasive, and unquestioned obedience to elders is expected. Haitians believe that some illnesses originate supernaturally or magically and may be treated with voodoo medicine. Dietetics professionals need to recognize and investigate these unique cultural differences.

Nonverbal behaviors also differ among cultural groups. Customs about touching, gestures, eye contact, and spatial relationships vary greatly.(8) While Americans believe in eye contact, other cultures may find this disrespectful. Rules about touching and space are culturally determined. Some cultures keep short distances between people, whereas others expect longer distances.(11) Signs of affection between men and women may be seen in the United States in public, but they would not be tolerated in other parts of the world.(9) Punctuality is important in the United States, but in parts of Asia and South and Central America, people are a more important priority than the clock, and the client may be late or miss an appointment.

Verbal behaviors may also be misunderstood. Slang has no meaning in other cultures. "How's it going?" is not a good choice for a greeting. "Do you understand?" will be answered "yes," for example, whether or not the person does understand. Instead, one can say, "Please tell me what you do not understand." Americans are among the most informal people worldwide, frequently calling both friends and strangers by their given names. Nearly all other cultures expect a more respectful approach with the use of the surname.(11) Americans are fairly direct, but direct questions may be deemed inappropriate or bring discomfort to those in other cultures.(9) In many world cultures, professionals are held in high regard for their expertise. Expecting individuals and families to be talkative and assertive may be unrealistic when the client is expecting a dependency role. A slower approach may be what a family prefers rather than a direct approach.(9) Launching into health and nutrition data gathering too soon may be perceived as intrusive and disrespectful.(11)

The family may be patriarchal, matriarchal, nuclear, or extended. Interactions among family members are culturally determined, and the roles of men and women may differ. A woman may not be allowed to speak openly or to work outside the home and may have to defer to a husband or mother-in-law. She may have little role in decision making in the family. As a result, counseling sessions may need to include the father, husband, or whomever is the family decision maker.(9)

Dietetics professionals need to develop cultural competence. Cultural competence consists of "ways of thinking and behaving that enable members of one cultural, ethnic, or linguistic group to work effectively with members of another."(9) It is a "unique category of awareness, knowledge, and skills" that enables a professional to succeed in cross-cultural counseling.(14)

A number of models of multicultural competence may be found in the literature. (9,14,15) One model for multicultural nutrition counseling competencies identified 28 competencies within the following three factors: (1) multicultural awareness, (2) multicultural food and nutrition counseling knowledge, and (3) multicultural nutrition counseling skills.(14)

Multicultural Awareness

Multicultural awareness is the first step toward multicultural competence in nutrition counseling.(14) An evaluation of our own cultural heritage and world view is the place to start to help in understanding those who are different. Each of us has a cultural, ethnic, linguistic, and racial identity.(9) For those in the dominant culture, however, our culture may not be at the level of self-awareness. We may be unaware of the ways in which our culture influences our behaviors and interactions with others. Awareness of our own values, beliefs, assumptions, biases, and prejudices must be brought to the level of conscious awareness before we can become cross-culturally competent. We can begin by examining our family and heritage including socioeconomic factors, beliefs, values, politics, religion, educational level, occupation, social and family factors, and the like. All of these shape our values, beliefs, and behaviors. Did you grow up hearing "God helps those who help themselves," for example, or "It's God's will." One must beware of thinking one's ways are the "best."

Cultural factors are major parts of a person's identity, as in foods served, ways holidays are celebrated, values, beliefs, spirituality, child-rearing practices, and expected family roles. Our cultural roots influence our attitudes and have a profound influence on our behaviors.(9) Values differ related to cooperation versus competition, activity versus passivity, youth versus age, importance of family versus friends, and independence versus interdependence. Americans encourage competitiveness, for example, but in the Asian culture competition is seen as self-serving and negative, whereas cooperation and teamwork are prized. We must appreciate and respect all cultural differences.

Multicultural Food and Nutrition Counseling Knowledge

For multicultural food and nutrition counseling knowledge, counselors must have a knowledge of the cultural food practices of various groups. Food choices, food preparation methods within a cultural context, knowledge of cultural eating patterns, family dynamics, and traditions during celebrations are important.(14) Information specific to each culture and community in which clients live is needed. You must determine the degree to which the family or individual follows the cultural tradition by consulting the individual.(11)

How can we learn about other cultures? We can visit their neighborhood ethnic food stores, ethnic restaurants in their neighborhoods, attend religious ceremonies in their places of worship, or other neighborhood events.(8) Workshops and training sessions on cultural food practices are available.(14) We can learn through their media, novels, newspapers, music, and some television shows. Reading about the role of foods in health and illness, approaches to health promotion, and treatment of disease and illness as well as beliefs about care and caregivers is another possibility.(10) We can examine their authentic recipe books and try cooking their foods. Conducting focus groups with group members may be helpful. Since there are differences within cultural groups, we need to talk not only about foods, but also about recipes, ingredients, portion sizes, and how food is prepared. If the counselor is unfamiliar with eating horsemeat, Korean kimchee, Indian ghee, or hummus, for example, he or she needs to ask about these foods when counseling others. Family foods and practices must be respected and incorporated into the dietary changes whenever possible.

The American Food Guide Pyramid may not be appropriate. A number of food pyramids for other cultures are available on the internet. The internet is the source of other information on cultural and diversity as well. (Websites are listed at the end of the chapter.)

Following are some phrases to consider using:

> **EXAMPLE:** *"I am not familiar with the way you cook ____ (name of food). Will you please share that information with me?"*
> *"Would you be my teacher and guide me about the foods you eat daily?"*
> *"What do people in your culture prefer for snacks?" (widens the focus to the whole group)*
> *"If you were explaining how to make that recipe to a friend, what would you say?"*
> *"You are the expert on your food choices. You can teach me a lot."*
> *You should reinforce any client response, such as saying the following:*
> *"Thank you for that information."*
> *"You are helping me to understand."*
> *Avoid saying, "I had a Mexican client last week and he told me . . . ."*

Multicultural Nutrition Counseling Skills

Multicultural nutrition counseling skills show the ability and experience to handle culturally appropriate interactions including nutritional and cultural assessments, culturally relevant treatment plans, and counseling sessions.(11) This factor includes the previous two skills of awareness and knowledge for the professional to perform adequately.(14)

The counselor may find that trust is more difficult to develop, but it is a key to success.(11) One must be credible in the eyes of the client. The gap between the professional and the client must be bridged whether the individual came voluntarily or involuntarily. You may develop rapport with conversation on neutral subjects. For example: "When did your family come to this country?" Develop the relationship first. "You are probably wondering what we are going to do. Let me explain." Then, explain the purpose, process, and the client's role as a cultural guide. Still the dietetics professional must be careful not to categorize people into groups, since each is a unique individual.

Clients may have problems with spoken and written English. The counselor needs to determine the language spoken in the home and the reading and writing proficiency. Some Spanish speakers, for example, may not read or write Spanish. A translator is needed to redo written handouts, and a skilled interpreter can help with oral information. Counselors should try to know some words or phrases in the client's language, such as a greeting and names of commonly eaten foods. Questions should be addressed to the client, not the interpreter, and counselors should focus on the client as answers are given. Using immediate family members and relatives as interpreters can be problematic. Using nonfamily members raises concerns with confidentiality. And a child as interpreter presents the problem of role reversal, which can lead to resentment and can change the family dynamics at home.(9)

Some families are monocultural; that is, they identify with one primary group. However, because of intermarriage, counselors may be seeing bicultural families that identify with two or more groups. What the client eats may depend on situational factors or what cultural identity he or she is responding to at the moment. More educated and middle class clients, for example, may move back and forth among groups easily.(9)

Cultural competence is essential for rendering effective nutritional services to clients. Campinha-Bacote describes multicultural competence as a "continuing journey."(15) Because of the diversity in the nation, she maintains that every client needs a "cultural assessment."

COUNSELING THROUGHOUT THE LIFE SPAN

Besides being diverse in their cultural and ethnic backgrounds, clients of the dietetics professional are diverse in ages as well. Many of the communication and education principles and strategies in other chapters of this book are appropriate for people of all ages; however, this section focuses specifically on preschool-aged children, school-aged children, adolescents, older adults, and those with limited literacy skills. Nutrition is a fundamental pillar of health and development across the entire life span. At all ages, the goal is to promote good nutritional practices to meet age-specific nutrient needs for optimum health and well-being, normal development, and prevention of disease.

Preschool-Aged Children

Professionals can work with parents and other caregivers in influencing children's eating behaviors. The goal of health and nutrition education for young people is to promote health and development and to prevent the chronic diseases of adulthood.(16) Children's food habits are learned through family food experiences, through education, and through personal experiences. In the preschool years, family and cultural practices are a major influence on what children eat.(17,18) As they mature in language and social skills related to eating, children experience meals as important social and family events.(19)

Another influence comes from watching television and media pressures on food selection begin to develop early.(18,19) Including Saturday cartoons, children watch an estimated 22 to 25 hours of television weekly but are unable to distinguish between the program and the commercials that are marketed to sell products.(18) A study of 2- to 6-year-old children found that even brief exposures to televised food commercials could influence preschool children's food preferences, leading children to try to pressure parents at the grocery store.(20)

A child who is a good eater as an infant may be a fair to poor eater as a toddler. Food jags may last a few days to months. The best approach is to provide only nutritious foods for meals and snacks and let the child decide how much and how often to eat. Too many juice boxes should be avoided, for example. The Dietary Guidelines for Americans and the National Cholesterol Education and Prevention Programs recommend that children over the age of 2 years should follow a diet that is made up of no more than 30% calories from fat and less than 10% from saturated fat.(21,22) The American Academy of Pediatrics Committee on Nutrition supports these goals.(19)

Some children may be in Head Start or other day care programs in which most nutrients are consumed away from home. About 60% of young children, or three of every five children age 5 years and younger, participate in some type of child care from persons other than their parents.(23) Studies show that parents/families and teachers working together can mutually reinforce learning about nutrition and make more of an impact than either working alone.(17) Recommended strategies for teaching nutrition include action stories, songs, videotapes, tasting parties, food preparation, vegetable and fruit gardens, puzzles, art projects, field trips, and health snacks. Modeling of healthful eating by adult role models and peers is especially help-

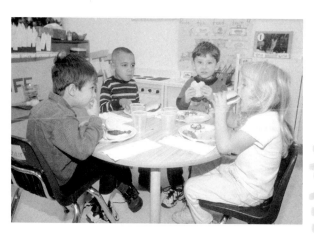

Food served at day care facilities contributes to total nutrition.

ful.(18) If parents do not eat fruits and vegetables, for example, it is less likely that their children will eat them. Parental intake may need exploring.

Nutritional assessment with a diet history, when needed, may take longer to accomplish at these ages. Amounts eaten with frequency may be difficult to determine and a 7-day food record is recommended.(18) Older children may be able to draw a picture of what they ate. Economic, psychosocial, cultural, and other factors need to be considered.

School-Aged Children (6—12 Years)

Childhood is the prime time of human development.(3) It may be easier to establish healthful dietary and exercise habits during childhood than later in life. The American Dietetic Association takes the position that "all children and adolescents should have access to adequate food and nutrition programs," including "nutrition education, screening, assessment, and intervention."(24) In these years, nutrition education seeks to teach children the knowledge needed to select healthy foods and also the analytical and evaluative skills necessary to examine food and nutrition information.(25) Since risk factors for some chronic diseases begin in youth, behaviorally focused nutrition education is appropriate, including cognitive learning (how to select a healthful diet), affective teaching (addressing motivation for change), and behavioral components (selecting new food choices). Incentives and rewards may be used. Studies show that interventions that focus on specific behavior changes result in more changes than a more general nutrition education approach.(25) Table 8-1 lists topics considered essential at the elementary, middle, junior high, and senior high school levels.

The dietetics professional needs to spend time assessing the child's family, cultural, social, physical, and psychological environment when dietary changes need to be made. Since a 6-year-old is very different from a 9-year-old, an evaluation of the developmental stage of the child according to theories of child psychology and of the child's cognitive level will help in planning any intervention.(25) The child's activity pattern including number of hours spent watching television or playing video games daily should be noted. The influence of peers and of the media increases. Children may be watching 23 to 24 hours of television weekly.(19) The appeal of food commercials is not to nutrition but to emotional and psychological appeals. Older children can understand that the purpose of food commercials is to sell a product and, with help, can begin to evaluate what they see.

The dietetics professional should bear in mind that breakfast has to be planned around school bus schedules and it may be skipped. The noon meal may be a bag lunch

---

TABLE 8-1   **Essential Topics to Teach Elementary Through Senior High School**

Food Guide Pyramid
Learning the benefits of healthful eating
Making healthful food choices for meals and snacks
Preparing healthy meals and snacks
Using food labels
Eating a variety of foods
Eating more fruits, vegetables, and grains
Eating foods low in saturated fat and total fat more often
Eating more calcium-rich foods
Balancing food intake and physical activity
Accepting body size differences
Following food safety practices

Additional topics at middle, junior high, and senior high school
Dietary Guidelines for Americans
Eating disorders
Healthy weight maintenance
Influences on food choices such as families, culture, and media
Goals for dietary improvement

Adapted from US Department of Health and Human Services. Healthy People 2010. McLean, VA, International Medical Publishing, 2000.

from home or the school lunch program, requiring choices to be made by the child, such as selecting either whole or skim milk. After-school snacks are required to meet the child's energy needs, although children in poverty may experience food insecurity. Children who become involved in competitive sports, such as little league baseball or soccer, may be receiving nutrition advice from a coach.(19) As the child gets older, peer influences on eating increase; yet the family is still a major influence on the child's early eating patterns.

Dietetics professionals recognize the need to include the family in the counseling sessions. Family nutrition counseling involves people who live in the same household, not just relatives in traditional family structures.(26) They may share common biological, social, cultural, psychological, and environmental spheres. The goal is to use the shared environment to influence nutrition and health for the better and to foster healthful food consumption practices. In some cases, the father, not the mother, is the person responsible for menu planning, purchasing, and preparation of food; most parents work outside the home. Children may prepare some of their own breakfasts, bag lunches, and after-school snacks using the microwave oven. With divorce, children may live with each parent at different times. The professional must be sensitive to family relationships.

If the family cooperates, social, psychological, and environmental support will assist in fostering the child's dietary changes. In families dealing with childhood obesity, an increasing problem, diabetes mellitus, or hyperlipidemias, for example, dietary changes often benefit everyone in the family. Changes in family food buying and food preparation influence the child's adherence to the regimen.(18)

Children, and even adolescents, are obviously highly dependent on their parents who control, to a great extent, the food served in the home. When only the correct, nutritious food is in the home, environmental cues to eat high-fat, high-calorie foods are reduced, and following the dietary regimen is enhanced.(26) Family members can serve as good role models for appropriate eating and encourage and reward healthful habits in the child.(18) Children frequently mimic their parents' food habits. If dad refuses broccoli, for example, so will Johnny. Parents who want their children to drink milk rather than coke need to set a good example. The counselor can negotiate changes in what is purchased and prepared by the family.

There are some barriers to family counseling. Some clients do not wish to involve certain family members; stepparents may refuse to participate; spouses and parents may be overly controlling and negative in dealing with the child; and mutually acceptable times for appointments may be difficult to arrange for several people.(26) In these cases, other sources of social support may have to be located.

Other concerns may be present. Parents may not be good role models or supportive of their children. They may use sweets and desserts as a reward or bribe. "Eat this and you can have dessert," for example. Siblings may tempt and tease a brother or sister who is not supposed to eat certain foods. Parents who take a food plan too literally create a stressful environment in the family, leading to food battles and conflicts. Nagging, criticism, and policing about food and weight issues should be replaced with positive reinforcement and praise when correct dietary behaviors are observed. One visit is insufficient for most family counseling.(26)

For the nutrition education of children, national objectives have been identified by government agencies including the Department of Health and Human Services, the Department of Education, and the Nutrition Education and Training (NET) program.(27) Objectives, priorities, and strategies for promoting healthy eating in children are recommended by NET. All states mandate or have initiatives to promote nutrition education in schools as a component of the curriculum. Examples of other agencies that commit resources to nutrition education of youth and adults include the National Cancer Institute (NCI) and the National Heart, Lung, and Blood Institute (NHLBI). The US Department of Agriculture's Team Nutrition website and others mentioned at the end of the chapter offer recommendations and activities for children.

In the earlier grades (K-3) family-based programs were found to be more effective, but not for middle or high school students.(25) In one case, worksheets, games, and other activities were mailed to homes so that the child and family could work on them jointly, which has been found to be a successful method of intervention.

Another study reported a survey of students in grades 5, 8, and 11.(27) The three topics students were most interested in learning about were weight control, how to improve their diets, and nutrition and disease, but interest varied by grade level.

In selecting ways in which they would like to learn about nutrition, fifth graders preferred games and food experiments most and information presented by the teacher least. Eighth graders preferred food preparation, but interest in any method was low. Videotapes and information from teachers were least preferred. Interest in food preparation and guest speakers increased by grade level.(26) The most popular methods and educational strategies actively involved students, whereas passive techniques were undesirable. Children and adolescents wanted to learn about nutrition topics that were consistent with their developmental stage.

Concerns about body image, appearance, and preoccupation with dieting start early. About one-third of children thought that their weight was too high, recognizing the cultural values of what is considered attractive. In the previous year, one-half had attempted weight loss.(27) The number of children who are overweight is of concern because it has more than doubled in the past decade. Approximately 11% of children are overweight.(28,29) Inactivity and parental overweight may contribute to overweight in children. The number of students who skip meals increases with grade level. Although chronic undernutrition is rare, up to 8% of 12-year-olds are estimated to experience food insecurity (limited access to nutritious food).

Children want learning to be fun.(30,31) Childhood is a time for play exploration and opportunities for learning. The play approach to learning has been recommended as an alternative to the social learning theory and behavioral approaches. The play approach, based on the theory of Jean Piaget, focuses on internal rather than external transaction, on intrinsic motivation, and on fun.(30,32)

In a school-based nutrition education program, fun was defined by intrinsic and extrinsic motivation. Intrinsic motivation was defined as performing a behavior for its own pleasure or purpose and was linked to an advanced stage of readiness to change. In contrast, extrinsic motivation was defined as performing a behavior to receive external rewards or pleasures, such as losing 5 pounds to receive a desired reward. Fun nutrition education materials were assessed if using fantasy, curiosity, and challenge to motivate.(33)

The fantasy of a play, game, or puzzle, for example, stimulates a level of curiosity. Sensory curiosity may be developed by music, bright colors, or visual effects, such as songs or videos. Cognitive curiosity may be created by varying levels of difficulty, competition, nutrition bingo, or scavenger hunts.

Materials such as the Food Guide Pyramid (Fig 8-1) and Nutrition Facts Label used to encourage dietary change do not use fantasy, curiosity, or challenge as fun activities directly. However, they can be linked, for example, by keeping a food diary and com-

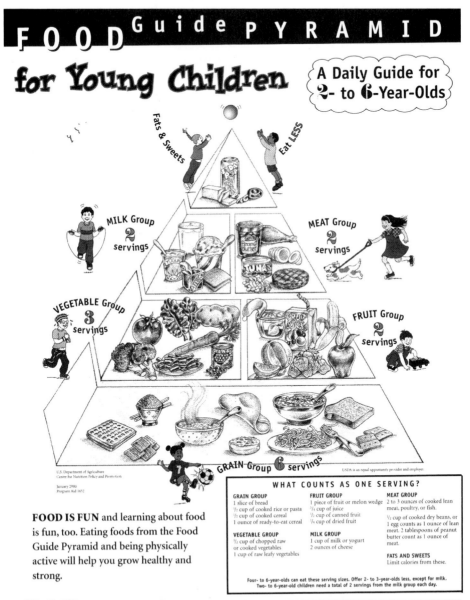

Figure 8-1 FOOD GUIDE PYRAMID FOR YOUNG CHILDREN.

paring it with the Pyramid, or comparing food labels for content such as fat, protein, sodium, or fiber. Students can guess the amount of a nutrient, such as fat, in groups of foods.

In the play approach, children actively explore and experiment with objects, materials, and knowledge. Active experimentation, hands-on experiences, and self-directed activities are recommended. Real-life situations, such as measuring quantities of food, recording and charting data, such as the amount of sugar in popular beverages or cereals, and communicating with others about food choices are examples. Experiments with new foods and methods of preparing them are appropriate.(30) Partnerships of children, schools, and families can promote health and well-being and influence lifetime food habits. Using the internet, a program called 5 a Day Virtual Classroom gave students the opportunity to counsel then-President Clinton about how to motivate children to eat five servings of fruits and vegetables daily (5 a Day).(34)

Children who have medical problems present a counseling challenge. In the management of children and adolescents with diabetes mellitus, involvement of families is essential. Parents can serve as resources and as support groups for other parents.(35) Needs can be assessed through telephone contacts, formal questionnaires, or informal information supplied at clinic visits. Games for use with diabetes are found in the literature.(36,37)

When dietary modifications are needed, the dietetics professional should try to choose words that children use and understand. The word "diet," for example, turns off most children as well as adults.(37) Food, food plan, food choices, meal plan, or menu are better words to use. The office environment can be made attractive with colorful, food models, magazine pictures, posters, food packages of commonly eaten foods, and

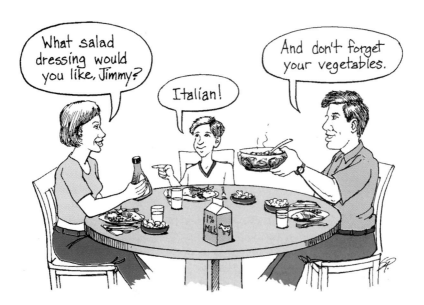

At all ages, parents should set a good example.

beverage glasses of various sizes and shapes. One group used food exchange playing cards, coloring placemats, and food models in teaching the diabetic exchange system.(36)

Another study assessed the effects of a home-based, parent-child autotutorial (PCAT) program for 4- to 10-year-old children with elevated low-density lipoprotein cholesterol (LDL-C).(38) The PCAT program, based on social cognitive theory, included 10 talking book lessons (audiotaped stories with accompanying picture books) and follow-up paper and pencil games for the children. A manual for parents was provided. The program was effective in helping children gain knowledge of "heart-healthy eating" and in reducing their dietary fat consumption and their plasma LDL-C levels.

A team approach using the classroom, school lunch program, athletic department, and activities in the home and the community help to teach children about nutrition. Although schoolteachers spend about 10 to 15 hours per year on nutrition education, one study found that 15 hours could only bring about changes in knowledge and that 50 hours were required to change attitudes and behaviors.(25) The school lunch menu, if available, may be used in teaching which foods to select.

Many successful programs include self-assessment of dietary intake to identify problem behaviors, setting personal goals for change, observing models (peers and adults) of desired behavior, enhancing self-efficacy though skill building, and incentives and reinforcement for change.(25) All children enjoy incentives for reaching goals. Experiential, active, and hands-on educational methods are recommended.

Six elements of successful nutrition education programming have been identified: (1) programs are behaviorally based and driven by theory; (2) for elementary school children, family members are involved in the program; (3) self-assessment of eating practices is included for middle school to senior high students; (4) behavior change programs intervene in the school classroom and lunchroom environments; (5) behavior change programs also intervene in the larger community; and (6) intensive instruction time is included.(39)

Adolescents (13–19 Years)

Adolescence is a time of rapid cognitive, physical, and psychosocial change with increasing nutrient needs. The growth spurt occurs in girls between 10 and 12 years of age, and in boys, about 2 years later.(19) Individuals vary in rates of physical growth, in the timing of the growth spurt, and in physical activity patterns from little activity to active involvement in sports. The dietetics professional needs to assess each person individually considering weight gain, physical growth, timing of the growth spurt, physiological maturation, and activity level as the first step before planning interventions, counseling, and education.

Balancing the demands of one's environment including work, school, social groups, and family is a challenge facing many of today's families.(40) The teen years are a time for weighing freedom and responsibility, for experimentation, for challenging people in authority, and for seeking self-identity and independence.(35,41) Food is often central to social life with peers, and adolescents have major problems with anything that makes them different from their peer group.(37) This can affect food choices at parties and sporting events, eating out, alcohol, smoking, and after-school snacks. Teens may skip meals, especially breakfast or lunch, eat more meals away from home, select their own snacks, replace milk with soft drinks, smoke, start drinking alcoholic beverages, and experiment with fad diets. Many have their own money to spend. In any week, 25% of preteens and 61% of teens eat with friends in fast-food restaurants.(42) In one-on-one counseling, personal decisions related to self-care can be explored between the dietetics professional and the adolescent. In working with groups, one may ask teens to discuss and share how they handle these situations.(43)

Dietary intakes of teens tend to be high in fat, sugar, salt, and fast foods but low in vegetables, fruits, fiber, and calcium and iron rich foods.(44,45) The connections between food choices and health may be discussed, since health and nutrition are not a primary influence on food practices in this age group.(43) Cognitive-behavioral therapy intervention strategies should target the affective domain, or feelings and attitudes, not just giving information to increase knowledge.(18) Adolescent attitudes and patterns related to food choices and physical activity should be explored, since they may persist into adulthood.(3) The foundation for the prevention of coronary heart disease prevention and osteoporosis, for example, by the promotion and maintenance of healthy lifestyles is important in adolescence and young adulthood.(44) Obesity is increasing in this age group and is associated with the risk of type II diabetes, discrimination and rejection by peers, and low self-esteem (refer to Table 8-1 for essential topics).(46).

Why do adolescents make the food choices they do? A study of adolescents assessed their perceptions of factors influencing their food choices. They included hunger and food cravings, appeal of the food such as taste, time considerations of both the adolescent and parents, convenience of the food, food availability, parental influences on eating behaviors (such as culture or religion), benefits of foods including health benefits, situation-specific factors, mood, body image, habit, cost, media influences, and vegetarian beliefs. Individuals were becoming more autonomous and influenced by the desire to fit the social norms of the peer group. The challenge for the counselor is to help individual adolescents incorporate healthful eating habits into their lifestyle.(47)

The study also examined adolescent barriers to healthy food choices. They found that eating healthfully was of low priority. Taste of food was of great importance, and healthy choices were not perceived to be as tasteful as other options. Up to one-third of eating takes place outside the home (i.e., at school, fast-food restaurants, vending machines, convenience stores, and the like).(44) When eating away from home, the better choices were not available or not appealing. Although almost all public schools participate in the school lunch program, many schools raise money by giving vending companies contracts to sell soft drinks, candy, chips, and other high-fat foods.(44) In addition, many a-la-carte food items are high in fat and energy and low in nutrients.(48) Factors influencing food choices need to be explored in the design of interventions if the interventions are to be effective in promoting change.(47)

A number of adolescent girls may become pregnant. If they have not completed the growth spurt, the nutritional needs of pregnancy are added to their normal needs.(19, 49) Counseling about eating healthful foods to achieve recommended weight gain during pregnancy is important. Nutrition is vital to the growth and development of the fetus and to the outcome of the pregnancy. Adolescents, however, are vulnerable to poor nutritional practices, and pregnant teens are at particular risk of having low-birth-weight babies.(25) Pregnancy may provide the counselor with an opportunity to encourage the vulnerable adolescent to improve her eating patterns since she wants to have a healthy baby.(18)

Girls are susceptible to other health hazards. Dieting is common and as a result, they may have marginal nutritional status.(19) Dissatisfaction with body image and weight is more common in girls than boys.(18,19) Up to 50% to 70% of teen girls are dissatisfied with their weight and body image.(44, 46) They desire a body image similar to popular peers, fashion models, or the excessively thin image promoted by the mass media. Idealized standards of attractiveness may make some refuse food, resulting in nutritionally inadequate intakes. In some, dieting may lead to anorexia nervosa and bulimia.(18) More than 5 million Americans suffer from eating disorders, of which an estimated 85% have their onset during adolescence.(50)

Those who become vegetarians may be vulnerable to nutritional deficiencies if their food intake is not balanced properly.(17) Some cultural and ethnic groups, such as Pakistanis, Chinese, and Seventh Day Adventists, regularly consume vegetarian diets and feed them to their children. Lacto-ovovegetarians meet their nutritional needs more easily than vegans.

Many teens are involved in competitive sports activities. A coach may be an influence on eating patterns as a way to improve athletic performance.(19) The professional should look for nutrition misinformation and fads with this group. In some sports, such as wrestling, for example, boys may be trying to lose weight by inappropriate means to wrestle at the top of a lower weight class. On the other hand, adolescent boys may be highly motivated to learn about nutrition to improve their athletic performance.

Promoting nutritional health across the life span can be a cooperative goal of many public and private agencies, as it is in the person's earlier years.(19) Many agencies have a nutrition education component. Examples are the Special Supplement Food Program for Women, Infants, and Children (WIC), the Food Stamp Program, the School Breakfast Program and National School Lunch Programs, the Nutrition Education and Training (NET) Program, and the Commodity Supplemental Food Program (CSFP).(49, 51) The US Department of Agriculture funds Team Nutrition to develop and disseminate to schools nutrition educational materials. For school nutrition education programs to produce changes in food attitudes and behaviors, at least 50 hours of instruction time are needed.(45) Federal, state, and local public health agencies employ nutritionists. As members of a health care team, they assess the community nutrition needs as well as provide services, such as maternal and child health. Other agencies,

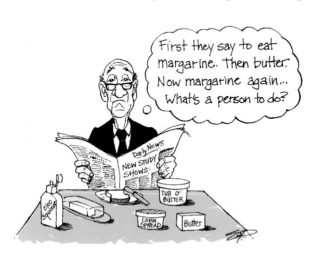

Many people are confused by conflicting media reports about food.

such as the American Heart Association and the American Dietetic Association, also have educational materials. However, the $10 million budget for Team Nutrition and $1 million for the National Cancer Institute's Five A Day for Better health Campaign are dwarfed compared with the $11 billion spent annually by the food industry on advertising.(44)

Older Americans

The aging of the US population presents challenges to families, policy-makers, and health care providers. Although many older adults enjoy a standard of living and increased life span unknown a century ago, this is not true of everyone. Because of immigration, the elderly population is becoming more ethnically diverse and is also racially diverse.(52) A comprehensive nutritional assessment of any older American considering the economic, psychosocial, cultural, health, physiological and lifestyle factors influencing food intake is necessary to complete the picture before planning a nutrition intervention.

Since there can be vast differences in older adults, the US census uses three age categories:(53)

Age 65 to 74—the young-old

Age 75 to 84—the old

Age 85 and over—the oldest-old and fastest-growing segment of older adults

In general, Americans are living longer after age 65 and living better than in earlier years. Although the young-old may still be working part-time and may be in relatively good health, for example, the oldest-old may be living in a nursing home owing to serious health problems and disabilities. In 2000, an estimated 35 million people—almost 13% of the population (one in eight people)—are 65 years or older. and these numbers are expected to continue increasing. This is a fast-growing segment of the population (Table 8-2).(52)

TABLE 8-2   Resident Population by Age (in thousands)

Age (years)	Number	Percent
Under 5	19,175,796	6.8
5–9	20,549,505	7.3
10–14	20,528,072	7.3
15–19	20,219,890	7.2
20–24	18,964,001	6.7
25–64	146,992,887	52.2
65–74	18,390,986	6.5
75–84	12,361,180	4.4
≥ 85	4,239,587	1.5

Source: US Census Bureau, American Fact Finder. http://factfinder.census.gov/_lang=en_vt_name=DEC_2000_SF1_U_DP1_geo_id=01000US.html.

Today's older Americans are generally better educated than previous generations, a factor that can influence socioeconomic status and health to a degree. Many continue to live in their own homes. Although the economic picture is good for most, there are significant disparities in income and wealth with some poverty. A large majority enjoy social contacts with friends and relatives including activities such as going to restaurants for meals.

An overwhelming majority of older adults rate their health is good or excellent.(53) But at more advanced ages, health and quality of life can be threatened by chronic diseases, depression, disability, and memory impairments. Hypertension, heart disease, diabetes, stroke, cancer, arthritis, and osteoporosis are examples of chronic health problems, and many older people have more than one health problem.

People 85 years and older are the most likely to live in nursing homes. Those in nursing homes tend to be more impaired functionally and may need assistance with eating. Malnutrition affects about two of every five elderly nursing home residents.(54)

The Gerontological Nutritionist (GN) dietetic practice group has developed practice standards for working with older adults.(55) More than half of the GN members work in nursing homes, and others are employed in community nutrition programs and hospitals. The members of GN "work with and through others while using their unique knowledge of food, human nutrition, and management as well as skills in providing services," including providing quality nutritional care, counseling, and services for older adults. The Consultant Dietitians in Health Care Facilities (CD-HCF) also work in long-term care and other settings. They have published standards of professional practice.(56)

Achieving and maintaining optimal nutritional status of the older population is a goal for nutrition counselors. However, obtaining the proper amount of nutrients can be a challenge, and the counselor needs to explore for those undergoing economic, physiological, social, and family changes, such as the following:(18,57)

- Although protein, vitamin, and mineral needs do not decrease and may increase in some cases, caloric needs decrease owing to changes in resting energy expenditure and decreased levels of physical activity, thus requiring a smaller quantity of food to be eaten that needs to be nutrient-dense.(53)
- Sense of taste and smell decline making food less appealing and influencing appetite and what people choose to eat. About 50% of older adults between ages 65 and 80 and 75% of those over age 80 have major loss of taste buds.(58,59) Declining vision and hearing are other sensory changes.(60)
- The failure of many older adults to have healthy diets or to engage in physical activity is of concern. A study using the Healthy Eating Index showed that 21% had diets rated as "good," 67% needed improvement, and 13% were "poor." Scores were low on daily servings of fruit and milk products.(52)
- Chronic diseases may require costly medications that may affect appetite and result in drug-nutrient interactions. Older adults use 35% of all prescription drugs and many over-the-counter drugs as well.(18,61)
- Income may be limited or fixed while health care and other expenses increase, resulting in food insecurity and economic problems. Approximately one out of six were poor or near poor in 1998.(53)
- Social isolation, loneliness, and bereavement due to loss of spouse decrease interest in cooking and eating.

- Physical disability and/or cognitive impairments (depression and dementia) may make shopping and cooking difficult. Lack of physical activity decreases muscle mass, which can affect mobility and strength. Approximately two-thirds of older adults do not exercise regularly.(53)
- Dental problems, dentures, or swallowing problems may limit food choices and intake.
- Physiological changes in digestion and absorption increase with age.(62)

Good nutrition is essential to the health, self-sufficiency, and quality of life of older adults. Enjoying food and maintaining the desire to eat reduce the risk of weight loss and undernutrition. The nutritional counselor should assess and identify potential problems and their effects on nutritional status. The counselor should establish individualized plans for intervention. Interventions need to be culturally and age sensitive. Nearly half of elderly people have low reading skills.(3) It may be necessary to go slowly, listening carefully and observing the spoken and unspoken needs. Health problems can vary by ethnic group; African Americans, Hispanics, and Asians have different problems.(63) For example, minorities generally come to old age with fewer economics resources.(52, 64) At present, 42% of US adults say they take daily vitamins, and 23% report they use herbal supplements; this is something to inquire about with all clients.(65)

Nutrition counselors should be aware of community programs to recommend to older adults. Examples are the food stamp program and the congregate/group meal program funded under the Older Americans Act, which funds meals at little or no cost in a social setting such as community or recreational centers, senior citizen centers, and churches. The program also funds Meals on Wheels, home-delivered meals to the frail elderly.(53,66)

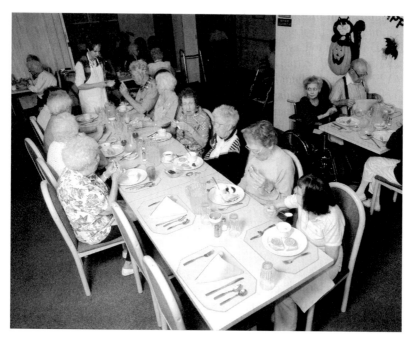

Older adults dine together at a community site.

LIMITED LITERACY

About 40 to 44 million people, or approximately 25% of the United States adult population, cannot understand materials written at a basic proficiency level.(67) Practitioners probably encounter these individuals more often than they realize, since such individuals hide the fact that they cannot read. The client may say: "I don't have my glasses with me and will read this later," "I broke my glasses," or another excuse. Another technique to identify such individuals is to hand them written materials upside down. Readers normally turn the paper right-side up, whereas nonreaders may not. Another approach is to ask the person to select a food from a list on the paper.

CASE STUDY 1

Judy R. is a new registered dietitian whose responsibilities at the medical center involve nutrition interviewing, counseling, and education on a frequent basis. Many of her patients are from cultural and ethnic groups other than her own. They are mainly Mexican, Puerto Rican, Thai, and Korean. She is finding it somewhat overwhelming to understand the variety of unfamiliar foods that they eat. This also inhibits her ability to provide appropriate food alternatives as she counsels people on modified diets. She wants to increase her effectiveness as a counselor.

1. What are possible suggestions for Judy so that she can improve her interviewing and counseling with patients from other cultural and ethnic groups?

CASE STUDY 2

Mrs. Smith, a widow, is 76 years old. She is 5'3" tall and weighs 150 pounds. She lives alone in an apartment. The arthritis in her knees and hands for which she takes aspirin or Tylenol tends to limit her mobility. She lives on a small pension and on Social Security. She mentions that her pension money does not go as far as it did 10 years ago, and her rent continues to increase annually.

Mrs. Smith walks to a small private grocery store three blocks from her apartment or to a convenience store two blocks away for food once or twice a week. During snowy winters, a daughter who lives an hour away takes Mrs. Smith to the store every 2 weeks. She eats cereal for breakfast and a sandwich or soup for lunch; she may do a small amount of cooking at the evening meal. She snacks on candy during the day.

1. What socioeconomic and lifestyle factors influence Mrs. Smith's food intake?
2. What physiological factors may influence her food intake that you would inquire about?
3. What federally funded programs would you explore with her?

Although low literacy people vary, they tend to be persons of lower socioeconomic status, those who dropped out of school, are learning disabled, are older, or are immigrants who do not yet know much English and may not read even in their native language.(67) It is important to identify these individuals, since poor reading skills are associated with poor health.(3,68)

The average reading level of US adults is around eighth-grade level, but fifth-grade level for enrollees in Medicaid. Typical health education print materials are often written at the 10th grade level or higher instead of an appropriate level for the audience—generally fifth-grade level.(3) You need to test written materials for readability and incorporate more visuals when educating people with low literacy.

Counselors should keep language simple and repeat important information. Dietary cholesterol and blood glucose, for example, are challenging terms to understand and are inappropriate for this audience. Sentences should be short (10–15 words) with one- and two-syllable words.(69) Paragraphs should be limited to three or four sentences. Then the counselor should ask the client to repeat what he has understood. Actual practice, such as planning a menu or a grocery shopping list, and role playing are helpful activities as well as using visual aids.

The Joint Commission on Accreditation of Healthcare Organizations (JCAHO) requires that steps be taken to ensure that patients and clients understand the oral and written information they receive.(67,70) An internet search finds a number of readability formulas, such as SMOG (Simplified Measure of Gobbledygook), Flesch, Fry, and others.(69) An example is www.cdc.gov/od/ads/smog.htm.

REVIEW AND DISCUSSION QUESTIONS

1. What is diversity? What are the ways in which people differ?
2. As a manager, what would you see as the goals and benefits of workplace diversity?
3. How can workplace diversity be evaluated?
4. What is culture?
5. Define assimilation, ethnocentrism, enculturation, and acculturation.
6. How does culture influence people?
7. What is cultural competence? What can a dietetics professional do to develop it?
8. In dealing with children, what factors should be assessed?
9. What educational and intervention strategies are recommended for children?
10. In dealing with adolescent boys and girls, what factors should be assessed?
11. What factors may make an impact on the diet and nutrition of older adults?
12. What strategies are helpful in educating older adults?

SUGGESTED ACTIVITIES

1. At your place of employment, determine what cultural and ethnic groups are represented. The Human Resource Department is a resource. Are all treated equally?
2. List the foods that you or your family prepare that are traditional for your group or heritage. Briefly describe them to others.

3. Select one cultural or ethnic group with which you are unfamiliar. Research their food choices and practices.

4. Find someone from a culture you would like to learn about. Ask the person to be your cultural guide or teacher. After developing a list of questions to ask in advance, interview the person to gather information on their food choices, practices, recipes, cooking methods, and foods for special occasions such as holidays, and beliefs about the relationship of food to health and disease.

5. Watch some children's television programs, and note the number and types of food advertising.

6. Interview a dietetics professional who works with children or adolescents about their nutritional problems.

7. Interview a dietetics professional who works in a public health nutrition program.

8. Interview the mother of a child to discuss eating problems and practices.

9. Interview a teenager about eating practices.

10. Buy a magazine read by teens. Assess the content of any articles on nutrition, food ads, weight control supplements, and the like.

11. Interview an older adult (age 65 or older) about food and eating practices.

12. Plan a 15-minute presentation on nutritious snacks for fifth graders.

WEB SITES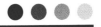

There are many diversity and multicultural sites on the internet, a number with links to other sites. A few suggestions follow:

www.diversityrx.org / promotes language and cultural competence to improve the quality of health care for minority, immigrant, and ethnically diverse communities

www.diversityresources.com / information on diversity issues in the workplace

www.doi.gov/diversity/ US Department of the Interior site with a site on workforce diversity

www.nal.usda.gov/fnic/etext/000010.html / the Food and Nutrition Information Center of the US Department of Agriculture; has cultural and ethnic food guide pyramids with links to other sites

www.ethnicgrocer.com / ingredients and recipes

http://monarch.gsu.edu/nutrition/download.htm / Georgia State University website; has downloadable materials in 37 languages including food pyramids and handouts for healthy adults, mothers and babies, mature adults, and children—all bilingual and copyright-free

www.semda.org/info/ the Southeast Michigan Dietetic Association site; has 16 or more food pyramids, which are copyrighted and may not be copied for commercial purposes without consent

http://ohioline.osu.edu/hyg-fact/5000 / information on eight cultural groups found under "Cultural Diversity" as well as information on nutrition in the life cycle

http://oregonstate.edu/dept/ehe/nu_diverse.htm / Oregon State University; information on cultural diversity

www.fda.gov/oc/opacom/kids / Food and Drug Administration site on children
www.fedstats.gov/kids/html / access to government web pages for elementary through high school
www.fns.usda.gov/tn / Team Nutrition site to empower children to make healthy food and activity choices
www.dole5aday.com / educational activities for school-age children on fruits and vegetables
www.hhs.gov/kids / Department of Health and Human Services and kids' activities
www.foodsafety.gov/~fsg/fsglang.html / information in other languages
www.fitness.gov / President's Council on Physical Fitness and sports site with links
www.foodsafety.gov/~fsg/fsglang.html / food safety information in over 30 languages
www.justmove.org / affiliated with American Heart Association; exercise diary
www.seniors.gov / health information for seniors with links
www.aarp.org/healthguide / American Association Retired Persons (AARP) site

REFERENCES

1. Profiles of general demographic characteristics 2000. US Department of Commerce, US Census Bureau, 2001.
2. The Hispanic population 2000. Census 2000 brief. US Department of Commerce, US Census Bureau, 2001.
3. US Dept Health and Human Services. Healthy People 2010. McLean, VA: International Medical Pub, 2000.
4. Arthur D. Recruiting, interviewing, selecting, & orienting new employees, 3rd ed. New York: American Mgt Assoc, 1998.
5. Keeping your edge. Managing a diverse corporate culture. Fortune 2001;143:S2.
6. Hudson NL. Management practice in dietetics. Belmont, CA: Wadsworth, 2000.
7. Griffin B, Dunn JM, Irvin J, et al. Standards of professional practice for dietetics professionals in management and foodservice settings. J Am Diet Assoc 2001;101:944.
8. Kittler PG, Sucher KP. Food and culture. Belmont, CA: Wadsworth, 2001.
9. Lynch EW, Hanson MJ. Developing cross-cultural competence, 2nd ed. Baltimore: Brookes Publishing Company, 1998.
10. Geissler DM. Pocket guide to cultural assessment, 2nd ed. St. Louis: Mosby, 1998.
11. Leigh JW. Communicating for cultural competence. Boston: Allyn & Bacon, 1998.
12. Gudykunst WB. Bridging differences: effective intergroup communication, 3rd ed. Thousand Oaks, CA: Sage Publications, 1998.
13. Position of the American Dietetic Association: food and nutrition misinformation. J Am Diet Assoc 2002;102:260.
14. Harris-Davis E, Haughton B. Model for multicultural nutrition counseling competencies. J Am Diet Assoc 2000;100:1178.
15. Campinha-Bacote J. A model and instrument for addressing cultural competence in health care. J Nurs Educ 1999;38:203.
16. Bronner YL. Nutritional status outcomes for children: ethnic, cultural, and environmental-context. J Am Diet Assoc 1996;96:891.

17. Contento I, Balch GI, Bronner YL, et al. Nutrition education for preschool children. J Nutr Educ 1995;27:291.
18. Worthington-Roberts BS, Williams SR. Nutrition throughout the life cycle, 3rd ed. St Louis: Mosby, 1996.
19. Committee on Nutrition. Pediatric nutrition handbook, 4th ed. Elk Grove Village, IL: American Academy of Pediatrics, 1998.
20. Borzekowski DLG, Robinson, TN. The 30-second effect: an experiment revealing the impact of television commercials on food preferences of preschoolers. J Am Diet Assoc 2001:101:42.
21. Dietary guidelines for Americans, 5th ed. USDA Home and Garden Bulletin No. 232. Washington, DC: USDA, 2000.
22. The report of the expert panel on population strategies for blood cholesterol reduction. National Cholesterol Education Program of the National Heart, Lung, and Blood Institute. Washington DC: HHS, 1990.
23. Position of the American Dietetic Association: nutrition standards for child-care programs. J Am Diet Assoc 1999;99:981.
24. Position of the American Dietetic Association: child and adolescent food and nutrition programs J Am Diet Assoc 1996:96:913.
25. Contento I, Balch GI, Bronner YL, et al. Nutrition education for school-aged children. J Nutr Educ 1995;27:298.
26. Dwyer J. Focus on family nutrition counseling: new ways to reinforce and extend eating behavior changes. Nutr Update 1991;1:1.
27. Murphy AS, Youatt JP, Hoerr SL, et al. Nutrition education needs and learning preferences of Michigan students in grades 5, 8, and 11. J School Health 1994;64:273.
28. Dwyer JT, Stone EJ, Yang M, et al. Prevalence of marked overweight and obesity in a multi-ethnic pediatric population: findings from the child and adolescent trial for cardiovascular health (CATCH) study. J Am Diet Assoc 2000;100:1149.
29. Position of the American Dietetic Association: dietary guidance for healthy children aged 2 to 11 years. J Am Diet Assoc 1999;99:93.
30. Rickard KA, Gallahue DL, Gruen GE, et al. The play approach to learning in the context of families and schools: an alternative paradigm for nutrition and fitness education in the 21st century. J Am Diet Assoc 1995;95:1121.
31. Evers CL. How to teach nutrition to kids. Tigard, OR: 24 Carrot Press, 1995.
32. Johnson SR, Mellin LM. Just for kids! San Francisco: Balboa Pub, 2001.
33. Matheson D, Spanger K. Content analysis of the use of fantasy, challenge, and curiosity in school-based nutrition education programs. J Nutr Educ 2001;33:10.
34. DiSogra L, Glanz K The 5 a day virtual classroom: an on-line strategy to promote healthful eating. J Am Diet Assoc 2000;100:349.
35. McKelvey J, Borgeren M. Family development and the use of diabetes groups: experience with a model approach. Pat Educ Counsel 1990;16:61.
36. Barry B. Games and activities to teach children about diabetes and nutrition. Diabetes Educ 1995;21:27.
37. Connell JE. Pizazz in the pediatric population. Diabetes Educ 1991;17:251.
38. Shannon BM, Tershakovec AM, Martel JK, et al. Reduction of elevated LDL cholesterol levels of 4- to 10-year-old children through home-based dietary education. Pediatrics 1994;94:923.
39. Little L, Achterberg C. Changing the diet of American's children: what works and why? J Nutr Educ 1995;27:250.
40. Neumark-Sztainer D, Story M, Ackard D, et al. The "family meal": views of adolescents. J Nutr Educ 2000;32:329.
41. Sturdevant MS, Spear BA. Adolescent psychosocial development. J Am Diet Assoc 2002;102:S30.

42. Patton S. Connecting with overweight kids. Today's Dietitian 2001;3:34.

43. Sigman-Grant M. Strategies for counseling adolescents. J Am Diet Assoc 2002;102:S32.

44. Story M, Neumark-Sztainer D, French S. Individual and environmental influences on adolescent eating behaviors. J Am Diet Assoc 2002;102,S40.

45. Hoelscher DM, Evans A, Parcel GS, Kelder SH. Designing effective nutrition interventions for adolescents. J Am Diet Assoc 2002;102,S52.

46. Lytle LA. Nutritional issues for adolescents. J Am Diet Assoc 2002;102:S8.

47. Neumark-Sztainer D, Story M, Perry C, et al. Factors influencing food choices of adolescents: findings from focus-group discussions with adolescents. J Am Diet Assoc 1999;99:929.

48. Calderon L. Promoting a healthful lifestyle and encouraging advocacy among university and high school students. J Am Diet Assoc 2002;102:S71.

49. Trissler RJ. The child within: a guide to nutrition counseling for pregnant teens. J Am Diet Assoc 1999;99:916.

50. Position of the American Dietetic Association: nutrition intervention in the treatment of anorexia nervosa, bulimia nervosa, and eating disorders not otherwise specified (EDNOS). J Am Diet Assoc 2001;101:810.

51. Boyle MA, Morris DH. Community nutrition in action: an entrepreneurial approach. Minneapolis: West Publishing, 1994.

52. Older Americans 2000: Key indicators of well-being. Federal Interagency Forum on Aging Related Statistics. Washington, DC: US Government Printing Office, 2000.

53. Position of the American Dietetic Association: nutrition, aging, and the continuum of care. J Am Diet Assoc 2000;100,580.

54. HCFA launches national nutrition and hydration awareness campaign. J Am Diet Assoc 2000;100:1305.

55. Shoaf LR, Bishirjian RO, Schlender ED. The Gerontological Nutritionists standards of professional practice for dietetics professionals working with older adults. J Am Diet Assoc 1999;99:863.

56. Vogelzang JL, Roth-Yousey LL. Standards of professional practice: measuring the beliefs and realities of consultant dietitians in health care facilities. J Am Diet Assoc 2001;101:473.

57. Chernoff, R. Geriatric nutrition: the health professional's handbook, 2nd ed. Gaithersburg MD: Aspen, 1999.

58. Hess MA. Taste: the neglected nutritional factor. Top Clin Nutr 1992;7:1.

59. Duffy VB. Smell, taste, and somatosensation in the elderly. In: Chernoff R, ed. Geriatric nutrition: the health professional's handbook, 2nd ed. Gaithersburg, MD: Aspen, 1999.

60. Wright KJ, Smickles-Wright A, Blood I, et al. Dietitians can and should communicate with older adults with hearing and vision impairments and communication disorders. J Am Diet Assoc 1997;97:174.

61. Blumberg J, Couris R. Pharmacology, nutrition, and the elderly: interactions and implications. In: Chernoff R, ed. Geriatric nutrition: the health professional's handbook, 2nd ed. Gaithersburg, MD: Aspen, 1999.

62. Salzman JR. The aging gut. In: Chernoff R. ed. Geriatric nutrition: the health professional's handbook, 2nd ed. Gaithersburg MD: Aspen, 1999.

63. Bernard MA, Lampley-Dallas V, Smith, L. Common health problems among minority elders. J Am Diet Assoc 1997;97:771.

64. Treas J. Older Americans in the 1990s and beyond. Population Reference Bureau, Washington, DC, 1995.

65. Diet & health: Ten megatrends. Nutrition Action Health Letter 2001;28:3.

66. Millen BE, Levine E. A continuum of nutrition services for older Americans. In: Chernoff R, ed. Geriatric nutrition: the health professional's handbook, 2nd ed. Gaithersburg MD: Aspen, 1999.

67. Weiss BD, Coyne C. Communicating with patients who cannot read. N Engl J Med 1997;337:272.
68. Albright CL, Bruce G, Howard-Pitney B, et al. Development of a curriculum to lower dietary fat intake in a multiethnic population with low literacy skills. J Nutr Educ 1997;29:215.
69. Kalista-Richards M. The dynamics of education: making a match. J Renal Nutr 1998;8:88.
70. Mayeaux EJ, Murphy PW, Arnold C, et al. Improving patient education for patients with low literacy skills. Am Fam Physician 1996;53:205.

9 Motivating Clients and Employees

After reading this chapter, you will be able to

1. define motivation and differentiate between intrinsic and extrinsic motivators.
2. discuss the motivation of patients and clients including variables motivating changes in food choices.
3. describe Maslow's and Herzberg's models of the motivation process.
4. compare the contemporary theories of motivation and find instances in which they complement one another

"I think I can. I think I can. I will."

Dietetics professionals need to know how to enhance and maintain the motivation of their clients and employees. This can be a challenging task. Before people can do things differently, make changes in their dietary practices, or work efficiently, they must have the motivation to do so.

Applying what is currently known regarding human motivation is vitally important in setting goals, planning behavior modification strategies, designing and executing educational programs and seminars, and counseling others individually or in groups. Professionals who understand motivational concepts and theories and have the skills to adapt them to particular situations significantly increase their chances of being instrumental and influential in helping others.

Because the exact nature of motivation cannot be scientifically validated, myriad differing opinions and definitions of motivation currently exist. Motivation can be defined as something that causes a person to act or the process of stimulating a person to action. It is concerned with the questions of why human behavior occurs. The word motivation is frequently used to describe processes that (*a*) arouse and instigate behavior; (*b*) give direction and purpose to behavior; (*c*) continue to allow behavior to persist; and (*d*) lead to choosing or preferring a particular behavior. Motivation concerns not only what people can do, but also what they will do. Recent studies appearing in the medical literature indicate continuous and ongoing study into the applications of motivation to health care.(1–8)

Motivation is complex, and many factors or variables, both intrinsic and extrinsic, influence the process at any one moment in time. Today's motivational influences may differ from tomorrow's, and short-term goals may take precedence over long-term ones. Having knowledge of how to work to get the most accomplished, of what to eat to become or remain healthy, or of what to do to cope with a current medical problem such as diabetes may easily be overpowered by other motivational factors. The problem is that being motivated to work, to make choices based on health, or to learn what one needs for appropriate cardiovascular or diabetes care involves long-term goals. Moreover, eating something such as chocolate cake or coming in late for work "just this once" meets a short-term goal of pleasure. Some people may delay the long-term for the immediate pleasure. Although there is a great deal of knowledge concerning motivation that is helpful, there are no miracle methods or universal answers to difficult motivational problems.(4,8)

Motivation can arise from factors that are either intrinsic (internal) or extrinsic (external), and these factors can affect the individual either positively or negatively. Intrinsic motivation arises from within people, according to their needs, desires, drives, or goals. People who desire to be promoted or patients who see recovery and better health as a personal priority after a heart attack have internal goals that motivate their behavior. External or extrinsic factors may supplement intrinsic motivation positively, or they may serve as barriers that have a negative impact on motivation. Examples of positive external factors enhancing motivation include support from others, praise, and material rewards. A person's motivation toward achieving dietary goals, however, may be hampered by social occasions or by family or friends who are not supportive and who offer improper foods.

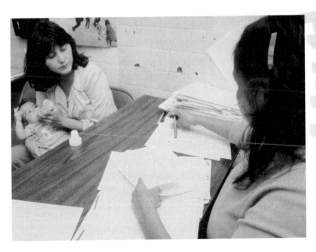

Parents may be motivated by concerns about child nutrition.

The dietetics manager influences the motivation of employees who must learn the procedures necessary to work effectively, do their jobs conscientiously without close supervision, and grow to improve in the work environment. The clinical dietitian must motivate not only staff but also clients, who may need to learn about such things as the effects of diet on prenatal care or the problems of sodium, cholesterol, or sugar in the diet.

This chapter discusses motivation in two contexts: as an aid to patient and client adherence and as an aid to managing staff. Although each area is treated separately, the same motivational principles and theories apply to both.

MOTIVATION OF CLIENTS AND PATIENTS

The goal of nutrition counseling and education is to change food and eating behaviors so that people select healthier diets. Food selection, however, is part of a complex behavioral system, which is shaped by a vast array of variables (see Chapter 1). The food choices of children are determined primarily by parents and by the cultural and ethnic practices of their group. Other influences include the price of food, taste of food, religion, geography, peer and social influences, advertising in the media, facilities available, food preparation and storage, skills of the consumer in food preparation, time factors and convenience, and personal preferences and tolerances. All these factors make food consumption a highly individual matter and resistant to change.(9,10)

As pointed out in other chapters in this book, counselors hope to provide clients with interventions and strategies to motivate changes in health-promoting and disease-preventing behaviors. However, no single theory or model is all-encompassing and ensures success. Instead, practitioners must be able to integrate a number of approaches and discern what may work with each individual. The motivational approaches referred to in this section have been discussed in more detail in other chapters of the book. This section combines the implications of the various approaches and models.

The purpose of all counseling is to enhance self-care and self-management. This, of course, depends on the person's readiness, willingness, and ability to undertake and maintain changes in eating practices.(8) Health-related decision-making is influenced by many factors.(11,12)

The Health Belief Model attempts to predict people's decisions about health behavioral change. Change is determined by the individual's belief: (1) that he or she is susceptible to an illness or disease; (2) that it would be serious to contract the illness or leave it untreated; (3) that changing dietary practices will be beneficial in reducing the risk; and (4) that barriers to taking action can be overcome.(8) The model is limited by the fact that behaviors such as eating are a matter of habit rather than decision making; that decisions to eat differently, such as to lose weight, may be made for reasons other than health; that health may not be a highly valued goal for some individuals; and that socioeconomic, psychological, and cultural factors may be more important to the person.(13,14)

The Transtheoretical Model or Stages of Change Model is helpful in pointing out that people are at one of several different stages of motivational readiness to change dietary practices from precontemplation (no intention of changing), to contemplation, preparation, action, and maintenance. At each stage, individuals use different processes or engage in various activities in making changes. Thus, the counselor can enhance motivation by recognizing the client's stage of change and using strategies appropriate to that stage. Decisions to change or move to a higher stage happen only when the pros outweigh the cons, or the benefits to the individual outweigh the costs and barriers. (6,7,15) An approach called motivational interviewing has been integrated into the Stages of Change Model.(16).

Bandura's work on self-efficacy looks at people's beliefs about their capabilities to be successful at changing a behavior such as food choices to reach the health outcomes desired. People who believe they cannot do something (precontemplators) do not make any effort to change. If self-efficacy is low for a behavioral change or goal, another goal should be selected. Self-efficacy is more relevant in the preparation, action, and maintenance stages of change. Those with high levels of self-efficacy will make a great deal of effort. Of four possible ways to increase self-efficacy in clients, the most effective is for the person to have small successes in reaching goals for change that can be followed by more small successes.(17)

Goal setting can enhance motivation to change. People without specific goals are not motivated to make lifestyle changes. If you did not have a goal to obtain a college degree, for example, so that you were prepared for an interesting career that paid you well enough to sustain the lifestyle you wanted (note that motivational factors are multiple rather than singular), would you spend 4 years of your life sitting in classes? Changes in food choices can be mutually negotiated into goals that are reasonable and measurable. The choices of goals should be selected by the client, not the counselor, and should be simple enough to ensure success. People self-evaluate their own progress against the goals and success increases self-efficacy.(18–20)

On the way to the goal, self-monitoring has been found to be helpful. Those who record food and exercise behaviors daily or for a period of time can see how well they are

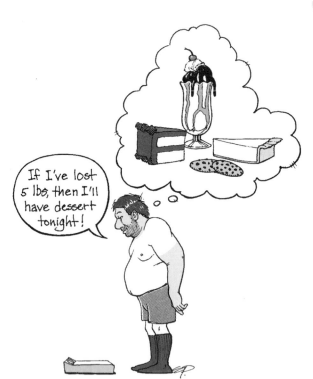

Nonfood rewards are needed.

doing. They can note patterns of eating. Whether counting fat grams or recording changes in blood pressure or blood sugar, the client finds valuable information and increases self-understanding.(18,19)

When the goal is reached, clients need to reward themselves with nonfood items, which are external motivators. As pointed out in Chapter 6, it is also helpful to decrease the stimuli or cues to eating in the environment and replace them with new and better cues. A behavioral program involves controlling the food and eating environment and rewarding oneself for successful change.(8,21)

No one is perfect, and there will be problems on the way to permanent change. Prochaska notes that people may recycle to earlier stages of change more than once.(2–6) If so, the counselor changes strategies, matching them to the stage. Before that happens, however, clients can be counseled about the possibility of high-risk situations, slips, lapses, and ways to avoid total relapse.(22)

During a lapse, the person's cognitions or thoughts may turn negative. Instead of thinking "I can do this" (positive cognitions increase self-efficacy), the client may be thinking "This is too hard. I want to eat whatever I want" (negative thinking decreases self-efficacy). Most people greatly underestimate the influence of thoughts or self-talk on motivation and behavior. Counselors can ask clients to self-monitor their self-talk before and after eating and work on cognitive restructuring.(22,23)

Social support can make an impact on motivation and dietary change as well. Is the family supportive of the change in food choices needed by one member? What are the cultural implications of the change? The support of significant others—family, friends, and the counselor—is helpful. Counselors may need to work with the family and within the cultural framework to ensure success.

Nutrition education is important in letting people know what to do. Yet, it is over-rated as a way to motivate people to change. Many people already know what they should eat and how much they should exercise. But they are not doing it. Nutrition education is necessary, but it is not sufficient alone to motivate and promote change in food choices.

SELF-ASSESSMENT

Ask yourself if you follow the Dietary Guidelines for Americans and exercise regularly.

Do the pros outweigh the cons?

What is your Stage of Change for eating and for exercise?

What motivates you?

The preceding models and concepts should be combined and woven into counseling approaches and strategies to motivate change in eating behaviors. The client needs both information and skills. A comprehensive approach emphasizing internal over external motivators is more likely to be successful.(8)

MOTIVATION OF EMPLOYEES

This section explores the concept of motivation as it relates to employees and examines theories of motivation and their behavioral implications for dietetics professionals. The reader should keep in mind that the forces instrumental in motivation are usually multiple rather than singular, that they differ in strength, and that more than one may be present at a given time.(24)

Maslow and Herzberg

Two early theorists who have made major contributions to the study of motivation are Abraham Maslow and Frederick Herzberg. Maslow correlated human motivation with individual desires. In his Hierarchy of Needs theory and "need-priority" model, he lists five universal needs to explain human motivation: physiological needs; the need for safety and security; social needs; the need for esteem; and the need for self-realization. For each need to become active as a motivating factor, the desire immediately preceding the need must be fulfilled. In simplified terms, Maslow would say that the way to stimulate motivation in individuals is to determine which of their wants is most unsatisfied and then to structure their work so that in the accomplishment of the work goal, they satisfy their personal goals as well.(25)

The most basic human requirements are physiological (Fig 9-1). Sickness and hunger tend to take precedence over all other human needs. Only after they are satisfied does a person experience the desire to satisfy other needs. Indigent persons who are able to take care of only their physiological necessities may work regardless of the working conditions for their own and their families' sustenance and shelter. After they have enough money to satisfy these essentials, however, working merely for nourishment and shelter is no longer adequate. At that point, the motivation to work arises from a drive to maintain safety and security.

In most organizations today, security needs are satisfied through work contracts, unions, governmental regulations, and various insurance plans. With the fulfillment of biological and security needs, the individual's urge for social affiliation and activity becomes the dominant unsatisfied need and should therefore be considered in the designing of work goals to motivate the employee. Social needs can be experienced as a desire to become a member of, and participate in, a recognized group: family, church, community, work, neighborhood business, union, and so forth. If the social need becomes satiated, the employees' motivation is stimulated by a desire for esteem and status, which is commonly experienced as the need to attain recognition for accomplishments.

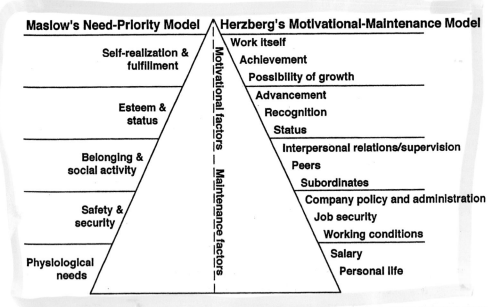

Figure 9-1 A COMPARISON OF MASLOW'S NEED-PRIORITY MODEL WITH HERZBERG'S MOTIVATION-MAINTENANCE MODEL. (ADAPTED FROM HERZBERG F. WORK AND THE NATURE OF MAN. CLEVELAND, OH: WORLD PUBLISHING CO, 1966; AND MASLOW AH. MOTIVATION AND PERSONALITY. NEW YORK: HARPER AND BROS, 1954.)

Although each of the five areas of needs becomes dominant at some time, the strongest motivator at a given moment is the one immediately above the last need satisfied. Once the requirement for esteem is no longer lacking, for example, the desire for self-realization becomes dominant. Self-realization is the highest human urge and the most self-centered. This drive for self-realization and the opportunity to grow as a person seems to be most effectively fulfilled only when most other needs are met. Now, during the twenty-first century, the need is commonly experienced as an urge for personal and professional growth that can best be satisfied through the work experience.

It is difficult for dietetics practitioners to apply Maslow's theory with any degree of certainty, although social scientists still recognize his hierarchy of needs as fundamental to designing an effective structure to facilitate motivation.(26) Unless, however, a practitioner has few others reporting to him or her, the task of getting to know subordinates well enough to infer their current need level accurately is not likely to be accomplished; furthermore, need intensity at each level can vary from day to day and sometimes from hour to hour. A person may be operating at the need level for increased esteem, suddenly have an accident, and become overwhelmingly concerned with the physiological needs of being able to feed the family if incapacitated and unable to work. In spite of the limited applications of Maslow's theory, however, it does provide insight into the process of motivation and can often be useful in designing jobs, selecting staff, and developing strategies to maintain enthusiasm and interest among employees.

Frederick Herzberg, a contemporary of Maslow's, is credited with the "two-factor theory of motivation" or the Motivation-Maintenance Model, which complements Maslow's theory and provides additional perspectives.(27) Herzberg reviewed previous theories and studies and attempted to ascertain the essence of motivation by asking employees what they liked about their jobs and what they disliked about their jobs. After examining the data, he determined that the answers to the first question ("What do you like about your job?") were "motivation factors," whereas the answers to the second question ("What do you dislike about your job?") were what he termed "maintenance factors" (Fig 9-1).

The five motivators Herzberg compiled in response to the first question were (1) the work itself, being personally involved in the work, with a sense of responsibility and control; (2) achievement, feeling personal accomplishment for having done a job well; (3) growth, experiencing the opportunity for challenge in the job and the chance to learn skills and knowledge; (4) advancement, knowing that the experience and growth will lead to increased responsibility and control; and (5) recognition or being recognized for doing a job well, resulting in increased self-esteem.(28)

Herzberg called the answers to the second question maintenance factors because he found that they maintained but did not improve current levels of production. Maintenance factors were physical conditions, such as lighting in the office and food in the cafeteria; security—a feeling of certainty about the future and of contentment; economic factors—salary and fringe benefits; and social factors—relationships with fellow workers and the boss.

Herzberg found that when the maintenance factors were poor, productivity decreased. Inadequate maintenance factors, then, hindered production, whereas adequate maintenance factors only maintained the current level. Thus, maintenance factors merely "satisfy" workers; they do not motivate them. Although Herzberg's theory first gained prominence in the 1960s, it remains the basis for current research in the area of motivation.(29) As indicated in Figure 9-1, Herzberg's motivational factors are similar to those at the top of Maslow's Need Priority Model, and his maintenance factors are toward the bottom of Maslow's model.

CONTEMPORARY THEORIES OF MOTIVATION

The theories of Maslow and Herzberg are well known but have not been consistently validated empirically. Several contemporary theories, however, do have a reasonable degree of valid supporting documentation. They are called contemporary theories not because they are only recently developed but because they represent the current state of the art in explaining employee motivation.

David McClelland's Theory of Needs

David McClelland's theory of needs focuses on three needs: achievement, power, and affiliation.(30–33) Some people are driven by the need to excel, to achieve in relation to a set of standards, and to strive to succeed. Others are driven by a need for power, the desire to make others behave in a way that they would not otherwise have behaved in. Still others are driven by a need for affiliation, the desire for friendly and close interpersonal relationships. McClelland suggests that determining an employee's major need structure is key to fitting that person into the right position. Although somewhat oversimplified, the theory posits that persons with high achievement needs might do particularly well managing themselves in sales, for example, but would not necessarily do well in management positions. Persons with high needs for power and recognition, however, would more likely be suited for management. Persons whose primary needs are in the affiliation area are best suited for the helping professions.

Although McClelland has conducted studies in the three need areas, most of the studies have focused on the area of achievement. McClelland has determined that high achievers prefer job situations with personal responsibility, feedback, and an intermediate degree of risk. When these characteristics are prevalent, high achievers are strongly motivated. A high need to achieve does not necessarily lead to being a good manager, especially in large organizations. People with high achievement needs are interested in how well they do personally and not in influencing others to do well.(30–33)

One promising phenomenon of McClelland's Achievement Theory is that employees have been successfully trained to stimulate their achievement need. Motivation specialists have been successful in teaching individuals to think in terms of accomplishments, winning, and success as well as helping them to alter behavior so as to act in a high achievement way by preferring situations in which they have personal responsibility, feedback, and moderate risks. Human resource professionals are optimistically hoping to learn that management can select a person with a high achievement need or develop its own candidate through achievement training.

Equity Theory

Equity theory is based on the belief that people compare their inputs and outcomes with those of others and then respond so as to eliminate any inequities. Employees might compare themselves with friends, neighbors, co-workers, colleagues in other organizations, or past jobs they themselves have had. Which referent an employee chooses is influenced by the information the employee holds about referents as well as by the attractiveness of the referent. If a dietetics practitioner, for example, were hired right out of college with a fair salary, challenging work, and an excellent opportunity to gain important experience, he or she would most likely be motivated to excel in the position until and unless someone he or she views as less competent is also hired to do the same work but for more money.

Based on equity theory, when employees perceive an inequity, they can be predicted to make one of six choices:(34)

1. Change their inputs (i.e., stop exerting so much effort)
2. Change their outcomes (i.e., increase their pay if paid on a piece-rate basis by producing a higher quantity of units of lower quality)
3. Distort perceptions of self (e.g., "I used to think I worked at a moderate pace, but now I realize that I work a lot harder than everyone else.")
4. Distort perceptions of others (e.g., "Mary's job isn't as desirable as I previously thought it was.")
5. Choose a different referent (e.g., "I may not make as much as my brother-in-law, but I'm doing a lot better than my Dad did when he was my age."
6. Leave the field (e.g., quit the job)(34)

The primary distinction of equity theory is its contention that people are concerned not only with the absolute amount of rewards they receive for their efforts, but also with the relation of this amount to what others receive. They make judgments as to the relation between their inputs and outcomes and the inputs and outcomes of others. When people infer an imbalance in their outcome-input ratio compared with others, tension is created. This tension provides the basis for motivation, since people strive for what they perceive as equity and fairness.

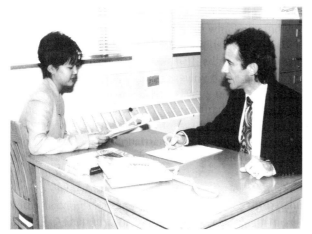

Managers can acknowledge the contributions of the employee.

Expectancy Theory

The Expectancy Theory, formulated by Victor Vroom, is based on the belief that the strength of a tendency to act in a certain way depends on the strength of an expectation that the act will be followed by a given outcome and on the attractiveness of that outcome to the individual. The expectancy theory is one of the most widely accepted explanations of motivation. Although it has its critics, most of the research evidence is supportive of the theory.(34–36)

The expectancy theory suggests that an employee is motivated to exert a high level of effort when he or she believes that effort will lead to a good performance appraisal; a good appraisal leads to organization rewards such as a bonus, a salary increase, or a promotion, and the rewards will satisfy the employee's personal goals.

Three relationships are focused on in this theory.

1. Effort-performance relationship: The probability perceived by the individual that exerting a given amount of effort will lead to performance.
2. Performance-reward relationship: The degree to which the individual believes that performing at a particular level will lead to the attainment of a desired outcome
3. Rewards-personal goals relationship: The degree to which organizational rewards satisfy an individual's personal goals or needs and the attractiveness of those potential rewards for the individual.(34)

Expectancy theory can be a useful tool in understanding why some dietetics employees are not motivated in their jobs and merely do the minimum necessary to get by. If, for example, an employee's motivation is to be maximized, an affirmative answer would be required for the three questions below:

1. If I give a maximum effort, will it be recognized in my performance appraisal?
2. If I get a good performance appraisal, will it lead to organization rewards?
3. If I'm rewarded, are the rewards personally attractive to me?

If the answer to any question is negative, less than maximum effort can be predicted according to the theory.

Motivation Through Enhancement of Self-Esteem

Key issues of the early twenty-first century are the attraction and retention of skilled workers, with shortages of human talent rather than surpluses characterizing the United States during this period. Baby boomers, those born between 1945 and 1964, are now beginning to retire; with fewer offspring, they are the parents of the new generation of workers, the "baby-bust generation." Because of fewer entrants to the job market in the early twenty first century, there may not be enough workers in the small cohort of people born after 1964 to fill the bottom level of the typical corporate pyramid. Increasingly, most of the workforce today is composed of post-baby boomers and recent immigrants. Both groups tend to define success in terms of power, prestige, and money, and senior management generally supports this definition as well. Managers face a challenge in responding creatively to these new demographics, and a major concern of the contemporary manager is to understand the new workforce and how to adapt its needs to those of the organization.(37)

Another employment issue results from the fact that the number of highly qualified people in the workforce is growing at a much faster rate than is the number of senior-level jobs. Consequently, supervisors must understand how to spot the plateau problem and deal with it effectively before the employees have no alternative but to quit the organization. The worker who has hit a career plateau often suffers from losses in productivity and/or self-esteem. When employees' careers have reached a plateau and the company does not want to lose them, they can redefine success so that the sense of having reached a plateau does not arise.(38) Success can be redefined, for example, through various forms of public recognition, such as company awards, plaques, and other forms of recognition.

A third reality of the early twenty-first century, particularly in the health professions, is that organizations have to continue to maintain as lean and as motivated a staff as possible to compete and to comply with governmental regulations. In the process of becoming "lean" by eliminating, "downsizing," "right-sizing," "merging," and combining as many positions as possible, those staff members who have survived may feel insecure, defensive, hostile, and fearful of losing their jobs and may object to having had their former positions changed or enlarged without any monetary compensation. They may be unwilling to extend themselves because of the inference that the organization does not care about them. The manager or supervisor who is attempting to "motivate" staff under these conditions has a considerable challenge. While monetary increases are being kept to a minimum, the manager is expected to obtain more work from fewer people, who are already feeling unappreciated and overworked. Given this depressing but not unrealistic scenario, the manager needs to know and to exercise every motivational option available.

Generally, members of the current workforce differ considerably from their predecessors. The values of both post–baby boomers and recent immigrants, for example, are distinctly different from those of their parents. These younger employees generally are more affluent and educated and are less willing to rely on authority figures. They have different perceptions of themselves and are generally unwilling to tolerate a disrespectful supervisory style. Workers indicate that what they want most are a heightened sense of self-esteem, realization, recognition, autonomy, responsibility, and managers who recognize their capacity for these achievements.(39) Although some employees can always be motivated by the hope of merit salary increases, contemporary managers will benefit most from knowing how to enhance their staff's self-esteem and confidence, a vital methodology for increasing motivation of contemporary employees.(40–42)

There have been numerous studies of motivation among health care workers, and much is known about the relationship between motivation and increased self-esteem or recognition.(43–49) For more than half a century, social scientists have been aware of the phenomenon of the "self-fulfilling prophecy," which suggests that people perform and develop according to others' expectations of them. In one study, students and instructors were selected randomly, and some instructors were told that they had been selected to have all the brighter students in their classes. Later tests did verify that these instructors had students who performed statistically and significantly better than those in classes where instructors had no previous expectations.(50) People who are told that they are incompetent and will be unable to achieve a specific goal or task, perform poorly compared with those who are told that they are competent and will be able to achieve the task, even though neither group has had previous experience with the task. A person's self-perceived ability, based on previous performance, is positively related to later performance. Success begets success, and failure begets failure.(39)

Unfortunately, an appreciation of the implications of this phenomenon for business and industry has only recently become apparent. Whenever supervisors acknowledge success in subordinates, they add to the likelihood that subsequent tasks will be performed successfully. For this reason, supervisors need to select carefully the right worker for the task, to provide adequate training to ensure employee success, and to assign work tasks that are manageable and accomplishable. Managers can enhance the self-esteem of employees by providing opportunities for their achievement, growth, recognition, responsibility, and control, which increase their motivation to improve or to continue to do well.

Motivation Through Setting Goals

Too often, subordinates believe that they are pleasing their supervisors only to learn that what they were doing was not what was desired or expected. Setting goals with subordinates as well as following up with subsequent periodic reviews provides feedback and promotes improved performance. Telling an employee, "Do your best," is useless. To the employee, who is faced with numerous alternatives for ways to spend his or her "working" time, this instruction can mean dozens of things. Setting goals complements the theories of Maslow and Herzberg. An effective way to assist others who wish to increase their esteem, growth, development, realization, and achievement is to teach them to be proactive in planning specific ways to accomplish more or to improve quality by setting goals.

The effect of setting goals on individual performance has been demonstrated. Theory and experiments support the proposition that supervisors should play an active role in setting goals with subordinates. Goals should be specific, clearly stated, and measurable.(34) When they fulfill these conditions, they provide a criterion for feedback, accountability, and evaluation. A person can be highly motivated by knowing the objective and working on a plan with the dietetics manager to accomplish it. The three identifiable elements in goal setting are (1) an action verb, (2) a measurable result, and (3) the cost and/or date by which the objective will be accomplished. Both employee and manager must agree on their mutual expectations and clarify the difference, for example, between "I want you to get your work done soon," and "I want to see an increase of 10% by June 16th." Perhaps the single most significant advance in the field of management has been the growth of participative management. A major advantage of goal setting, a form of

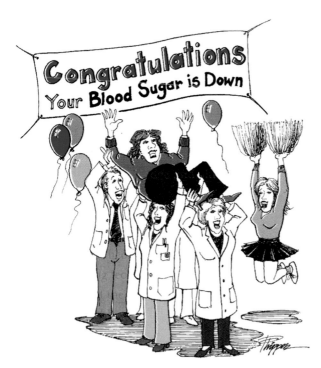

The counselor should reinforce the client positively.

participative management, is that it directs work activities toward organizational goals and forces planning.

People who have specific and challenging goals tend to perform best. Goals seen as "sure things" may discourage motivation as much as those that are believed to be impossible. The best goals—those that inspire quality performance—are those that are perceived as difficult and challenging but attainable. A major proposition, supported experimentally, is that employees who set or accept harder goals perform at levels superior to those who set or accept easier goals.(51, 52)

Regardless of whether the goal is actually set by the manager or the employee, the two parties need to agree. When staff members feel that they are actively participating in setting their own goals, even if the supervisor originally proposes the goals, they are more solidly motivated to perform with distinction than if they feel that they are merely being told what to do.

Motivation Through Reinforcement

Reinforcement, knowing how to encourage desirable behavior and to discourage undesirable behavior, is related to motivation. One way to increase the likelihood that a performance or behavior will recur is to follow the performance with a positive event, such as praise for a job well done. A positively reinforced response is more likely to recur simply because it pays off.

Another type of reinforcement is the removal of something negative after the performance. In this case, the persons are likely to repeat the behavior because something they dislike is taken away as a consequence of the behavior. This removal or elimination of adverse conditions is referred to as negative reinforcement. A hospital dish washer, for example, who is constantly being checked by the manager and who has been able to decrease dish breakage by 30% from the previous month, will be motivated to continue improving if the manager not only praises the dishwasher but also checks this employee less often during the following week. The manager can then encourage the desired action by removing an unfavorable condition—the frequent inspections.

Two strategies that may discourage a given behavior are punishment and extinction. Reprimanding an employee for being late is an example of formal punishment. Although punishment is often used to eliminate undesirable behavior, its value is questionable because of its negative side effects. Punishment can make an employee hostile and prone to retaliation. If the punishment is perceived as unwarranted by employees, they may resume the undesirable behavior as soon as punishment stops. The way to overcome the employee's feelings of resentment when punished is to provide frequent constructive feedback each time an infraction occurs. In that way, when formal punitive action is taken, the employee perceives it as warranted and rational.

The other basic technique for decreasing the likelihood of a behavior is extinction. With extinction, the undesirable performance is neither punished nor rewarded; it is simply ignored. Ignored behaviors tend to diminish and ultimately to become extinguished as a result of a consistent lack of reinforcement. For example, a manager who never acknowledges an employee's suggestions is actually encouraging the employee to stop sending them. Although its use may be unintentional, extinction is an effective technique for terminating behavior. A manager should be aware of the potentially negative consequences of ignoring desired behavior. Managers through carelessness can unintentionally extinguish motivated performances.

SUMMARY OF RECOMMENDATIONS

Managers should give recognition to the employees in the presence of their peers. Recognition provides positive feedback and builds a worker's confidence and self-esteem. Organizations can benefit from involving their employees in the decision-making process. The more that the employees are involved, the higher the level of their performance and satisfaction. Employees who participate in making decisions feel a sense of ownership and commitment.

Managers at all levels reduce stress and increase efficiency and motivation when they negotiate with employees with clearly defined goals and objectives. The more that employees understand what they are expected to do, the more highly motivated they become. Supervisors should give respect and dignity to their staff. The more they respect the rights and privileges of employees, the better the employees feel about themselves and the more they produce. Managers must become familiar with reinforcement techniques, training themselves to recognize and comment on good work to reinforce it. Ignoring good work may lead to extinction of desired behavior. Top management needs to instill in lower-level management an appreciation of the human

---

CASE STUDY 1

John, age 30, has been hired as an assistant cook at a small hospital. He has 1 year of previous experience cooking at a nursing home. The head cook and dietetics manager have participated in training John for the past 4 months.

1. What can the head cook and dietetics manager do to maintain and increase John's level of motivation?

CASE STUDY 2

Martha M. was recently diagnosed with mild type II diabetes mellitus. She is 50 years old, 5'6", and 180 pounds. A homemaker, she is married to an electrician, and their only child is away at college.

The dietetics counselor has taken a nutrition history and is considering alternative ways to motivate Martha to make changes in her food choices and eating practices.

1. What internal and external factors can the counselor explore to motivate Martha to change her eating practices?

Note: Students may want to consult Diabetes Care and Education Dietetic Practice Group. Scope of practice for qualified dietetics professionals in diabetes care and education. J Am Diet Assoc 2000;100:1205.

resources of the organization, supporting the development of increased self-esteem, recognition, and growth among all staff.

This chapter has emphasized the complexity of motivation and has discussed its behavior implications for dietetics professionals. Practitioners are involved daily with motivation of both staff and clients. Understanding motivational concepts and being able to use the strategies and techniques associated with them can add immeasurably to the professional's effectiveness. The chapter has provided a brief background on numerous theories of motivation, including endnotes referring to supportive studies. Attempts to validate most theories, however, have been complicated by methodological, criterion, and measurement problems. As a result, many published studies that purport to support or negate a theory must be viewed with caution.

REVIEW AND DISCUSSION QUESTIONS

1. What processes is the word "motivation" used to describe?
2. Give an example of positive external factors that enhance motivation.
3. Explain intrinsic motivation and give examples.
4. Discuss ways to motivate patients and clients.
5. List Maslow's need-priority model.
6. Compare Maslow's and Herzberg's theories.
7. Explain the equity theory and the expectancy theory.
8. List ways to enhance employee self-esteem.

SUGGESTED ACTIVITIES

1. List the factors that motivate you to go to work or to continue with your present job. Explain your reactions in terms of the Maslow and Herzberg models.
2. Interview someone who is on a diet, and determine the positive and negative influences on motivation.
3. Examine the forces that motivate you to learn something new. Are they related to your desire to remain physically well, secure, well-liked and respected, or are they related to your desire to prepare yourself for taking on additional responsibility, having more control, and achieving realization and actualization?
4. Indicate why the following statements would have a negative impact on an employee's motivation and how they might be amended so that they maintain the employee's self-esteem.
   A. That job has been done incorrectly! What do I have to do to get you to understand?
   B. I'm tired of listening to you complain. Just keep still and do your job.
   C. You will probably make a mess of this, but there isn't anyone else to do it.
   D. If you would listen, you would understand.
   E. You can't be serious about that suggestion.
5. For each of the following examples, list the reinforcement technique used and the feelings it might produce in the employee.

A. **Employee:** Mrs. Jones, since you told us to be on the lookout for problems with equipment, we have discovered two more.
   Dietetics professional: Yes, but I'm looking for Helen now. Have you seen her?
B. **Employee:** Mrs. Jones, I've finished all the work in the kitchen and have begun to rearrange the cabinets.
   Dietetics professional: You mean it took you all this time just to do that?
C. **Dietetics professional:** Mary, I am putting you on suspension for 3 days.
D. **Dietetics professional:** Mary, I want you to know that I appreciate how effectively you work with others. Several people have told me how thorough you are in using the new procedures.

WEB SITES

http://www.ucc.vt.edu/stdysk/motivate.html / motivation suggestions
http://www.academicpress.com/l&m / learning and motivation
http://www.cba.uri.edu/Scholl/Papers/Self_Concept_Motivation.HTM / work motivation
http://www.d.umn.edu/student/loon/acad/strat/motivate.html / goal setting
http://www.motivationalinterview.org / motivational interviewing.

REFERENCES

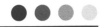

1. Berg-Smith SM, Stevens VJ, Brown KM, et al. A brief motivational intervention to improve dietary adherence in adolescents. Health Educ Research 1999;14:399.
2. Smith DE, Heckemeyer CM, Kratt PP, et al. Motivational interviewing to a improve adherence to a behavioral weight-control program for older obese women with NIDDM. Diab Care 1997;20:52.
3. Shinitzky HE, Kub J. The art of motivating behavior change: the use of motivational interviewing to promote health. Public Health Nurs 2001;18:178.
4. Miller WR. Motivational interviewing: research, practice, and puzzles. Addictive Behaviors 1996;21;835.
5. Rosal MC, Ebbeling CB, Lofgren I, et al. Facilitating dietary change: the patient-centered counseling model. J Am Diet Assoc 2001;101:332.
6. Prochaska JO, Norcross JC, DiClemente CC. Changing for good. New York: Avon Books, 1994.
7. Greene GW, Rossi SR, Rossi JS, et al. Dietary applications of the Stages of Change Model. J Am Diet Assoc 1999;99:673.
8. Brownell KD, Cohen LR. Adherence to dietary regimens 2: components of effective interventions. Behav Med 1995;20:155.
9. Gabaccia DR. We eat what we are: ethnic food and the making of Americans. Cambridge MA: Harvard University Press, 1998.
10. Capaldi ED. Why we eat what we what: the psychology of eating. Washington, DC, Am Psych Assoc, 1996.
11. Glasgow RE, Eakin EG. Issues in diabetes self-management. In Shumaker SA, Schron ED, Ockene JK, McBee WL eds. The handbook of health behavior change, 2nd ed. New York: Springer Pub, 1998.
12. Gillis BP, Caggiula AW, Chiavacci AT, et al. Nutrition intervention program of the Modification of Diet in Renal Disease study: a self-management approach. J Am Diet Assoc 1995;95:1288.

13. Clark NM, Becker MH. Theoretical models and strategies for improving adherence and disease management. In: Shumaker SA, Schron EB, Okene JK, McBee WL, eds. The handbook of health behavior change, 2nd ed. New York: Springer Pub, 1998.
14. Rosenstoc IM. Historical origins of the health belief model. Health Educ Monographs 1974;2:328.
15. Prochaska JO, Velicer WF. The transtheoretical model of health behavior change. Am J Health Promot 1997;12:38.
16. DiClemente CL. Motivational interviewing and the stages of change. In: Miller WR, Rollnick S, eds. Motivational interviewing: preparing people to change addictive behaviors. New York: Guilford Press, 1991.
17. Bandura A. Exercise of personal and collective efficacy in changing societies. In: Bandura A, ed. Self-efficacy in changing societies. New York: Cambridge University Press, 1995.
18. Cullen KW, Baranowski T, Smith SP. Using goal setting as a strategy for dietary behavior change. J Am Diet Assoc 2001;101, 562.
19. Strecher VJ, Seijts GH, Kok GJ. Goal setting as a strategy for heath behavior change. Health Educ Q 1995;22:190.
20. Diabetes Care and Education Practice Group. Scope of practice for qualified dietetics professionals in diabetes care and education. J Am Diet Assoc 2000;100:1205.
21. Holli BB. Using behavior modification in nutrition counseling. J Am Diet Assoc 1988;88:1530.
22. Marlatt GA, George WH. Relapse prevention and the maintenance of optimal health. In: Shumaker SA, Schron EB, Okene JK, McBee WC, eds. The handbook of health behavior change, 2nd ed. New York: Springer Pub, 1998.
23. Nash JD. The new maximize your body potential: lifetime skills for successful weight management. Palo Alto CA, Bull Pub, 1997.
24. Owen AV. Management for doctors: getting the best from people. BMJ (England), 1996;310:648.
25. Maslow AH. Motivation and personality. New York: Harper & Bros, 1954.
26. Clark K. Simply motivate. Industrial Society 1989;22:26.
27. Herzberg F. Work and the nature of man. Cleveland: World Publishing Co, 1966.
28. Kivimaki M, Voutilainen P, Koskinen P. Job enrichment, work motivation, and job satisfaction in hospital wards. J Nurs Mgt (England)1996;3:87.
29. Herzberg F. Innovation: where is the relish. J Creative Behavior 1987;21:179.
30. McClelland DC. The achieving society. New York: Van Nostrand Reinhold, l961.
31. McClelland DC. Power: the inner experience. New York: Irvington, l975.
32. McClelland DC, Winter DG. Motivating economic achievement. New York: Free Press, l969.
33. McClelland DC. Toward a theory of motive acquisition. Am Psychol 1965;10:321.
34. Robbins SP. Organizational behavior, 8th ed. Englewood Cliffs, NJ: Prentice Hall, 2001.
35. Van Eerde W, Thierry G. Vroom's expectancy models and work-related criteria. Academy of Mgt J 1997;3:154.
36. Heneman HG, Schwab, DP. Evaluation of research on expectancy theory prediction of employee performance. Psychological Bulletin 1979;12:1.
37. Wendling W. Responses to a changing work force. Personnel Administrator 1988;33:50.
38. Modic S. Motivating without promotions. Industry Week 1989;238:24.
39. Rosenbaum BL. How to motivate today's workers. New York: McGraw-Hill, 1982.
40. Knippen J, Green TB. Building self-confidence. Supervisory Mgt 1989;34:22.
41. Dutton K, Brown JD. Global self-esteem and specific self-views as determinants of people's reactions to success and failure. J Pers Soc Psychol 1997;73:139.
42. Abel MH. The role of self-esteem in typical and atypical changes in expectations. J Gen Psychol 1997;124:113.

43. deVries H. Motives for protective behavior against carcinogenic substances in the workplace. J Occup Environ Med 2000;42:88.

44. Linden H, Wayne J, Sparrowe R. An examination of the mediating role of psychological empowerment on the relations between the job, interpersonal relationships, and work outcomes. J Appl Psychol 2000;85:407.

45. Umiker W. Front-line training. Health Care Mgt 2000;18:14.

46. Schneider R, Casey J, Kohn R. Motivational versus confrontational interviewing. J Behav Health Serv Res 2000;27:60

47. Sheldon K, Elliot A. Personal goals in social roles. J Pers 2000;68:51.

48. Flenert G. How measurement systems act as employee motivators. Hosp Mater Manage Q 2000;21:69

49. Griffin M, Neal A. Perceptions of safety as work: a framework for linking safety climate to safety performance, knowledge, and motivation. J Occup Health Psychol 2000;5:347.

50. Rosenthal R, Jacobson L. Pygmalion in the classroom. New York: Rinehart & Winston, 1968.

51. Robbins S, Hunsaker P. Training in interpersonal skills, 2nd ed. Englewood Cliffs, NJ: Prentice Hall, 1996.

52. Bohlander G, Snell S, and Sherman A. Managing Human Resources, 12th ed. Cincinnati, South-Western Publishing Co, 2001.

10

Principles and Theories of Learning

After reading this chapter, you will be able to

1. compare and contrast theories and strategies for learning.
2. explain several types of consequences.
3. identify strategies that enhance long-term memory.
4. discuss learning styles and teaching styles.
5. list the stages involved in the adoption of innovations.

N utrition education falls within the realm of practice of all dietetics professionals. Consumers are faced with a multitude of confusing and conflicting media messages, so nutrition education focuses on health promotion and the prevention of chronic diseases. The goal is behavior change toward a more healthful diet. It is essential for people "to achieve and maintain optimal nutritional health."(1)

The foundation for effective education efforts is based on theory. Theory is important in the planning, implementation, and evaluation of education. In general, the more effective programs are based on appropriate theories.(2)

LEARNING AND LEARNING THEORIES

What is learning? Learning may be defined as a change in a person as a result of experience or the interaction of a person with his or her environment.(3) The changes may be in knowledge, skills, attitudes, values, and behaviors, and they are relatively permanent outcomes brought about by the experience. As you read this chapter, for example, you are learning something. Other than learning by reading, the practitioner's problem is determining how to present people with the right stimuli and experiences on which to focus their attention and mental effort so that they acquire new knowledge, skills, attitudes, and behaviors.

How do people learn? How do they retain what they learn? The field of educational psychology studies questions about learning, learners, and teaching. Its major focus is on the processes by which knowledge, skills, attitudes, and values are transmitted from teachers to learners.

In the workplace, dietetics professionals are involved with training and educating new employees and retraining current workers. Educational programs are also planned for other health professionals, students, interns, residents, paraprofessionals, and therapists.

Client education is a process of influencing behavior, producing changes in knowledge, attitudes, values, and skills required to improve and maintain health. Although it may begin with imparting information, this is not sufficient to achieve behavior change. Changes in attitudes and behaviors beneficial to health status are necessary.

Dietetics practitioners are concerned with discovering the most effective methods of teaching to influence the dietary behaviors of clients and the work behaviors of employees. Although theory alone does not guarantee effective education, applying theories to planning and implementing interventions does.

Education can be directed at several levels: the individual level such as one-on-one or group classes; the social network such as family; and the community level such as society at large, the media, or grocery stores. The 5 a Day for Better Health program is an example of a community level educational program.

Effective use of theory takes practice in helping people make changes in their eating practices and environments. Yet it results in more effective interventions.

No single theory explains behavior. Health behaviors are too complex to be explained by a single theory.(4) Theories may overlap and the professional may need to use more than one in an intervention.(5)

The social and behavioral sciences provide many of the health education models. They can be found in other chapters, such as the Health Belief Model in Chapter 9, the Transtheoretical or Stages of Change Model in Chapter 5, motivational interviewing in Chapter 4, behavior modification in Chapter 5, and social cognitive theory in Chapter 7. All of these can be applied to nutrition interventions in appropriate circumstances. The educator must select the most important strategies and methods for each situation.

To explain how people learn, psychologists have developed several learning theories. This chapter discusses behavioral learning theory, cognitive theory, memory, a model of adult learning or andragogy, learning styles, and adoption of innovations. Over time, the boundaries between some of these theories have become less distinct.

BEHAVIORAL LEARNING THEORIES

Behavioral learning theories are explanations of learning that are limited almost exclusively to observable changes in behavior, with emphasis on the effects of external events on the individual.(3) Theorists are interested in the way in which pleasurable or painful consequences of behavior may change the person's behavior over time. This approach is based on the belief that what we learn has readily identifiable parts and that identifiable rewards and punishments can be given to produce the learning.(6) The teacher's role is to arrange the external environment to elicit the desired response.(7)

Most educational interventions to reduce the risk of chronic diseases incorporate behavioral change strategies based on social learning theory and behavioral self-management.(2) Behavioral learning theories evolved from the research of several individuals including Ivan Pavlov on classical conditioning; Edward Thorndike, who noted that the connections between stimuli and subsequent responses or behaviors are strengthened or weakened by the consequences of behavior; and B.F. Skinner's work on operant conditioning.(3,8) Other information on their research may be found in Chapter 6.

Based on the Pavlovian approach, association theory suggests that a stimulus event cues or elicits a response in the learner. Teaching or conditioning, therefore, involves arranging the stimulus and response events. This is a teacher-centered approach with passive learners.

Skinner's work focused on the relationship between the behavior and its consequences. Skinner believed that many human behaviors are operants, not merely respondents. The use of pleasant and unpleasant consequences following a particular behavior is often referred to as operant conditioning.(3,8) Learning involves three related events: the stimulus, a response, and a reinforcer. The teacher must manage all three events. The desired target behavior must be followed by reinforcement for the behavior to continue. Thus, reinforcers such as small objects must be identified and given if the desired response is present. This is also a teacher-centered approach with a passive learner.

In the following sections, four consequences of a behavior are discussed: positive reinforcement, negative reinforcement or escape, punishers, and extinction. In addition, shaping and the timing of reinforcement are examined.

Positive Reinforcers

One of the most important principles of behavioral learning theory is that behavior changes according to its immediate consequences. Pleasurable consequences are called "positive reinforcers" or rewards and may be defined as consequences that strengthen and increase the frequency of a behavior.(3) Examples are praise for a job well done, good grades received in school, money in the form of a salary increase, and token reinforcers such as stars or smiley-face stickers on a chart. When behaviors persist or increase over time, one may assume that the consequences are positively reinforcing them. The pleasure associated with eating, for example, is a positive reinforcer, ensuring that people will consume their favorite foods again and again.

These reinforcers are highly personal, however, and none can be assumed to be effective at all times. The behavior of an employee who has a poor relationship with a supervisor, for example, may not be affected by the supervisor's praise. And the professional's praise of a client who has followed a dietary regimen may not matter to that specific individual. The person must value the reinforcer to increase the frequency of a desired behavior. The professional can explore the things that an individual considers positive reinforcers and can help arrange such reinforcement in the person's environment. Knowledge of results is also an effective secondary positive reinforcer. Clients and employees should know their stage of progress. If they know they are doing something properly, that knowledge reinforces the response.

The way in which praise is given is also important, and the person doing the praising must be believable.(3) The praise should recognize a specific behavior, so the person clearly understands what he or she is being recognized for. "Good job" as a praise

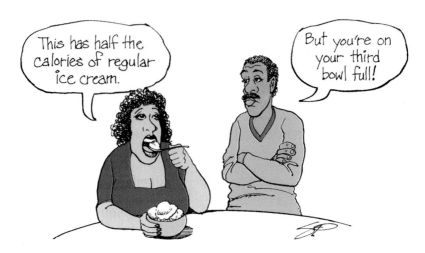

Pleasurable consequences reinforce eating behaviors.

is not as effective as saying specifically, "Thanks for completing the extra project on time. I appreciate it."

Negative Reinforcers/Escapes

Reinforcers that are escapes from unpleasant situations are called negative reinforcers. These also strengthen behaviors because they withdraw from unpleasant situations.(3) Overeating may be reinforcing if the individual escapes, for example, feelings of loneliness, unhappiness, fatigue, and the like. Or, an employee may escape the supervisor's wrath by behaving correctly. If some action allows you to stop, avoid, or escape something unpleasant, you are likely to repeat that action again when faced with a similar situation.

Punishers

Negative reinforcers, which strengthen behaviors, should not be confused with punishers, which weaken behaviors. Unpleasant consequences, punishers, decrease the frequency of or suppress a behavior.(3) Punishment may take one of two different forms. One type is to remove positive reinforcers that the person already has, such as a privilege. A second form of punishment involves the use of unpleasant or adverse consequences, as when a person is scolded for improper behavior. Punishment can make a person avoid the situation in the future, so scolding a client who has not lost any weight is not appropriate.

Extinction

What happens when reinforcers are withdrawn? A behavior weakens and eventually disappears, a process called extinction of a behavior.(3) If a person starts an exercise program or dietary change, for example, and there are no continuous positive reinforcers, that person may decrease the new behavior and eventually end it.

When behaviors are undesirable and the reinforcers for it can be identified and removed, the behavior also may become extinct. An employee's boisterous behavior, for example, may change if the supervisor and other employees ignore the person and do not give him or her the attention he or she is seeking. Instead, the supervisor will want to reinforce positively nonboisterous behavior in this person.

Shaping

The decision of what and when to reinforce in a client or employee is also important. Does one wait until the desired behavior is perfect? No! Most people need reinforcement along the way to something new. Reinforcing each step along the way to successful behavior is called shaping, or successive approximations.(3) It involves reinforcing progress rather than waiting for perfection. When client or employee goals can be broken down into a series of identified steps or subskills, positive feedback may be given as each step or subskill is mastered or accomplished.

Timing Reinforcement

An important principle is that positive consequences that are immediate are more effective than those that are delayed. The connection between the behavior and the consequences is better understood in the person's mind. As a result, the dietetics professional needs to identify with the client or employee not only what is positively reinforcing to that person, but also a time schedule for dispensing that reinforcement for proper behaviors. This concept also explains why it is difficult for people to change their eating behaviors. Usually, the positive consequences of the change, such as weight loss or better health, are in the future, whereas eating disallowed foods is positively reinforcing immediately. It tastes good or hunger is reduced. Eating is intrinsically reinforcing, that is, a behavior that is pleasurable in itself.

The frequency of reinforcement has also been studied. In the early part of a behavior change, continuous reinforcement after every correct response helps learning. Later on, a variable or intermittent schedule of reinforcement is preferable. When rewards are overused, they lose their effect, so that after an individual has had some rewarded successes, rewards should be given less frequently. Table 10-1 summarizes some of the implications of the theories discussed in this chapter.

SOCIAL COGNITIVE THEORY

Social cognitive theory expanded the behaviorist view. Psychologists found that operant conditioning offered too limited an explanation of learning and overlooked important social influences.(3) Albert Bandura believed that the observation of and imitation of other people's behavior, that is, vicariously learning from another's successes and failures, had been ignored. He maintained that people learned not only from external cues,

TABLE 10-1 Implications of Learning Theories and Models

Theory/Model	Implications
Behavioral theory	Find out what reinforcers are valued
	Tell the person their stage of progress
	Use positive reinforcement
	Praise specific, not general, behaviors
	Reinforce progress on the way to mastery
	Use continuous reinforcement, then intermittent
	Ignore undesirable behaviors
	Avoid punishment
Social learning	Be a good role model
	Provide other good role models
	Avoid negative models
	Have new skills demonstrated and practiced
Cognitive theory	Explore prior knowledge
	Gain and maintain attention
	Ask questions
	Use goal setting
	Use repetition and review
	Make information meaningful
	Organize information
	Link new information to the memory network
Learning styles	Identify preferences for styles
	Offer several methods/techniques of learning
Adult learning	Adults are self-directed
	Recognize prior experience
	Use participatory methods
	Orient learning to problems and projects
	Use goal setting

but also from observing models or "modeling." People who focus their attention on watching others are constructing mental images, analyzing, evaluating, remembering, and making decisions that affect their own learning. Professionals need to be aware of this and to be good role models themselves. If we do not eat nutritiously and exercise regularly, for example, how can we expect others to do so? Children model after their parents eating practices.

When Oprah Winfrey lost weight the first time, many of her viewers started on the same diet to model after her success. It is preferable, of course, if the model is an attractive, successful, admired, and well-known individual. Then people will imitate the behavior, hoping to capture some of the same success.

In group learning situations, clients and employees can learn from good role models. In demonstrating the operation of kitchen equipment to a new employee, part of the learning comes from watching the trainer. Then the employee imitates what he or she has seen. In group classes for individuals making dietary modifications due to heart disease, for example, people may be influenced to make dietary changes by modeling after the success stories of others in the group.

We also learn vicariously from watching negative models. When we see that something does not work or we disagree with it, we decide not to imitate it. Seeing an obese person can trigger this type of reaction in some people. "I'll never be like that" may be a response. People judge behaviors against their own standards and decide which models to follow. Sometimes, employees model after others who take shortcuts and do not follow proper procedures. For example, if the supervisor takes extra long breaks and lunches, employees may conclude that this behavior is permissible.

When the professional wants people to model knowledge or skills they are acquiring, it is important to have them practice and demonstrate the skill, not just rehearse it mentally. This shows whether or not they are modeling correctly. For example, the practitioner may want a client who is learning to make different food choices to plan several menus to model the new knowledge and skill. A new employee who can demonstrate the proper use of equipment is modeling correctly. If the individual is correct, feedback and positive reinforcement such as praise should be given; self-efficacy and motivation are then enhanced. If the person is only partially correct, using "shaping," one may give positive reinforcement for the correct portion and then assist in altering the rest. Mentoring another person is another example of using these principles as the mentor models and guides new roles and behaviors.

Each learner is more effectively counseled by the professional who has an understanding of the person's unique circumstances, style, and context so that the professional can personalize an intervention strategy for learning. Each person is at a different developmental life stage with degrees of motivation. Family and social contexts vary. A multicultural society requires the awareness of group customs, traditions, and acceptable counselor approaches.

COGNITIVE THEORIES

Cognitive psychologists studying learning focus on mental activities, such as thinking, remembering, and solving problems that cannot be seen directly. Rather than observable changes brought about by external events, cognitive learning theories are explanations of learning that focus on internal, unobservable mental processes that people use to learn and remember new knowledge or skills.(3) Learning processes that are less visible, such as thinking, perceiving, remembering, creating, forming concepts, and solving problems are the domain of cognitive learning. The teacher's role is to structure the content of the learning experiences.(7)

Which is easier to learn—the formulas for the essential amino acids or the Food Guide Pyramid? Which is easier to remember—a phone number used yesterday for the first time or the food that was eaten for dinner last evening? The difference is between rote learning, which requires memorizing facts not linked to a cognitive structure, and learning and remembering more meaningful information without deliberately memorizing it. Both are necessary.

TABLE 10-2 Learning Theories and Strategies

	Behavioral	Social Learning	Cognitive	Andragogy
Teacher's role	Arrange environment to get desired response Arrange reinforcement	Serve as role model Arrange for other role models	Structure content or problems with essential features Organize knowledge	Facilitator Plan, implement, evaluate jointly Provide resources
Management	Teacher-centered	Learner-centered	Learner-centered	Learner-centered
Learner participation	Passive/active	Active Imitate models	Active, solve problems Test hypotheses	Active
Motivation	Rewards motivate External	Both external and internal	Internal Use goal setting	Internal
View of learning	Rote learning Subject matter approach Practice in varied contexts	Observation of others	Insight learning Understanding Internal mental process	Performing tasks Solving problems Goal-oriented
Strategies	Stimulus-response Behavioral objectives Task analysis Competency-based Computer-assisted learning	Social roles Discussion Mentoring Role playing	Inquiry learning Discovery learning Simulation Learning to to learn	Oriented to problem solving and task performance

The cognitive view sees learning as an active internal mental process of acquiring, remembering, and using knowledge rather than the passive process influenced by the external environmental stimuli of the behaviorists.(3) Individuals pursue goals, seek information, solve problems, and reorganize information and knowledge in their memories. In pondering a problem, the solution may come as a flash of insight as people reorganize what they know.

The cognitive approach suggests that an important influence on learning is what the individual brings to the learning situation, that is, what he or she already knows.(3) Prior knowledge is an important influence on what we learn, remember, and forget. Remembering and forgetting are other topics in cognitive psychology. Table 10-2 compares the theories discussed in this chapter.

Discovery learning is an example of a cognitive instructional model. When people learn through their own active involvement, they discover things for themselves. This approach, using experimentation and problem solving, helps people to analyze and absorb information rather than merely memorize it.(3) The professional can provide problem situations that stimulate the client to question, explore, and experiment. Examples of questions are: What can you eat for breakfast? In a restaurant? On trips? What does the food label tell you? The person has to discover the answers.

MEMORY

There are many theories of memory that explain how the mind takes in information, processes it, stores it, retains it, and retrieves it for use when needed. Cognitive-perception theories see learning as an all-or-none event rather than incremental. Past perceptions already are stored in memory for future use. If the learner has no prior experience to draw upon (a perceptual deficit), a frame must be created with the help of the educator. With prior experience, a frame exists already. If the current frame is incorrect, a different frame must be created. Through the use of questions and listening, the dietetics professional can discover the learner's frame of reference and build on it. Strategies must fit the client's frame of reference. Teaching involves managing real or vicarious experiences until the learner develops insight, outlooks, or thought patterns.(9) This is a teacher-student-centered approach with cooperative and interactive inquiry and problem solving.(10)

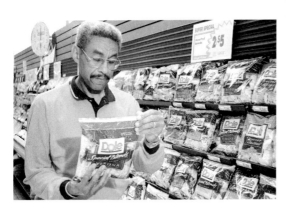

People learn through active involvement.

Other interventions are based in cognition-rational/linguistic learning theory.(10) Experiences become encoded in memory. As a result, people can organize, modify, or combine memories resulting in new knowledge or higher levels of thinking. Reasoning skills allow analysis of experiences and prediction of future outcomes. Most behavior results from the cognitive analysis of knowledge, so thoughts are believed to precede a person's actions.

The consumer information processing theory addresses processes by which a consumer takes in and uses information in decision making. The theory points out that people have a limited capacity to process, store, and retrieve information at any one time. In making decisions, they seek only enough information to make a choice quickly. Thus, information should be organized, limited, and matched to the comprehension level of the individual, who can then process it with little effort. For example, people may look for the frozen dessert with the lowest fat content, store the information about their satisfaction with the product, and decide whether or not to purchase it again.(11)

To enhance memory and reasoning, teaching requires providing labels for new experiences and structures. Problems may be treated as cognitive deficits requiring new structures. Clients with defeating self-statements and cognitive distortions, for example, require cognitive restructuring that rules out the current incorrect structure and introduces a new one (see Chapter 7).

The dietetics professional wants people not only to acquire information, skills, and attitudes, but also to remember them and use them. Since people are bombarded with information all day long from family, friends, coworkers, supervisors, newspapers, magazines, television, and radio, how do they remember it all? They don't. Much is immediately discarded.

Psychologists agree that people must make sense of new information to learn and remember it. Some information enters working or short-term memory until it is used, such as the time of an appointment; then it is forgotten. Of course, nothing even enters short-term memory until the person pays attention to it, that is, focuses on certain stimuli and screens out all others.(3) Therefore, the dietetics professional needs to think first of obtaining and then maintaining a client's or employee's attention. Otherwise, the individual may be thinking about something else.

There are various ways to gain a learner's attention, such as the use of media or bright colors, raising or lowering one's voice, using gestures, starting a discussion with a question, explaining a purpose, repeating information more than once, and saying, "this is important." Gaining someone's interest in a topic at hand and indicating its importance to him or her as well as putting it in the context of what the person already knows is helpful. The professional should try to indicate how it will be useful or important.(3)

Asking questions arouses curiosity and interest. Ask a new employee, "What do you know about the meat slicer?" Or, ask a new client with heart disease, "What do you know about saturated fats?" Ask why they think learning this information is important to them. This forces the person to focus attention.

Working Memory

The human mind is like a computer. It receives information, performs operations on it to change its form and content, stores it, and retrieves it when needed.(3) Not all information or stimuli are selected for further processing, but some is focused on at a given moment.

After the person attends to something new, it enters working memory. There are limits, however, to the amount of new information that can be retained at one time and on the length of time it will be retained, probably 5 to 20 seconds.(3) Repeating something new over and over, such as the name of a person you have just met, helps to keep information longer in short-term memory. But if you meet five new people at once, this can be too much new information to handle. Besides repetition, you may attempt to associate new information with information currently in long-term memory. Chunking, or grouping individual bits of information, also helps. For example, the telephone number 467-3652 becomes 467 36 52. Because of memory limits, it is helpful to give not only oral information, but also a written dietary regimen to a client or a written task analysis to an employee, since details are forgotten quickly.

Long-Term Memory

On a computer a person takes the input and "saves" it onto a diskette or hard drive to be retrieved later. To move new information from working memory to long-term memory, a person tries to organize it and integrate it with information already stored there. Here, the professional needs to make clear to clients and employees what is important and probably repeat it more than once. It takes time and effort to reflect, to grasp the implications, to interpret and experience, and to guide an internal representation of new knowledge in the brain.(3)

The ability to recall rote information is limited, whereas meaningful information is retained more easily. The implication for planning educational sessions for clients and employees is to make the information meaningful to the individual, present it in a clear and organized manner, and relate it to what the individual already knows and has stored in memory. The person can then connect it to other known information and apply it if necessary.

Which is easier to store and later retrieve—something one hears, something one sees, or something one both sees and hears? People retain visual plus verbal images better. Some people use imagery to aid retention by picturing something in the mind.(3, 8) Can you picture the Food Guide Pyramid, for example?

There are various strategies to help people remember. The professional can summarize in the middle and at the end of a presentation. Repetition and review are helpful. You may put an outline on an overhead transparency to organize information. Get people involved talking with active, not passive situations. Present information in a clear, organized fashion, not as isolated bits of information. Then, ask the person to translate the information into his or her own words or solve a problem with it, such as plan a menu.

People also remember stories, metaphors, and examples better than isolated facts. In teaching employees about food sanitation, for example, stories of actual outbreaks of foodborne illness are helpful. When teaching about modified diets, examples of actual client cases may be used. In discussion of fiber with a client, examples of whole grain breads and cereals and fruits and vegetables may be discussed. Learning requires people to make sense of information, to sort it in their minds, to fit it into a neat and orderly pattern, and to use old information to help assimilate the new.

Long-term memory requires connections of new knowledge to known information. Information is probably stored in networks of connected facts and concepts. Each piece of information in our memory is connected to other pieces in some way. We remember things by association. The word "apple," for example, may be associated with fruits, red, or tree. You would be unlikely to associate it with cat.

Following is an example of a partial knowledge network on water-soluble vitamins:

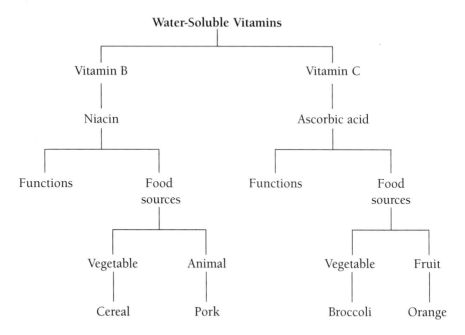

If a person already has the above network and learns something new about vitamin C, such as that raw cabbage is a good food source of vitamin C, it is easy to file it into the existing network by association. If, however, a persons knows nothing about vitamin C, it would be much more difficult to file the new information into long-term memory. The result is that it may be forgotten.

Following is an example of a knowledge network on food sanitation:

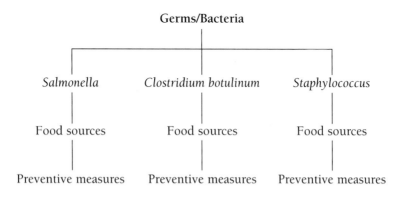

For food service workers, the term "germs" may be more meaningful than "pathogenic bacteria." Probably, they have not heard the term pathogenic bacteria. One wants to add new information to their existing network. If the above is their network, one can more easily add to it a new germ they have not heard of before, such as E. coli (Escherichia coli) or hepatitis A.

Dietetics professionals should spend time finding out what the person already knows, the words he or she uses, and the topics in the knowledge networks; should ask a lot of questions; and should then help the person to link new information into the existing network. Material that is organized well is much easier to learn and remember than material that is poorly organized. Our motivation to learn is intrinsic or internal as we seek to make sense of what is happening in our world.(6)

Organizing around concepts also helps the learner to organize vast amounts of information into meaningful units. Following is an example of organizing around the concept of meals:

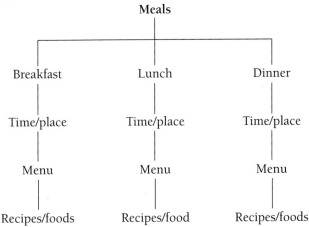

Using questions from time to time helps people learn by asking them to assess their understanding of what they are hearing or reading.

When teaching about concepts, one needs to use a lot of examples. What mental picture or ideas does the client or employee have if the professional discusses "cholesterol," "saturated fatty acids," "blood glucose," "microorganisms," "grams" as a weight, "ounces" of meat, "quality assurance," and the like. Finding out what words people use in the content of their current knowledge network helps in using examples with them.

TRANSFER OF LEARNING

In human resource management as well as in other situations, the question frequently asked is "Did the training transfer?" In other words, can an individual take the knowledge, skills, attitudes, and abilities learned in the training situation, remember them, and apply them effectively on the job in a new situation or in a dissimilar one.(3) Transfer of learning cannot be assumed. It depends partly on the degree of similarity between the situation in which the skill or concept was learned and the situation to which it is applied. The implication is that one should teach people to handle the range of situations that they are likely to encounter most frequently at work (employees) or at home (clients). The practitioner needs to give many examples from the range of problems that the person may encounter in using the knowledge or skills learned.(12) When people do use their new knowledge and skills to solve problems, transfer of training is indicated.

For a client on a modified diet, for example, it is not enough to teach which foods to eat and avoid, but also how to transfer that information into planning menus, reading food labels, adapting current or using new recipes, eating in restaurants or while traveling, and the like. Using knowledge or skills to solve problems, such as what to do in a restaurant, helps people to apply what they learned. Can a person with diabetes, for example, calculate what half of an exchange of fruit is if one exchange of orange juice is one-half cup? Can you? In school, one would multiply $\frac{1}{2} \times \frac{1}{2} = \frac{1}{4}$.

The dietetics professional cannot assume that learning transfers. For employees, it is best to teach them in the actual situation they will encounter. Cashiers, for example, need to be trained on the equipment they will be using as well as how to handle all types of transactions. When training does not transfer to the job, possible reasons are that trainees found the training irrelevant, that they did not retain it, or that the work environment or supervisor does not support the newly learned behavior.(12)

Since most people consider that it is "bad" to be wrong, and "good" to be right, some people may avoid answering questions or solving problems for fear of being wrong, with the psychological discomfort this brings. The implication is that one should handle incorrect answers carefully, with every effort to preserve the person's self-image and avoid making the person feel dumb. If the answer is partially correct, concentrate on that part. If totally wrong, you may say, for example, "Perhaps I did not phrase my question well." Then you can rephrase it. A relaxed atmosphere and a non-critical professional are important.

ANDRAGOGY

Besides behavioral and cognitive theories of learning, others have explored the differences between adults and children as learners. If you as a dietetics professional can explain how adults learn, you should be able to arrange for it to happen. When the dietetics professional accepts responsibility for teaching clients, patients, or employees, it is natural to think back to your own past experiences of being taught. Most educational experiences were the result of pedagogy, which may be defined as the art and science of teaching children.(13, 14) The teacher was an authority figure, and students were dependents who complied with assignments.

Adult education has challenged some of the basic ideas and approaches of pedagogy. Malcolm Knowles has focused attention on beliefs about educating adults, and instead of pedagogy, uses the term "andragogy." He maintains that the basic assumptions regarding adult learners differ from those regarding children. He sees adults as mutual partners in learning.(7) Following are Knowles' major assumptions for adult learners:(13–15)

1. Adults become aware of a *need to know*. They seek to learn what they consider important, not what others think is important.
2. In adulthood, the *self-concept* changes from being a dependent to being a self-directed learner. Adults have autonomy in the learning situation.
3. *Expanding experiences* are a growing resource for learning and can be shared with others.
4. *Readiness to learn* is based on the developmental issues in adults' lives. Learning should be relevant to their needs.

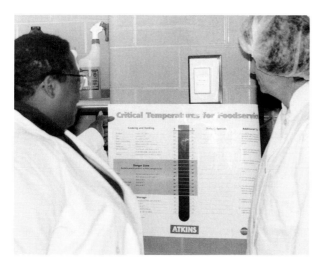

Adults are ready to learn when they have a need for learning.

5. Adult learning is *problem-centered* rather than subject-centered, with a present-oriented focus not a future-oriented focus. Adults pursue learning that can be applied immediately to solve a problem.
6. *Adult motivation* to learn comes more from internal than from external sources.

Need to Know

Before learning something new, adults must become aware of a need to know about it.(13) They need to understand where they are now and see a need to reach a higher level of knowledge or skill. This may, for example, improve the quality of their health and lives. Employees may work more efficiently.

Self-Concept

Childhood is a period of dependency. As a person matures, the self-concept changes, and the individual becomes increasingly independent and self-directed. Eventually, people make their own decisions and manage their lives.(13) Once people become adults, they prefer to be independent and self-directing in learning experiences. Any educational experience in which a person is treated as a dependent child is a threat to the self-concept. Negative feelings may result, and resentment, resistance, or anxiety will interfere with learning.

Experience

Compared with children, adults have more experiences and different kinds of experiences that they bring to new learning situations. This background is a resource for learning. Ignoring the adult's quantity and quality of experiences may be misinterpreted as a sign of rejection. Employees may have had previous work experience which should be referenced.

A client who has had diabetes for 5 years, for example, has a wealth of experience that should be recognized when the dietetics professional discusses dietary changes. To ignore this prior experience and start from the beginning may annoy, bore, or possibly antagonize the client and may place obstacles in the way of the learning process. Teaching methods such as lectures are de-emphasized in adult education in favor of more participatory methods that tap a person's wealth of experience, such as group discussion, problem-solving activities, role playing, simulation, and the like.

Practical applications that apply learning to the individual's day-to-day life are appropriate. Focus group members planning a worksite cholesterol education program, for example, were "adamant about the importance of activities that allowed them to participate actively."(16) They wanted programs on snack ideas, easy breakfasts, dining out, fast foods, brown-bag lunches, easy recipe substitutions, and evaluating cholesterol information. A review of over 200 nutrition education interventions found that the educational process requires active participation and decision making on the part of the learner not only in activities such as food tasting, but also in the analysis of his or her dietary practices and the setting of goals.(2)

Readiness to Learn

Readiness to learn differs for children and adults. Children are assumed to be ready to learn because there are subjects they ought to know about and there are academic pressures from teachers and parents to perform. Adults have no such pressures and are assumed to be ready to learn things required to perform their social roles in life—as spouses, employees, parents, and the like—or to cope more effectively in some aspect of their lives.

Education of adults should be appropriate to the individual's readiness or need to know something, and the timing of learning experiences needs to coincide with readiness. People seek information and are ready to learn when they are confronted by problems that they must solve. For example, new employees may be ready to learn about their job responsibilities, but not necessarily about the history of the company. Clients may not be ready to learn about dietary changes until they have accepted the fact that their medical conditions and future health require it.

Orientation to Learning

A child's learning is oriented toward subjects, whereas an adult's learning is oriented toward performing tasks and solving problems. These different approaches involve different time perspectives. Because children learn about things that they will use some time in the future, the subject matter approach may be appropriate. Adults approach learning when they have an immediate need to learn because of a problem to solve or a task to perform. The implication is that learning should be applied to problems or projects that the person is currently dealing with. Adults learn what they want to learn when they want to learn it, regardless of what others want them to learn.

Motivation

Children are motivated primarily by external pressures from parents and teachers, by competition for grades, and the like. The more potent motivators for adults are internal ones, such as recognition, promotion at work, self-esteem, the desire for a better quality of health and life, and the like.

From an examination of various educational theories, Knowles described the appropriate conditions for learning to take place.(13,14) He suggested that learners should feel the need to learn something and should perceive the goals of any learning experience as their own personal goals. Before undertaking new learning, adults need to know why they need to learn it. Adults should participate actively in planning, implementing, and evaluating learning experiences to increase their commitment to learning, and the process should make use of the person's life experiences. The physical and psychological environment needs to be comfortable, as discussed in the next chapter. The relationship between the professional and the learner should be characterized by mutual trust, respect, and helpfulness, and the environment should encourage freedom of expression and the acceptance of differences.(14)

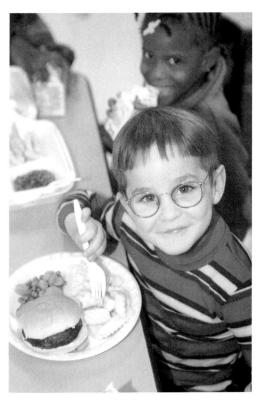

Children learn from experience and the example set by adults.

The professional who accepts the assumptions of andragogy becomes a facilitator of learning or a change agent rather than a teacher. The practitioner involves the learner in the process of learning and provides resources for assisting learners to acquire knowledge, information, and skills, while maintaining a supportive climate for learning.

In summary, there is no single educational theory or model for dietetics practitioners to use to facilitate learning and behavioral change. However, the theory that the professional prefers will undoubtedly influence the way he or she teaches and the relationship with clients and employees. Table **10-2** summarizes the learning theories and strategies. Individuals and groups are more likely to be motivated if the information presented emphasizes the personal consequences of behaviors, as mentioned in the Health Belief Model, and is appropriate to the individual's stage of change. Positive reinforcement appropriate to the needs and interests of the individual should be arranged.(2)

LEARNING STYLES AND TEACHING STYLES

Learning Styles

People have preferred learning styles. People's learning styles play an important role in how effectively they deal with new information. Each of us has a unique learning style and teaching style. Think for a minute about the ways you learn best or how you process and remember new information. If you remember your own school experiences, you preferred some teaching methods to others and processed and retained for a longer period of time material presented in your preferred style.

A unique learning style differentiates people in terms of preferences for content, methods of delivery, learning environment, and teaching techniques. Learning-style preferences are defined as "preferred ways of studying and learning, such as using pictures instead of text, working with other people versus alone, learning in structured or in unstructured situations, and so on."(3) Emphasis is placed on the learner and the learning environment.

Different styles of learning reflect the fact that learners differ in their preferences for and ability to process the content of various instructional messages. Brilliant individuals who do well learning new information from reading, for example, may be all thumbs in a hands-on experience enjoyed by others (tactile learners). Others are visual learners. And some learn well by listening to lectures (auditory learners); those who do not enjoy this method may like learning in a group discussion. Their own discussion can enhance remembering. These preferences influence how easy or difficult learning is for the individual, and therefore they have important implications for educators. They have been described as "hear-learners," who are thinking about the topic at hand; "see-learners"; "feel-learners," who make judgments based on feelings; and "do-learners," who prefer active experimentation.(17)

Components of style that influence learning include cognitive, affective, and environmental factors. Cognitive factors are the person's preferences in thinking and problem solving. Those who think through an experience tend more to abstract dimensions of reality. They reason and analyze what is happening. Others who sense and feel (affective) tend to prefer learning by way of more concrete, actual, hands-on experiences and are more intuitive. Some learn best by thinking through ideas; others learn best by testing theories and learn through self-discovery or by listening and sharing ideas.

In addition to perceiving differently, people process information in different ways. Some are reflective, watching what is happening and thinking about it. Others are doers who prefer to jump right in and try things. In learning to use a computer, for example, some prefer to read the directions first and others just try different things. In a study environment, some require absolute silence to process information, others can block out sound, and still others prefer sound and turn on a radio or stereo when studying and learning. The learner's style preference may vary from situation to situation, affected by the subject matter or skill to be learned.

Learning styles are a function of personality.(18) One's personality can affect the preference for style of intervention. Extroverts, for example, enjoy a group environment for learning, whereas introverts prefer to listen, go away, and try things out. Sensors need facts and details, whereas intuitives prefer the big picture and want to have a hand in getting there. Thinkers like brief, concise, logical information, and feelers want a way to change that won't negatively affect themselves and others. Judgers believe rules give structure to what they do, whereas perceivers find self-monitoring to be too structured.

Instruction can be improved and learners are likely to perform better if the professional identifies the learner's preferred learning style and makes the instructional environment compatible. To measure learning styles, researchers have developed a variety of inventories. Though perhaps helpful, they have been criticized for lacking reliability and validity.(3) Learning preferences may be too complicated for a simple test or inventory.(19)

The instructor can attempt to diagnose learning style by observing how people learn or by asking them questions about their preferences, such as: "Do you prefer to read, to view, to listen, or to have actual experiences?" "Do you prefer to learn alone or in groups?" Whether training employees or designing adult nutrition education programs, professionals should offer new information in a variety of ways, since people learn in different ways—by thinking though ideas reflectively, by hands-on experiences, by solving problems, by experimentation, by trial-and-error, by viewing material, and by self-discovery. Since preferred style varies with the situation, offering alternative techniques and methods that reflect the variety of ways in which people acquire knowledge and skills allows the learners to learn in their preferred mode at least some of the time.

Teaching Style

Teaching style is a related matter that affects learning significantly. Teaching style refers to the sum of what one does as a teacher—the preferred instructional methods, activities, organization of material, interactions with learners, and the like. People may be categorized as either teacher-centered or learner-centered.(20) The teacher-centered approach is associated more with Skinner and assumes that learners are passive and that they respond to stimuli in the environment. In the learner-centered approach, such as Knowles' andragogy, individuals are assumed to be proactive and to take responsibility for their actions. Focus is on the learners and their needs rather than on the subject matter.

Some evidence suggests that teachers tend to select learning activities based on how they themselves prefer to learn, but they should be focusing on the learner's preferred style. Do you teach in the same way you were taught? Do you see yourself as the expert or as a facilitator? Good teachers seek to improve their styles and search for better ways to adapt to the styles of the learners.(19)

DIFFUSION OF INNOVATIONS

The diffusion of innovations theory is important in the larger social environment in the community where people may, for example, rely on the mass media as a source of information. The theory addresses how new ideas and practices are communicated and spread to members of the social system—both planned and spontaneous. The process by which adults adopt new ideas and practices, such as healthy eating patterns, involves five stages in the innovation-decision process:(21)

1. **Knowledge of the innovation**. A person becomes aware of a new idea, practice, or procedure.
2. **Persuasion**. A person forms a favorable or unfavorable attitude toward the innovation based on perceived characteristics of the innovation.
3. **Decision to adopt or reject**. A person engages in activities that lead to a choice to adopt or reject the innovation based on trial.
4. **Implementation of the new idea.** The person puts it into use.
5. **Confirmation of the decision.** A person seeks reinforcement of the decision already made and evaluates it over time.

The nutrition labeling on foods, for example, and the Food Guide Pyramid require a series of steps from knowledge of its existence to forming an attitude about it as a source of information, a decision to adopt or reject its use, implementation and use, and confirmation of continuing. Nutrition education and employee education are incomplete until stage 5 is reached. People learn only what they want to learn and adopt new behaviors to satisfy the basic needs of survival or to achieve some personal goal.

The characteristics of the innovation influence whether or not someone is persuaded in stage 2. Innovations are more readily adopted if they provide a relative advantage over current practices; if they are compatible with current beliefs, values, habits, and practices; if they are simple (complexity) to understand and to do; if they can be tried (trialability); and if results can be observed (observability).(22)

CASE STUDY 1

"I am about ready to give up on this batch of new trainees," Ross said to his boss in frustration.

"I thought you liked training the entry-level employees, Ross," replied Bob, the Department Director.

"I do, but it seems as if this latest batch of trainees just is not retaining the information. Now they get 2 additional days of classroom training before going on-the-job for a total of 5 days of instruction. Before I changed the program they only got 3 days of classroom training and then 2 days on-the-job. They have 2 extra days of lecture now. I just don't understand what is wrong with these people."

1. Where is the problem: with the trainees, the trainer, or the training program?
2. What impact did changing the training schedule have on the trainees?
3. How should a training program be designed to provide more effective results?

CASE STUDY 2

John Richards has been referred for counseling because of his high blood pressure. He is 65 years old and of normal weight with normal serum cholesterol. Six months ago, his wife died and he lives alone in the family home. His physician recommended a diet restricted in sodium with an increase in fruits and vegetables. If dietary changes are successful, he may not need medication.

1. What types of things would you ask Mr. Richards about before educating him on the dietary changes he needs to make?
2. What principles from the chapter would you use to help his memory of the changes you plan to tell him about?

It may be unrealistic to expect new behaviors to be adopted from short-term educational endeavors. A dietary program with the achievement of one or two goals for change rather than total change may not be what the professional considers best, but limited benefits may be preferable to total abandonment of the dietary regimen.

Other comprehensive community-based planning systems, such as Social Marketing and the Precede-Proceed Model can be found in the literature.(5,23)

REVIEW AND DISCUSSION QUESTIONS

1. Compare and contrast the behavioral and cognitive theories of learning in terms of what is learned, the role of reinforcement, and the like.
2. Explain the four types of consequences and their effect on behaviors.
3. What effect does the timing of reinforcement have?
4. How can you encourage persistence in a client's or employee's behavior?
5. What is modeling?
6. How can you reinforce yourself after reading this chapter?
7. Can you remember today anything you learned yesterday?
8. What makes information easy for you to learn and remember?
9. What strategies enhance long-term memory?
10. How do adults differ as learners from children?
11. What steps are involved in adopting innovations?
12. What are learning styles and teaching styles?

SUGGESTED ACTIVITIES

1. Match these types of consequences with the examples A. through C following them:

   _____positive reinforcement

   _____negative reinforcement

   _____punishment

   A. "With the diet you are on, you should know better than to eat fried chicken and French fries."
   B. "Employees who learn the new procedures this afternoon will not have to take any work home to study this evening."
   C. "Congratulations on your success. I'm proud of you."
2. Extinction occurs as a result of which of the following?
   A. Not rewarding a response.
   B. Punishing a response.
3. According to cognitive learning theory, which of the following statements is true?
   A. Learning involves associations that are arbitrary.
   B. Learning involves specific information being organized into more generalized categories.
   C. Learning involves observing and modeling after others.

4. Cognitive educators believe that
   A. New information and knowledge should be presented in an organized fashion considering prior knowledge.
   B. New knowledge and information should be presented separately from prior knowledge.
   C. It does not matter how new knowledge is presented as long as rewards are given.
5. Discuss in small groups each person's examples of experiences with positive reinforcement, negative reinforcement, punishment, and extinction.
6. Discuss in groups the techniques or methods that individuals use in enhancing their memories of new information.
7. Discuss in groups the individuals' learning styles and environments people prefer for learning.

WEB SITES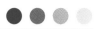

http://tip.psychology.org/theories.html / **learning theory links**
www.learningstyles.org / **Institute for Learning Styles Research**
www.learningstyles.org/survey/index.html / **Perceptual Modality Preference Survey**
www.premiumhealth.com/memory/links.htm / **resources on memory**
www.demon.co.uk/mindtool/memory.html / **memory techniques**

REFERENCES

1. Position of the American Dietetic Association: Nutrition education for the public. 1996;96:1183.
2. Contento I, Balch GI, Bronner YL, et al. Chapter 5. Nutrition education for adults. J Nutr Ed 1995;27:312.
3. Woolfolk AE. Educational psychology, 8th ed. Boston: Allyn & Bacon, 2001.
4. Glanz K, Lewis FM, Rimer BK, eds. Health behavior and health education: theory, research, and practice. San Francisco: Jossey-Bass, 1997.
5. Glanz K, Rimer BK. Theory at a glance: a guide for health promotion practice. National Cancer Institute, US Dept Health & Human Services, 1995.
6. Caine G, Caine RN. The brain, education, and the competitive edge. Latham, MD: Scarecrow Press, 2001.
7. Merriam SB, Caffarella RS. Learning in adulthood: a comprehensive guide, 2nd ed. San Francisco: Jossey-Bass, 1999.
8. Elliott SN, Kratochwill TR, Littlefield J, Travers JF. Educational psychology, 2nd ed. Madison, WI: Brown & Benchmark, 1996.
9. Gerber S. Where has our theory gone? Learning theory and intentional intervention. J Counsel Dev 2001;79:282.
10. Rankin SH, Stallings KD. Patient education: principles & practice. Philadelphia: Lippincott Williams & Wilkins, 2001.
11. Glanz K. Current theoretical bases for nutrition intervention and their uses. In: Coulston AM, Rock CL, Monsen ER, eds. Nutrition in the prevention and treatment of disease. San Diego: Academic Press, 2001.
12. Wexley KN, Latham GP. Developing and training human resources in organizations. Englewood Cliffs, NJ: Prentice Hall, 2002.

13. Knowles MS, Holton EF, Swanson RA. The adult learner: the definitive classic in adult education and human resource development, 5th ed. Houston: Gulf Publishing Company, 1998.
14. Knowles MS. The modern practice of adult education. New York: Association Press, 1970.
15. Knowles MS. Andragogy in action. San Francisco: Jossey-Bass, 1984.
16. McCarthy PR, Lansing D, Hartman TJ, Himes JH. What works best for worksite cholesterol education? Answers from targeted focus groups. J Am Diet Assoc 1992;92:978.
17. Heffler B. Individual learning style and the learning style inventory. Educ Studies 2001;27:307.
18. Wennik RS. Changes from within: improving lifestyle habits using personality type. J Am Diet Assoc 1999;99:666.
19. Apps JW. Mastering the teaching of adults. Malabar, FL: Krieger Publishing Company, 1991.
20. Conti GJ. Identifying your teaching style. In: MW Galbraith, ed. Adult learning methods: a guide for effective instruction, 2nd ed. Malabar, FL: Krieger Publishing Company, 1998.
21. Rogers EM. Diffusion of innovations, 4th ed. New York: Free Press, 1995.
22. Oldenburg B, Hardcastle DM, Kok G. Diffusion of innovations. In: Glanz K, Lewis FM, Rimer BK, eds. Health behavior and health education: theory, research, and practice. San Francisco: Jossey-Bass, 1997.
23. Gielen AC, McDonald EM. The Precede-Proceed Planning Model. In: Glanz K, Lewis FM, Rimer BK, eds. Health behavior and health education: theory, research, and practice. San Francisco: Jossey-Bass, 1997.

Planning Learning

It is the position of the American Dietetic Association (ADA) that optimal nutrition and physical activity can promote health and reduce the risk of chronic disease.

Journal of the American Dietetic Association 1998;98:205

To prepare future practitioners for their role in nutrition education, health promotion, and disease prevention, the American Dietetic Association (ADA) requires educational programs to include competencies in nutrition education. For dietitians and dietetic technicians, these include knowledge of educational theory and techniques, methods of teaching, and the use of oral and written communications in presenting an educational session for a group. Since up to 50% of chronic disease mortality can be attributed to lifestyle factors that can be changed, the dietetics professional must be competent in planning and implementing appropriate interventions.(1)

The previous chapter examined principles and theories of education. Dietetics practitioners draw on educational theory and models of human behavioral change to plan, implement, and evaluate educational interventions and programs to measure their effectiveness.(2) Other chapters discuss nutrition counseling approaches that seek to change eating behaviors. During every counseling session, the dietetics professional has the opportunity to provide information to clients about some aspect of food and nutrition important to the informed decisions of the individual.

TEACHING, LEARNING, AND EDUCATION

Teaching is a major job responsibility of all dietetics professionals whether they specialize in clinical, community, education, consultation, or management areas of practice. Health care facilities accredited by the Joint Commission on Accreditation of Healthcare Organizations (JCAHO), the largest health care accrediting body in the United States, are required to provide the patient, family, and/or significant others with education specific to their needs and to document in the medical record.(3,4) Practitioners are expected to be effective teachers. Chambers noted that "a well-informed and well-intentioned dietitian who lacks the communication skills necessary for effective nutrition instruction is not competent."(5)

Where do we teach? We teach one-on-one or in groups both in formal and informal settings. The locations may be a health care setting—either inpatient or outpatient—long-term care facility, home care, public health and government programs such as WIC (Women, Infants and Children), food industry, academia, worksites, schools, health clubs, supermarkets, internet, media, health fairs, and community programs.

Whom do we teach? Besides patients, clients, and employees, we teach parents, caregivers, family members, health care professionals, such as nurses and physicians, students, interns and residents, teachers, paraprofessionals, therapists, health department personnel, athletes, consumers, food service personnel, and the public.(6)

In the workplace, managers are expected to provide dietetics and food service staff with the information they need to succeed through training, continuing education, and staff development.(7) Many practitioners are responsible for the supervision of employees. Human resource orientation, training, and development programs are necessary for these subordinates. The goal of training is to have employees know their job responsibilities and to update knowledge and skills. An employee's on-the-job performance must meet standards acceptable to the organization, and it is the responsibility of the manager to ensure that training needs are recognized and met. The fact that an employee knows proper procedures, but may not always follow them, is an indication of the difficulty involved in getting a person to change.

In the patient care arena, dietetics professionals educate clients and patients about normal nutrition and about diet modifications necessitated by such medical problems as cardiovascular disease and diabetes. The professional may one day be teaching a 50-year-old man about fatty acids and cholesterol in foods, the next day teaching an 18-year-old pregnant woman about prenatal nutrition, and the next day teaching an athlete about nutritional needs before, during, and after exercise. Nutrition education cannot improve a person's health unless the results influence the purchase and consumption of foods and beverages and change eating behaviors.

Nutrition education has been defined as, "a process by which we assist people in making decisions regarding their eating practices by applying knowledge from nutrition science about the relationship between diet and health."(8) Some clients have considerable dietary knowledge. Others may need to know that food choices are related to health; that improving choices can benefit health; that changes can be made without disrupting the family; and that eating still can be pleasurable.(9)

Nutrition education has also been defined as "any set of learning experiences designed to facilitate the voluntary adoption of eating and other nutrition-related behaviors conducive to health and well-being."(10) Patient and client education focuses on "self-management" training that promotes independent living. It is the cornerstone of medical nutrition therapy for individuals. Ongoing nutrition self-management education is recommended for individuals with diabetes as well as for those other medical problems.(11) The professional assists people to develop the knowledge, skills, and motivation necessary for making appropriate decisions about healthful food choices to promote optimum health.

The goal of nutrition education is to influence people to change to more healthful diets and ultimately to sustain behavioral change.(12) The practitioner provides information to increase people's knowledge and skills but also assists individuals to integrate this knowledge into new attitudes, dietary choices, and behaviors in their total environment. Improved dietary behaviors can reduce the risk of chronic diseases as well as improve nutritional adequacy, health, and well-being. The changes may sound simple: to decrease consumption of certain foods (such as fats and oils), to increase consumption of others (fruits, vegetables, and whole grains), to shop for different foods (reduced in fat), to read food labels (for fat, calories, sodium, fiber, and so on), to change cooking methods (bake instead of fry), to order different foods at a restaurant (baked potato instead of French fries), and the like. But these changes are not simple to accomplish. They are complex!

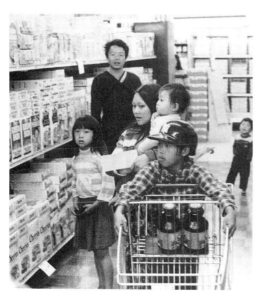

Cultural and ethnic groups may have different needs for learning.

The internal and external forces that shape people's eating habits are long-standing and create barriers to successful, long-term change. Nevertheless, the ultimate criterion for nutrition education effectiveness is behavioral change in food and health habits. The dietetics professional must be a facilitator of positive behavioral change in the educational process. Studies have found that interventions that used educational methods directed at establishing goals for behavioral change were more successful than those directed at disseminating information with the assumption that the information would lead to changes in behaviors and attitudes.(10)

The terms "teaching" and "learning" have different meanings. Some people have the mistaken notion that if they teach something, the audience or individual learns automatically and will transfer the learning to appropriate situations. The practitioner may teach a pregnant woman about the Food Guide Pyramid, for example, tell her why it is important to use in menu planning, and give her printed handouts. A passive learner who has not participated actively in the learning may not make any connection between what was taught and her own food choices or menu planning. Knowledge alone cannot guarantee a change in food choices.

To change behavior, dietetics professionals should endeavor to motivate and further the adoption of better practices. Although knowledge is a prerequisite for change, knowledge in itself does not lead to a different behavior. Research has shown that knowledge accounts for "4% to 8% of the variance in eating behavior, leaving 92% to 96% of the behavior to be accounted for by other influences."(13) Knowledge may be modified by psychosocial, cultural, and environment barriers that weaken dietary change.(14) A person may be knowledgeable about a healthy diet but lack commitment or perseverance. A client may be familiar with the sodium-restricted diet, for example, but still may consume salted pretzels.

Teaching factual information should not be mistaken for education. The term "teaching" suggests the educator's assessment of the need for knowledge and the use of techniques to transfer knowledge to another person. Education is the process of imparting or acquiring knowledge or skills in the context of the person's total matrix of living. Education should assist people in coping with their problems and challenges as they adapt to circumstances.

Learning refers to the cognitive process through which people acquire and store knowledge, attitudes, or skills and change their behavior owing to an educational experience. The change in behavior may be related to knowledge, attitudes, beliefs, values, skills, or performance.

Government agencies are a source of much health information that is useful to us in educating others.(15,16) Government provides science-based nutrition, food, and health guidance to the public. Examples are the Food and Drug Administration (FDA) Nutrition Facts Label on foods, the US Department of Agriculture (USDA) Food Guide Pyramid and Dietary Guidelines for Americans, and the National Institutes of Health (NIH) National Cholesterol Education Program materials, and others. There are also public-private partnerships, such as the 5-a-Day for Better Health campaign that follows the principles of social marketing theory, as well as information from industry and trade groups.(2) Relevant websites are listed at the end of this chapter.

ENVIRONMENT FOR LEARNING

An educational environment has two components: the psychological environment and the physical environment. Both are important to enhancing teaching and learning.

Psychological Environment

The psychological climate for learning is important, and it is determined by the approach of the dietetics professional. A supportive and friendly environment with a tolerance for mistakes and a respect for individual and cultural differences makes people feel secure and welcome. Openness and encouragement of questions create an informal atmosphere. People should be known by their names, and respect for their opinions should be demonstrated.

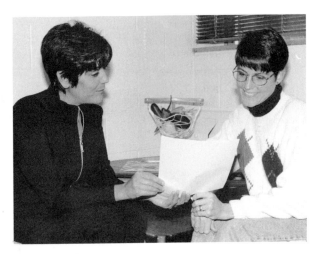

One should create an environment conducive to learning.

In group teaching of clients or employees, participants should be encouraged to introduce themselves and to get to know one another at the first session. Collaboration and mutual assistance rather than competition should be promoted, and initial feelings of anxiety should be minimized to promote learning. The professional who creates this informal, supportive, and caring environment for adult learners can obtain better results than one who creates a formal, authoritative environment. Since some adults have negative memories of their early experiences in school—for example, if they were disrespected or failed classes—a physical or psychological climate that reminds them of their past unpleasant experiences will create barriers to learning.(17)

Physical Environment

Comfort should be provided with appropriate temperature, good lighting, ventilation, and comfortable chairs to create conditions that promote learning rather than inhibit it. Noise from a radio, television, telephone, or people talking may be distracting and may interfere with a client's, patient's, or employee's attention. People should be able to both see and hear. Interaction is facilitated by seating groups of people in a circle or around a table where everyone has eye contact, rather than seating people in row upon row of chairs.

The remainder of this chapter includes a model or framework for planning, implementing, and evaluating learning. The first three steps, which are (1) preassessment of the learner or needs assessment, (2) planning performance objectives, and (3) determination of the content, are examined along with information on grouping people together for learning. (Discussion of the additional steps in the learning process follows in Chapter 12.)

STEPS TO EDUCATION

Successful educational efforts that meet the needs of the adult learner include a number of interactive steps. The framework and components are as follows:

1. Assessment of the needs of the individual or group
2. Planning of performance objectives that are measurable and feasible and can be accomplished in a stated period of time considering the domains of learning

3. Determination of the content based on the preassessment and the objectives
4. Selection of methods, techniques, materials, and resources appropriate to the objectives and the individual or group
5. Implementation of the learning experiences (intervention) and provision of opportunities for the person to practice new information
6. Evaluation of progress and outcomes performed continuously and at stated intervals, including rediagnosis of learning needs
7. Documentation of the outcomes and results of education

NEEDS ASSESSMENT

The first step in education is to conduct a preassessment or needs assessment with the client or employee. (Nutritional assessment is discussed in Chapter 3). *Preassessment* is a diagnostic evaluation performed by gathering data before instruction for the purpose of establishing a starting point. It serves to classify people regarding their current knowledge, skills, abilities, aptitudes, interests, personality, educational level, degree of literacy, age, gender, occupation, culture, lifestyle, health problem, and psychological readiness to learn. Each person is unique. Also assessed is the Stage of Change according to the model in Chapter 5.

Previous information learned must be assessed to determine the current level of knowledge or skill. A need for learning may be defined as a gap between what people know now and what they should know as well as the difference between how employees should perform and how they actually do perform or what they are doing.

| Desired knowledge, skill, attitude, or performance | − | Current knowledge, skill, attitude, or performance | = | Need for learning |

If preassessment determines that a person already has some prior knowledge and experience, such as a client with long-term diabetes who knows how to count carbohydrates, more advanced material is indicated. Determine in advance how much the person already knows, since it would waste everyone's time to repeat known information and could lead to boredom or lack of attention on the part of the learner. A number of questions need to be asked. Does the client have the intellectual skills and reading skills to understand the instruction? Educational planning should be based on the dietetics professional's preassessment of the client's or employee's knowledge, skills, ability, and lifestyle factors, compared with what the practitioner thinks the individual needs to know or do.

In determining what the person already knows, preassessment may be handled by oral interviewing. You may inquire: "Have you been on a diet before?" "Can you tell me what foods are good sources of potassium?" "Can you explain the relationship between your diet and your health?" "What foods are high in sodium? Fat?" The line of questioning should be based on what the person needs to know or would like to know. Interviewing may be used with employees as well. "Have you ever used a meat slicer before?" "Can you show me how you set tables at the restaurant where you worked previously?"

Psychological preassessment is also necessary because the dietetics professional must understand the client's or employee's attitudes toward health and nutrition, willingness to change, motivation, and readiness to learn, which influence his or her behavior. Attitudes are thought to be predispositions for action and change. Despite our efforts, people often do not make the changes recommended by health professionals. Problems may not be caused by deficits in knowledge, but the cause and solution may be found in the affective domain or in the individual's attitudes, values, and beliefs.

Eating behaviors are the result of many motivations, and having nutrition information does not necessarily mean that it will be applied to better food choices.(2) For example, the hospitalized patient who has just learned of a confirmed diagnosis of chronic illness is unlikely to learn much about medical nutrition therapy at that moment. The patient may be thinking: "Why me?" "What did I do to deserve this?" "How will this affect my job? My lifestyle? My marriage?"

A new employee may feel high levels of anxiety that may interfere with learning for the first few days on the job. Anxiety may arise whenever a superior trains a subordinate. "What does the superior think about me?" "I will appear to be dumb if I don't understand, so I had better pretend I do understand." These feelings are barriers to learning that must be recognized, reduced, or eliminated before teaching.

Motivation can enhance learning and behavior change as well as be a consequence of it.(17) The practitioner or environment is the source of extrinsic rewards, such as positive reinforcement or praise from the counselor, family, or friends, or a promotion or salary increase for an employee. Adults, however, are highly pragmatic learners wanting practical information leading to knowledge or skill about how to do something that they find important and value. Their interest, voluntary involvement, and persistence are measures of intrinsic motivation to learn. To tap into clients' intrinsic motivations, the dietetics professional must first seek to understand their environment, attitudes, values, and needs. The reader should refer to other chapters that discuss motivation in more detail.

In more formal situations, a preassessment questionnaire or test may be developed and administered. The purpose of a test is to evaluate the person's knowledge and capabilities before instruction begins and to identify what the person already knows. Pretest results may be compared later with post-test results after instruction has been completed. Preassessment is most necessary when the dietetics professional is unfamiliar with the knowledge, ability, and values of the client, patient, or employee. At the community level, a survey questionnaire, a focus group, or a telephone interview survey may be used. The focus group interview technique was useful, for example, in determining preferred methods for receiving nutrition information of low-income women.(18) (More information on focus groups is in Chapter 12.)

In business, training and development programs are planned to meet current and future goals and objectives of the organization. Training provides specific skills under the guidance of established personnel so that employees meet quality standards acceptable to the organization. Training is needed, for example, by new employees and by current employees accepting new assignments, such as after a promotion or transfer. A need for training is described as the difference between a person's actual and desired knowledge, skill, or performance or the gap between current and desired results.(19)

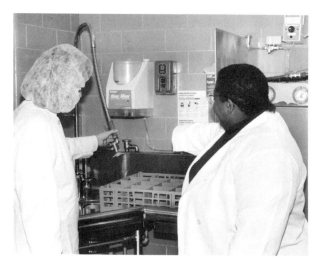

Training needs assessment may be handled in a number of ways, for example, by directly observing the work; by structured interviewing of managers or employees about needs and problems; by seeing what is done correctly and especially what is not; by examining reports of accidents, incidents, grievances, turnover, productivity, and quality control and assurance; and by administering employee attitude surveys.(20) You may ask: "What are the knowledge, skills, abilities, and attitudes that employ-

Objectives for learning should be planned around what the employee needs to know.

ees need to perform their jobs successfully?" This assessment deals with ends, not the means to the ends, which are selected later.

PERFORMANCE OBJECTIVES

Developing precise statements can help to organize one's thinking regarding the purpose of instruction, that is, what is to be learned. The professional needs to decide what is to be learned before selecting the optimal methods, techniques, and tools to accomplish it. References to statements are found in the literature under the terms "behavioral objectives," and "measurable objectives." The term "performance objectives" is used in this chapter. Written performance objectives are helpful tools in planning, implementing, and evaluating learning.

A well-stated performance objective communicates the intended outcome of instruction for the patient, client, employee, or audience. It specifies the people's behavior or degree of competence after instruction is complete. Writing performance objectives has many advantages. It results in less ambiguity regarding what is to be learned. Also, clear performance objectives make it possible to design and implement instruction, select appropriate instructional materials, and assess or evaluate whether or not the objectives are achieved. Both the practitioner and the individual benefit from clearer instructions. When people know what they are supposed to learn, it does not come as a surprise. They should not be kept guessing about what should be learned or about what is important. This is a waste of their time. More broad-scope goals may also be written for a whole program.

Thus, initial effort is devoted to delineating the tangible outcome of instruction for the individual or what he or she will be able to do, rather than to the methods or processes of learning. First, define the ends and then explore the means to the ends.

The statement specifies the desired behavior of the trainee at the end of training, that is, what the trainee will know or be able to do after participating. If clear, measurable objectives are not known, the professional cannot select content or materials for instruction. You cannot select an educational video, for example, without knowing what it is to accomplish. As pointed out by Robert Mager, "if you're not sure where you're going, you're liable to end up someplace else."(21)

Objectives should focus on the person learning, not on the health educator. The following objective is poorly stated: "The dietetics professional will teach the client about his diet." Note that this statement focuses on what the practitioner will do and not on what the client or learner will do. The following is preferred because it focuses on the client: "After instruction [when], the client [who] will be able to plan appropriate menus using the sodium-restricted diet as a reference [what]."

Mager wrote one of the most useful guides for writing performance objectives.(21) A key to writing measurable performance objectives is the selection of the verb that describes the desired outcome. Some verbs are vague and subject to misinterpretation, as in the following objectives:

To know (is able to know which foods contain potassium)

To understand (is able to understand that foods high in potassium should be consumed daily when certain medications are prescribed)

To appreciate (is able to appreciate the importance of following the dietary instructions)

In the written objective for "to know," it is not clear whether "knowing" means that the client will purchase foods high in potassium, be able to tell a friend which foods are high in potassium, or recognize them on a list. "Understanding" could mean being able to recall reasons, being able to read an article about it, or being able to apply knowledge to one's own situation. The meanings of knowing, understanding, and appreciating are vague and unclear.

Instead, select verbs that describe what the person is able to do after learning has taken place. Note that the phrase "after learning [when], the individual [who] is able to [do what]" is understood to precede the phrase, since one is describing what the person will be capable of doing. Another method involves starting with the action verb. The first two examples are rewritten from the unsatisfactory objectives in the previous list. Better verbs to use are summarized in Table 11-1 and include the following:

To recall (is able to name five good food sources of potassium)

To explain (is able to explain why foods high in potassium should be consumed)

To write (is able to list the groups in the Food Guide Pyramid)

To compare (is able to compare the nutrient needs of an adult woman with those of a pregnant woman)

To identify (is able to identify on the menu those foods which are permitted)

To solve or use (is able to plan menus including five servings of fruits and vegetables daily)

TABLE 11-1	Verbs Describing Performance

Verbs to Use

analyze	discuss	prepare
apply	distinguish	produce
assemble	evaluate	recall
calculate	explain	recite
cite	identify	recognize
classify	illustrate	recommend
compare	interpret	repair
complete	list	select
construct	measure	solve
contrast	name	state
define	operate	summarize
demonstrate	plan	use
describe	practice	write

Vague Verbs

appreciate	feel	learn
believe	grasp	like
comprehend	hope	realize
discern	know	understand

To demonstrate (is able to demonstrate the use of the mixer or is able to select low-fat foods at the grocery store)

To operate (is able to slice meat on the meat slicer)

Mager noted that three characteristics improve written objectives: (1) performance, (2) conditions, and (3) criterion.(21) The "performance" tells what the learner will be able to do after instruction is given. The second characteristic describes under what "conditions" the performance is to occur. Finally, a "criterion" tells how good the individual's performance must be to be acceptable. Table 11-2 summarizes the three-part system for writing objectives. Conditions and criterion may not be included in all objectives. In general, the more that can be specified, the better the objective and the more likely that the patient, client, or employee will learn what the dietetics professional intends.

Performance

The performance component of an objective describes the activity that the individual will be doing. The performance may be visible or heard, such as listing, reciting, explaining, or operating equipment, or invisible, such as identifying or solving a problem. Although overt or visible performance may be seen or heard directly, invisible or covert performance requires that the individual be asked to do something visible or audible to determine whether the objective is satisfied and learning has taken

TABLE 11-2 Mager's Three-Part System for Objectives: Client and Employee Examples

Part	Question	Client Example
Learner behavior	Do what?	Plans a menu for a day
Conditions	Under what conditions?	Given a list of permitted foods
Criterion	How well?	With no errors

Part	Question	Employee Example
Learner behavior	Do what?	Measures sanitizer in a bucket
Conditions	Under what conditions?	When cleaning the work area
Criterion	How well?	Using the exact concentration recommended

place. In invisible performance, one adds an "indicator behavior" to the objective, for example:

Is able to identify the parts of the meat slicer (on a diagram or verbally)

Is able to plan a day's menu based on the Food Guide Pyramid

Identifying is invisible until the learner is asked to identify the parts on a diagram or to recite them verbally, which are indicator behaviors. The major intent or performance should be stated using an active verb, and an indicator should be added if the performance cannot be seen or heard.

Conditions

Once the performance is clearly stated, you may ask whether or not there are specific circumstances or conditions under which the performance will be observed. The conditions describe the setting, equipment, or aids associated with the behavior. With what resources will the individual be provided? What will be withheld? Conditions are in parentheses in the following examples:

(Given the disassembled parts of a meat slicer) is able to reassemble the parts in correct sequence.

(Given a standard menu) is able to calculate the appropriate carbohydrate in the foods.

(Given a list of foods including both good and poor sources of potassium) is able to identify the good sources.

(Given a standard menu) is able to select low-sodium foods for a complete day.

(Without looking at the diet instruction form) is able to describe an appropriate dinner menu.

(Without the assistance of the practitioner) is able to explain the foods a pregnant woman should eat on a daily basis.

Although every objective may not have conditions, there should be enough information to make clear exactly what performance is expected.

Criterion

Once the end performance is described and the conditions, if any, under which it will be observed, a criterion may or may not be added. The criterion describes a level of achievement, that is, how well the individual should be able to perform. Possible standards for measuring performance include speed, accuracy, quality, and percentage of correct answers.(21) A time limit can be used to describe the speed criterion. The following are examples:

Is able to type (50 words per minute)

Is able to reassemble the meat slicer (in 5 minutes or less)

Is able to complete a diet history (in 20 minutes)

For objectives that require the development of skill over a period of time, you must determine how much time is reasonable in the initial learning period as opposed to the time when the skill is well developed. A new employee cannot be expected to perform a task as rapidly as an experienced person.

Another standard is accuracy. Accuracy should communicate how well the person needs to perform for his or her performance to be considered competent. Examples include:

Is able to type 50 words per minute (with 5 errors or less)

Is able to identify good sources of potassium (with 80% accuracy), when given a list of foods including both good and poor sources

Is able to plan a menu for a complete day (with no errors) when given a copy of a sodium-restricted diet

Is able to calculate the carbohydrate in the diabetic diet (within 5 grams)

When the person is expected to perform with a degree of accuracy, include this in the objective.

The dietetics professional should also examine quality to assess what constitutes an acceptable performance. It is easier to communicate quality when objective standards are available to both the individual and the practitioner. Any acceptable deviation from the standards can then be determined. The following are examples of such standards:

Is able to reassemble the meat slicer (according to the steps in the task analysis)

Is able to measure the amount of sanitizer (according to the directions on the label of the container)

Is able to substitute foods on a diabetic menu (using carbohydrate counting)

In these examples, the quality of performance has been stated according to a known standard.

SELF ASSESSMENT

Plan several performance objectives for clients or employees including some with conditions and criteria.

DOMAINS OF LEARNING

Learning encompasses knowledge, attitudes, and skills. After developing skill in writing measurable performance objectives, consider the range of learning objectives that may be written. Objectives have been organized into domains, taxonomies, or classification systems to focus on precision in writing, and you may examine the range of possible outcomes desired from instruction. There are three basic types of objectives: (1) cognitive (knowledge), (2) affective (attitudes and values), and (3) psychomotor (skills). Each is a hierarchy from the simple to the complex. Figure 11-1 shows their interrelationship.

Cognitive Domain

A taxonomy of educational objectives in the cognitive domain was published by Bloom and colleagues.(22) The cognitive domain involves the acquisition and utilization of knowledge or information and the development of intellectual skills and abilities. The cognitive domain has six major levels or categories and a number of subcategories as shown in the following:

1.0 KNOWLEDGE
    1.1 Knowledge of specifics
    1.2 Knowledge of ways and means of dealing with specifics
    1.3 Knowledge of the universals and abstractions in a field
2.0 COMPREHENSION
    2.1 Translation
    2.2 Interpretation
    2.3 Extrapolation
3.0 APPLICATION
4.0 ANALYSIS
    4.1 Analysis of elements
    4.2 Analysis of relationships
    4.3 Analysis of organizational principles

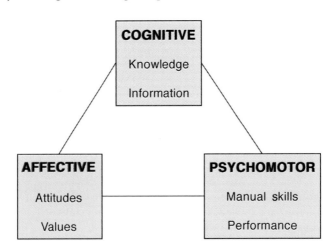

Figure 11-1 **THE INTERRELATIONSHIP OF OBJECTIVES.**

5.0 SYNTHESIS
    5.1 Production of a unique communication
    5.2 Production of a plan, or proposed set of operations
    5.3 Derivation of a set of abstract relations
6.0 EVALUATION
    6.1 Judgments in terms of internal evidence
    6.2 Judgments in terms of external criteria

The classes are arranged in a hierarchy from simple to complex, from concrete to more abstract. The objectives in any one class are likely to be built on the behaviors in the previous class. The subcategories help to define further the major headings and make them more specific.

The dietetics professional needs to think beyond the simplest levels of knowledge and also to write objectives at higher, more complex levels. Without examining the possibility of writing higher-level objectives, you may tend to think only in terms of knowledge and comprehension, which are the easiest objectives to write. The client or employee may then be denied the opportunity of applying knowledge or using it in problem solving and will be reduced to memorizing facts. In nutrition education, for example, knowing facts is necessary, but the client also needs the ability to analyze food labels, to synthesize all information learned so that she may tell others about it, and to evaluate nutritional information in making wise food choices. In the following discussion of the six levels in the taxonomy, examples of objectives are given.

Knowledge

At the lowest levels in the cognitive domain, knowledge involves the remembering and recall of information without necessarily understanding it. This includes the recall of specific bits of information, terminology, and facts, such as dates, events, and places, chronological sequences, methods of inquiry, trends over time, processes, classification systems, criteria, principles, and theories. Table 11-3 suggests verbs describing performance in the cognitive domain.

    EXAMPLE: *Is able to list foods high in sodium.*

Comprehension

The second level, comprehension, is the lowest level of understanding. It involves knowing what is communicated by another person and being able to use the information communicated. The use of information may include restatement or paraphrase, interpretation, summarization or rearrangement of the information, and extrapolation or extension of the given information to determine implications or consequences.

    EXAMPLE: *Is able to explain (verbally or in writing) why certain foods are not recommended on the diabetic diet.*

Application

At the level of application, a person is able to use information, principles, concepts, or ideas in concrete situations. Knowledge is understood sufficiently to be able to apply it to solve a problem.

    EXAMPLE: *Is able to plan a sodium-restricted menu for the day.*

TABLE 11-3   Verbs Describing Performance—Cognitive

Level	Verbs to Use
Knowledge	cites, defines, describes, identifies, labels, lists, matches, memorizes, names, outlines, recalls, recites, repeats, reproduces, selects, states
Comprehension	converts, defends, discusses, distinguishes, estimates, explains, generalizes, gives examples, paraphrases, predicts, recognizes, rewrites, selects, summarizes, translates
Application	applies, assembles, calculates, changes, computes, demonstrates, designs, manipulates, modifies, operates, plans, practices, prepares, produces, shows, solves, translates, uses
Analysis	analyzes, compares, differentiates, discriminates, distinguishes, identifies, illustrates, interprets, investigates, outlines, relates, researches, separates, solves, studies
Synthesis	assembles, categorizes, classifies, combines, compiles, composes, creates, designs, diagnoses, explains, formulates, generates, manages, organizes, plans, recommends, revises, rewrites, summarizes, writes
Evaluation	assesses, appraises, compares, concludes, contrasts, criticizes, critiques, discriminates, evaluates, judges, justifies

Analysis

Analysis entails the breakdown of information into its parts to identify the elements, the interaction between elements, and the organizing principles or structure. Relationships may be made among ideas.

> E X A M P L E : *Is able to analyze the nutrition labeling on a food product for fat content.*

Synthesis

Synthesis requires the reassembling of elements or parts to form something new. You may assemble a unique verbal or written communication, a plan of operation, or a set of abstract relations to explain data.

> E X A M P L E : *Is able to explain the low-cholesterol diet accurately to a friend.*

Evaluation

At the highest level in the cognitive taxonomy, evaluation is the ability to judge the value of materials or methods in a particular situation. Such judgment requires the use of criteria, which may be internal criteria, such as logical accuracy or consistency, or external criteria, such as external standards.

> E X A M P L E : *Is able to evaluate a nutrition article from the daily newspaper.*

Affective Domain

The affective domain deals with changes in attitudes, feelings, values, beliefs, appreciation, and interests. Often, the dietetics professional wants a client or employee not only to comprehend what to do, but also to value it, accept it, and find it important. Attitudes and beliefs about food are widely recognized as important determinants of a person's food choices, and we want people to value good nutrition and select healthful foods. When imparting information fails to bring about behavior change, the common response is to redouble efforts to teach facts and explain why something should be done. Instead, an examination of the person's attitudes and values should be pursued.

The affective domain involves a process of internalization from least committed to most committed. It categorizes the inner growth that occurs as people become aware of, and later adopt, the attitudes and principles that assist in forming the value judgments that guide their conduct. For the client learning about prenatal nutrition, the dietetics professional may desire the woman not only to be knowledgeable (cognitive domain) about the proper foods to eat during pregnancy, but also to value the knowledge so much (affective domain) that she eats nutritious foods and practices good nutrition. Note that an objective in one domain may have a component in another. Cognitive objectives may have an affective component, and affective objectives may have a cognitive one.

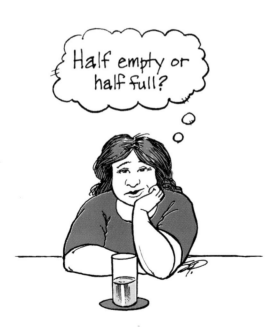

One's outlook may be positive or negative.

Affective objectives are more nebulous and resist precise definition; therefore, evaluation of their achievement is more difficult. The practitioner may find it a formidable task to describe affective behaviors involving internal feelings and emotions, but they are as important as overt behaviors. Because affective objectives are more difficult to express, most written objectives express cognitive behaviors.

Krathwohl and colleagues published a taxonomy of educational objectives in the affective domain.(23) It includes five categories and a number of subcategories:

1.0 RECEIVING (ATTENDING)
    1.1 Awareness
    1.2 Willingness to receive
    1.3 Controlled or selected attention
2.0 RESPONDING
    2.1 Acquiescence in responding
    2.2 Willingness to respond
    2.3 Satisfaction in response
3.0 VALUING
    3.1 Acceptance of a value
    3.2 Preference for a value
    3.3 Commitment
4.0 ORGANIZATION
    4.1 Conceptualization
    4.2 Organization of a value system
5.0 CHARACTERIZATION BY A VALUE OR VALUE COMPLEX
    5.1 Generalized set
    5.2 Characterization

The ordering of classes describes a process by which a value progresses from a level of mere awareness or perception to levels of greater complexity until it becomes an internal part of one's outlook on life that guides or controls behavior. This internalization may occur in varying degrees and may involve conformity and high commitment or nonconformity. At higher levels, behavior may be so ingrained that it is unconscious rather than a conscious response, and responses may be produced consistently in the absence of external authorities and in spite of barriers. Thus, a client may eventually select healthful foods, or an employee may wash his or her hands without thinking about it at the conscious level. Table 11-4 suggests verbs describing performance in the affective domain.

Receiving

At the lowest level of the affective domain, the learner is willing to receive certain phenomena or stimuli. Receiving represents a willingness to attend to what the professional is presenting. The person may move from a passive level of awareness or consciousness to a neutral willingness to tolerate the situation rather than to avoid it and then to an active level of controlled or selected attention despite distractions.

    E X A M P L E : *Is able to focus attention on instructions on a diabetic diet.*

Responding

The second level is responding, which indicates a desire on the part of the individual to become involved in, or committed to, a subject or activity. At the lowest level of responding, the client or employee may passively acquiesce, or at least comply, in response to the professional or manager. At a higher level, a willingness to respond or voluntarily make a commitment to a chosen response is evident. Finally, a feeling

TABLE 11-4	Verbs Describing Performance—Affective

Level	Verbs to Use
Receiving	asks, attends, chooses, describes, follows, gives, identifies, listens, replies, selects, uses
Responding	answers, assists, complies, conforms, cooperates, discusses, helps, participates, performs, practices, presents, reads, recites, reports, responds, selects, tells, writes
Valuing	completes, describes, differentiates, explains, follows, imitates, joins, justifies, participates, proposes, reads, selects, shares, supports
Organization	accepts, adheres, alters, arranges, combines, compares, defends, discusses, explains, generalizes, identifies, integrates, modifies, organizes, prefers, relates, synthesizes
Characterization	acts, advocates, communicates, discriminates, displays, exemplifies, influences, performs, practices, proposes, questions, selects, serves, supports, uses, verifies

of satisfaction or pleasure in response involves an internalization on the part of the individual.

E X A M P L E : *Is willing to read diet materials with interest and ask questions.*

Valuing
At the third level, valuing, the individual believes that the information or behavior has worth. The person values it based on a personal assessment. When the value has been slowly internalized or accepted, the client or employee displays a behavior consistent with the value. When something is valued, motivation is not based on external authorities or the desire to obey, but on an internal commitment. The person may demonstrate acceptance of a value, preference for a value, or commitment and conviction.

E X A M P L E : *Is able to select a nutritious meal from the cafeteria line.*

Organization
At the level of organization, the individual discovers situations in which more than one value is appropriate. Individual values are incorporated into a total network of values, and at the level of conceptualization, a person relates new values to those he or she already holds. New values must be organized into an ordered relationship with the current value system. Perhaps a client has valued eating whatever he or she wants. If the dietetics professional is teaching a client a new diet, the client has to learn a new value (different foods) and change an old one (some of the current eating choices).

E X A M P L E : *Is able to discuss plans for making different, healthful food choices.*

Characterization

The highest level, characterization, indicates that the person has internalized the values for a sufficient time to control behavior and acts consistently over time. A generalized set is a predisposition to act or perceive events in a certain way. At the highest level of internalization, beliefs or ideas are integrated with internal consistency.

> **EXAMPLE:** *Is able to select only those foods permitted on the diet at almost all times.*

Behavioral change in the affective domain takes place gradually over a period of time, whereas cognitive change may occur more rapidly. Affective change may take days, weeks, or months at the higher levels.

SELF ASSESSMENT

Plan a performance objective for each level in the affective domain on a similar topic.

Psychomotor Domain

The psychomotor domain involves the development of physical abilities and skills. Knowledge and attitudes are interrelated and may be necessary to perform these skills. For example, a person cannot drive a car or operate a meat slicer, tasks requiring manual skills, without some basic knowledge of the equipment. The authors who developed the cognitive and affective domains did not develop a taxonomy for the psychomotor domain, but more than one has been published.(24,25) Table 11-5 suggests verbs describing performance at the various levels of the psychomotor domain. The performance of physical ability proceeds to increasingly complex steps. Simpson's seven levels and subcategories are as follows:(24)

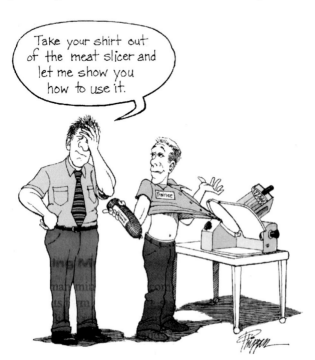

Both knowledge and skills are needed in operating equipment.

TABLE 11-5	Verbs Describing Performance—Psychomotor

Level	Verbs to Use
Perception	attends, observes, perceives, recognizes, watches
Set	demonstrates, positions, prepares, senses, touches, uses
Guided response	calculates, computes, cuts, imitates, performs, practices, repeats, replicates, tries
Mechanism	assembles, calibrates, cleans, disassembles, operates, performs, practices, prepares, repairs, uses, washes
Complex overt response	cooks, demonstrates, executes, interviews, masters, performs
Adaptation	adapts, changes, develops, modifies, organizes, produces, solves
Origination	instructs, operates, originates, uses

1.00 PERCEPTION
    1.10 Sensory stimulation
        1.11 Auditory
        1.12 Visual
        1.13 Tactile
        1.14 Taste
        1.15 Smell
        1.16 Kinesthetic
    1.20 Cue selection
    1.30 Translation
2.00 SET
    2.10 Mental set
    2.20 Physical set
    2.30 Emotional set
3.00 GUIDED RESPONSE
    3.10 Imitation
    3.20 Trial and error
4.00 MECHANISM
5.00 COMPLEX OVERT RESPONSE
    5.10 Resolution of uncertainty
    5.20 Automatic performance
6.00 ADAPTATION
7.00 ORIGINATION

Perception
The lowest level of the psychomotor domain is perception. It involves becoming aware of objects by means of the senses—hearing, seeing, touching, tasting, and smelling—and by muscle sensations or activation. The individual must select which cues to respond to in order to perform a task. The person then must mentally translate the cues received for action.

E X A M P L E : *Is able to recognize a need to learn how to use the meat slicer.*

Set

Set is the second level and suggests a readiness for performing a task. In addition to being set or ready mentally, the employee must be ready physically by correct positioning of the body, and emotionally, by having a favorable attitude or willingness to learn the task.

E X A M P L E : *Is able to position oneself to use the meat slicer.*

Guided Response

The third level of the psychomotor domain is guided response. The professional or trainer guides the employee during the activity, emphasizing the individual components of a more complex skill. The subcategories include imitation of the practitioner and trial and error until the task can be performed accurately. Performance at this level may initially be crude and imperfect.

E X A M P L E : *Is able to practice the steps in using the meat slicer under supervision.*

Mechanism

Mechanism, the fourth level, refers to habitual response. At this stage of learning, the employee demonstrates an initial degree of proficiency in performing the task, which results from some practice.

E X A M P L E : *Is able to use the meat slicer properly.*

Complex Overt Response

The fifth level, complex overt response, suggests that a level of skill has been attained over time in performing the task. Work is performed smoothly and efficiently without error. Two subcategories are resolution of uncertainty, in which a task is performed without hesitation, and automatic performance. Performance is characterized by accuracy, control, and speed.

E X A M P L E : *Is able to demonstrate considerable skill in using the meat slicer with a variety of foods.*

Adaptation/Origination

Adaptation requires altering manual skills in new but similar situations, such as in adapting slicing procedures to a variety of different foods on the meat slicer. The final level, origination, refers to the creation of a new physical act, such as slicing something that has not been done before.

In understanding the psychomotor domain, it may be helpful to recall the process of learning to drive an automobile, responding to the physical and visual stimulation, feeling mentally and emotionally ready to drive, learning parallel parking by trial and error under the guidance of an instructor, developing a degree of skill, and finally starting the car and driving without having to think of the steps. With time, sufficient skill is developed so that the person can adapt quickly to new situations on the road and create new responses automatically.

Using the taxonomies ensures that the objectives of learning are not limited to the lowest levels, that is, to the recall of facts, or to the cognitive domain only. The taxonomies assist the dietetics professional in thinking of higher levels of knowledge, which may be more appropriate behaviors for the learner. They also serve to remind the practitioner that there are interrelationships among the three domains. The professional should be concerned not only that clients can plan menus using their diets, but also that they think that the food choices are important enough to their health to follow them. Employees need not only to know proper sanitation procedures, for example, but also to value them if they are going to practice optimum sanitary procedures regularly.

> **SELF ASSESSMENT**
>
> Plan several performance objectives in the psychomotor domain on a similar topic.

DETERMINING THE CONTENT

A close examination of the objectives helps to identify the content of the instruction. The objective states what the patient, client, or employee will be able to do when instruction is complete and directs attention to the appropriate content. The preassessment may have eliminated certain objectives as unnecessary, and those that remain should be examined in planning content. Some people may need to start at the lowest level in the taxonomy, whereas those who have already mastered the lower level objectives are ready for those at higher levels.

ORGANIZING TRAINING GROUPS

Learning may take place individually or in groups. Groups are advantageous in that they save time and money and provide opportunities for people to share experiences. Those who are successful in making dietary changes can model behaviors and discuss information with those who have been unsuccessful in coping. The more complex the information to be learned, the greater the need to discuss it in groups.

Even when one person is involved, the dietetics professional should consider whether or not others should be present. In nutrition counseling and education, the individual responsible for purchasing the food and preparing the meals should be present. When a child is placed on a modified diet, such as a diabetic diet, usually the mother or caregiver requires instruction as well, since her cooperation is essential to the child's successful adherence to the diet and management of the disease.

Training sessions for employees may be organized in several ways. Frequently, all new employees are grouped together for initial orientation and training. Although current employees may be grouped by age, educational level, amount of experience, or job title, the best grouping probably occurs when employees with similar learning needs are together. Wait staff, for example, may require sessions on sanitary dish and utensil handling while cooks may need classes on sanitary food handling. The learning needs of employees differ according to their job content and level of current knowledge. The preassessment should show differences in knowledge levels and should assist in making grouping decisions.

Another question is whether supervisors should be grouped in the same classes as their employees. One disadvantage of such a grouping is that the employees may be reluctant to participate by asking questions when the superior is present. The final decision rests on the size of the group. There is more opportunity for individual participation in small groups of 10 to 15 than in groups of 30 to 50 or more.

This chapter has explored the initial steps in planning learning. After needs assessment has been completed, performance objectives should be written in the

CASE STUDY 1

Joan is the dietetics professional responsible for employee education at a worksite. She moderated a focus group interview consisting of 10 employees. The purpose was to determine the employees' concerns about nutrition and health. At the top of the list of concerns was the relation of diet and fats to heart disease.

1. The follow-up focus group will determine more precisely the employees' needs and interests related to the topic. What questions would you ask the focus group?
2. What objectives could you write for an educational presentation to employees on the topic?

CASE STUDY 2

The dietetics professional is responsible for the school lunch program at a large urban high school with over 3,000 students. In her first 6 months on the job, she noted that some students did not eat a well-balanced diet and discarded portions of their meals, leading to a waste of food.

Before planning any nutrition education, she decides to identify what seems to be the problem in selecting better food choices.

1. What approaches can she consider to assess regarding the reasons why high school students are not eating nutritiously?
2. What information should she collect?
3. What approaches to nutrition education might she try with high school students eating lunch in the cafeteria?

cognitive, affective, and psychomotor domains. Either individual or group instruction may be organized. The content of instruction is determined from an examination of the objectives. Chapter 12 explores the remaining steps in the framework for education.

REVIEW AND DISCUSSION QUESTIONS

1. How do you define teaching and learning?
2. What are the three parts of Mager's learning objectives? What question does each answer?
3. What are the three domains of learning objectives? What are the levels in each domain?
4. How are the objectives in the three domains interrelated?
5. What in-service topics would be appropriate for food service employees in the three domains? For clients?
6. How should the physical and psychological environments be arranged?
7. What are the steps to education?
8. What are the reasons for conducting a preassessment or needs assessment?

SUGGESTED ACTIVITIES

1. Make a list of questions you would ask in the preassessment of knowledge of some subject with which you are familiar.
2. Write three performance objectives using active verbs to describe behavior.
3. Write examples of performance objectives containing conditions and a criterion.
4. Write examples of objectives in various levels of the cognitive, affective, and psychomotor domain. Note overlap from one domain to another.
5. Decide which of the following performance objectives are measurable as opposed to nonmeasurable.
   A. Presented with a menu, the patient will be able to circle appropriate food selections according to his or her diet.
   B. At the close of the series of classes, the clients will be more positively disposed toward following their diets.
   C. After counseling, the patient will know which foods he or she should eat and which not to eat.
   D. The patient will be able to explain the diabetic diet to her husband.
6. Examine the following objectives and decide whether each concerns primarily the cognitive, affective, or psychomotor domain.
   A. All clerical staff should be able to type 50 words per minute without errors.
   B. Given a series of objectives, the student will be able to classify them according to the taxonomies in the chapter.
   C. At the end of the session, clients will request more weight control classes.

WEB SITES

www.astd.org / **American Society of Training and Development**
www.tcm.com/trdev / **training links**
www.eatright.org / **American Dietetic Association**
http://navigator.tufts.edu / **Tufts University rates nutrition web sites**

REFERENCES

1. Position of the American Dietetic Association: The role of nutrition in health promotion and disease prevention programs. J Am Diet Assoc 1998;98:205.
2. Position of the American Dietetic Association: Total diet approach to communicating food and nutrition information. J Am Diet Assoc 2002;102:100.
3. Krasker GD, Balogun LB. 1995 JCAHO standards: development and relevance to dietetics practice. J Am Diet Assoc 1995;95:240.
4. Rankin SH, Stallings KD. Patient education: principles & practice, 4th ed. Philadelphia: Lippincott Williams & Wilkins, 2001.
5. Chambers DW, Gilmore CJ, Maillet JO, Mitchell BE. Another look at competency-based education in dietetics. J Am Diet Assoc 1996;96:614.
6. Acosta PB, Ryan AS. Functions of dietitians providing nutrition support to patients with inherited metabolic disorders. J Am Diet Assoc 1997;97:783.
7. Witte SS, Escott-Stump S, Fairchild MM, Papp J. Standards of practice for clinical nutrition managers. J Am Diet Assoc 1997;97:673.
8. Anderson JEL. What should be next for nutrition education? J Nutr 1994;124:1828S.
9. Brownell KD, Cohen LR. Adherence to dietary regimens 2: comments on effective interventions. Behav Med 1995;20:155.
10. Contento I, Balch GI, Bronner YL, et al. Executive summary. J Nutr Educ 1995;27:279.
11. American Diabetes Association position statement: Evidence-based nutrition principles and recommendations for the treatment and prevention of diabetes and related complications. J Am Diet Assoc 2002;102:109.
12. Position of the American Dietetic Association: Nutrition education for the public. J Am Diet Assoc 1996;96:1183.
13. Fleming PL. Nutrition education and counseling. In: Paige DM, ed. Clinical nutrition, 2nd ed. St. Louis: Mosby, 1988.
14. Harnack L, Block G, Subar A, et al. Association of cancer prevention-related nutrition knowledge, beliefs, and attitudes to cancer prevention dietary behaviors. J Am Diet Assoc 1997;97:957.
15. Position of the American Dietetic Association: Food and nutrition misinformation. J Am Diet Assoc 2002;102:260.
16. Mark S, Krause C. Federal role in nutrition education, research, and food assistance for women and their families. J Am Diet Assoc 1999;99:671.
17. Wlodkowski RJ. Enhancing adult motivation to learn: a comprehensive guide for teaching all adults, rev ed. San Francisco: Jossey-Bass, 1999.
18. Reed DB, Meeks PM, Nguyen L, et al. Assessment of nutrition education needs related to increasing dietary calcium intake in low-income Vietnamese mothers using focus group discussions. J Nutr Educ 1998;30:155.
19. Kaufman R. Needs assessment and analysis. In: Tracey WR, ed. Human resources management & development handbook, 2nd ed. New York: American Management Association, 1994.

20. Bohlander G, Snell S, Sherman A. Managing human resources, 12th ed. Cincinnati: South-Western, 2001.

21. Mager RF. Preparing instructional objectives: a critical tool in the development of effective instruction, 3rd ed. Atlanta: CEP Press, 1997.

22. Bloom BS, Engelhart M, Furst E, et al. Taxonomy of educational objectives. Handbook I: Cognitive domain. New York: David McKay, 1956.

23. Krathwohl D, Bloom BS, Masia B. Taxonomy of educational objectives. Handbook II: Affective domain. New York: David McKay 1964.

24. Simpson E. The classification of educational objectives in the psychomotor domain. IL Teacher of Home Econ 1966;10:110.

25. Harrow A. A taxonomy of the psychomotor domain. New York: David McKay, 1972.

CHAPTER 12

Implementing and Evaluating Learning

After reading this chapter, you will be able to

1. explain the advantages and disadvantages of various educational methods and techniques.
2. discuss the educational methods and techniques appropriate in the cognitive, affective, and psychomotor domains.
3. compile a task analysis.
4. list the ways in which instruction can be organized and sequenced.
5. identify the purposes of an educational evaluation.
6. explain several types of evaluation.
7. prepare a lesson plan.
8. compare and contrast formative and summative evaluation, norm-referenced and criterion-referenced evaluation, and reliability and validity.
9. plan, implement, and evaluate an educational presentation for a specific, target audience.

How does the dietetics professional successfully educate clients and employees? With clients, the practitioner seeks to promote health and reduce the risk of chronic disease; with employees, the practitioner seeks to enhance their ability to do their jobs. The initial steps in planning learning, as discussed in Chapter 11, include a preassessment of the learner's current knowledge and competencies; the development of performance objectives in the cognitive, affective, and psychomotor domains; and the determination of the content to be learned.

This chapter discusses the selection and implementation of appropriate learning activities for the cognitive, affective, and psychomotor domains. Plans for the evaluation of the outcomes of learning and for documentation are also discussed, since these steps are essential for completing the educational process.

SELECTING AND IMPLEMENTING LEARNING ACTIVITIES

Various methods and techniques of educational presentation are available to deliver the material to be learned to the audience. Techniques are the ways that the instructor organizes and presents information to learners to promote the internal processes of learning.(1) They establish a relationship between the teacher and the learner and between the learner and what he or she is learning. They include lectures, discussions, simulations, demonstrations, and the like. All are not equally effective in facilitating learning, and each has its advantages and disadvantages, its uses and limitations as summarized in Table 12-1.

In deciding on the method that will be most effective, the dietetics professional may be guided by several factors, including the educational purpose the method serves, learner preference or style, needs, group size, facilities available, time available, cost, and one's previous experience or the degree of success with the techniques.(2) The practitioner must consider what is effective for different populations, such as those from different cultural and ethnic groups, socioeconomic groups, educational and literacy levels, and age groups such as teens so that desired outcomes are reached.

In addition, an examination of the performance objectives may suggest which approach is most appropriate, since methods and techniques differ for the cognitive, affective and psychomotor domains All factors being equal, the practitioner should select the technique that requires the most active participation of the learner and includes strategies for effective behavioral change. As Confucius said:

I hear and I forget,
I see and I remember,
I do and I understand.

Motivation

Adults are highly pragmatic learners who want practical information that leads to knowledge, a skill, or an understanding of how to do something, and they need to apply what they have learned.(3) Adults need to know that the information is important to them and to value it. This will enhance their intrinsic motivation to learn.

A common measure of motivation is persistence.(3) People work longer and harder and with more intensity when motivated than when not motivated. If information is valued or perceived to be needed, this calls forth energy and intrinsic motivation and can enhance self-efficacy. Dietetics professionals can ask clients or employees what they know now and what they need to know or do so that they can first understand the individual. Motivation is enhanced by praise and positive reinforcement as the individual learns.

The dietetics professional must also be concerned that clients and employees remember and retain what they learn. Studies show that the more actively a person is involved in the learning process, the better the retention. Figure 12-1 shows that reading and hearing information are not as productive as both seeing and hearing or, better yet, discussing information or doing something with it.

TECHNIQUES AND METHODS

Lecture

The lecture is the presentation technique that is most familiar to people. It has been used for years as a method of informing and transferring knowledge—the lowest level

TABLE 12-1 Strengths and Weaknesses of Teaching Methods

	Strengths	Weaknesses
Lecture	Easy and efficient Conveys most information Reaches large numbers Minimum threat to learner Maximum control by instructor	Learner is passive Learning by listening Formal atmosphere May be dull, boring Not suited for higher-level learning in cognitive domain Not suited for manual learning
Discussion Panel Debate Case study	More interesting, thus motivating Active participation Informal atmosphere Broadens perspectives We remember what we discuss Good for higher-level cognitive, affective objectives	Learner may be unprepared Shy people may not discuss May get side-tracked More time-consuming Size of group limited
Projects	More motivating Active participation Good for higher-level cognitive objectives	Size of group limited
Laboratory experiments	Learn by experience Hands on method Active participation Good for higher-level cognitive objectives	Requires space, time Group size limited
Simulation Scenarios In-basket Role playing Critical incidents	Active participation Requires critical thinking Develops problem-solving skills Connects theory and practice More interesting Good for higher-level cognitive and affective objectives	Time consuming Group size limited unless on computer
Demonstration	Realistic visual image Appeals to several senses Can show a large group Good for psychomotor domain	Requires equipment Requires time Learner is passive, unless can practice

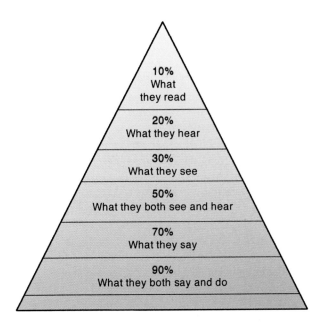

Figure **12-1 WHAT PEOPLE REMEMBER.**

in the cognitive domain—from the teacher to the learner. It is especially useful in situations with a large number of learners, a great deal of information to be communicated, and a limited amount of available time.(4) Examples are a class on sanitation for food service employees or on cholesterol and fat in relation to heart disease for worksite employees or medical center clients.

In spite of the advantages of efficiency, a major drawback of lectures is that there is no guarantee that the material is learned and remembered or that food choices and eating behaviors will change. This is because the individual is a passive participant whose learning depends on listening skills. Lecture may be the least effective technique for use with adults. A review of over 200 nutrition education interventions found that often there was a mismatch between stated goals related to dietary change and the use of a didactic, information-based educational methodology.(5)

Although well-educated people may respond positively to lectures because of long experience with this approach, those with less education or those from other cultures may learn better with other methods. Their attention to lectures may wane quickly as they tune out, especially if the lecturer is not an effective speaker or if the lecture is dull, and new information may be rapidly forgotten. A focus group of clients with limited literacy skills, for example, considered lectures an ineffective way to obtain nutrition information and preferred more hands-on activities where they could share ideas and experiences.(6) Furthermore, lectures do not meet the requirements of adult education, or "andragogy," for self-directed learning and problem-solving approaches. When lectures are used, it is advisable to limit the number of concepts presented, use examples and summaries frequently, add visual aids, provide ample time for a question-and-answer or discussion period, and provide resources for further study.

Discussion

In discussion techniques, whether on a one-to-one basis or in groups, individuals are active participants as they examine their own thinking and internalize knowledge through the exchange of ideas and through their verbal responses. Discussion may be guided by the dietetics professional's raising open-ended questions, problems, or key issues so that clients or employees make comparisons or work to draw conclusions. Or, discussion may be more group-centered if the participants are fairly well acquainted. With a series of classes on weight reduction, for example, clients could discuss and share what they have done to change their food choices, recipes, and shopping habits. The basis for discussion may be common experiences, problem solving, topics that were preannounced so that the group has prepared, or case studies of real-life situations, which are developed.

Facilitated group discussion was preferred over lecture in WIC (Women, Infants, and Children) clinic settings. Clients shared their knowledge, problems, and experiences with other group members through discussion facilitated by a dietitian. The discussions developed clients' self-perceived skills and self-efficacy.(7) Debates and panel discussions, in which several people of notable competence and specific knowledge of a topic informally discuss or debate the topic in front of a larger group, are other approaches.

For best results, seating should be arranged in a circle so that everyone can see and hear one another and so that the practitioner can participate as a member of the group. Smaller groups of 10 to 15 people offer more opportunity for participation as learners explore their thoughts, values, and experiences, think critically, and influence others.

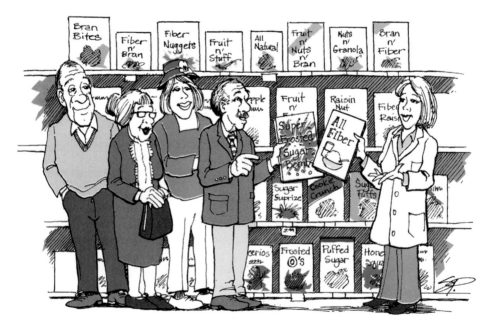

People prefer hands-on learning to lectures.

Discussion is more time-consuming than lecture, but it can be more interesting for learners, and thus more motivating, especially with higher-level cognitive objectives and with affective objectives when attitudes and values need to be explored. Discussion and oral summarization facilitate and promote the person's acquisition and retention of information, since we remember what we say out loud. When people study alone or are passive listeners, some cognitive processing may not take place.

Simulation

Simulations of real-life situations are active ways to develop learner knowledge, skills, behaviors, and competencies.(8) Several means of representation may be used, such as scenarios, in-basket exercises, critical incidents, and role-playing. These methods involve learning by actively doing something, in other words, experiential learning rather than learning by listening or watching. Active learner involvement enhances optimum transfer of learning.

Simulation may be based on scenarios or models of real-life problem situations. Clients on sodium-restricted diets, for example, could take restaurant menus and determine what they should order. Learners use a process of inquiry in exploring a problem, developing decision-making and evaluative skills. Food service employees could discuss food temperatures and HACCP (Hazard Analysis Critical Control Points) procedures through preparation, holding, service, and leftovers.

In-basket exercises test the person's ability to handle day-to-day challenges. The technique has been used, for example, to simulate a supervisor's decision-making ability in handling problems that arrive in the in-basket on the desk each day. Written memos, notes, requests, or reports are given to an individual and require a decision.

Critical incidents also require the learner's responses to specific situations. Emergencies such as fires and electrical blackouts or unusual incidents are used, and the learner has to provide a solution in handling the situation or problem.

Role playing, in which two or more persons dramatize assigned parts or roles simulating real-life situations, is another possibility.(3) Role playing allows learners to practice new behaviors in relatively safe environments, and it can be used to work through real problems. This is followed by discussion of the problem, ideas, feelings, and emotional reactions, as, for example, the handling of an employee disciplinary problem or learning to say no when offered disallowed foods. Though time consuming, simulations may be helpful in providing opportunities for individuals to make a connection between theory and practice, to engage in critical thinking as active participants, and to develop problem-solving and coping skills. Simulation may be used with cognitive, affective, and psychomotor objectives.

Demonstration

A demonstration may be used to show how something is done or to explore processes, procedures, equipment operation, techniques, ideas, or attitudes. It is often concerned with acquiring a combination of knowledge and skill and is useful for cognitive and psychomotor objectives.(8) Learning to prepare low-fat recipes and learning how to use a

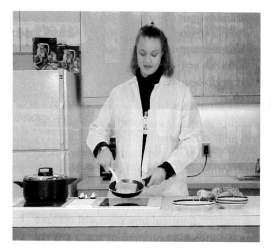

*A demonstration is one approach
to presentations.*

meat slicer are examples of when demonstration is appropriate. Usually, the client or employee observes as the dietetics professional makes the presentation or models the skill, although a participant volunteer may be used. The demonstration may be a dramatic learning experience if it holds the individual's attention and may be appropriate for any type of learning objective.

If skills are demonstrated, the person will need ample opportunity to practice the task or skill soon after and evaluate the performance after passively watching the instructor. Job Instruction Training, discussed later in this chapter, is an example of the use of demonstration to achieve mastery. Sometimes, duplicate work operations are set up independent of the work site and are used for training.

Computer-Assisted Instruction

Computer programs can be used with employees and clients. Computer-based training is used by over half of US organizations with 50 or more employees.(9) A WIC program used client-directed, interactive, multimedia software to deliver nutrition education to a high-risk, low-income population. Positive changes in knowledge, attitudes, or behavioral intentions, and a high level of client acceptance were found.(10)

Audiovisual Aids

According to an old Chinese proverb, "one picture is worth more than 1,000 words." An effective media presentation can enhance learning by providing variety and improving memory through visual stimulation. The appropriateness of such material to the learning situation, and to the individual or group, should be considered. A videotape of your own setting, for example, would probably foster better learning among employees than one that is purchased. Such materials are an adjunct to learning and should not be considered the total learning experience. (Chapter 15 discusses media in more detail.)

Techniques for Different Domains of Learning

For learning in the cognitive domain, most of the preceding techniques may be effective. There are additional factors to consider in fostering learning in the affective and psychomotor domains. From a review of 80 studies of nutrition education interventions, there appeared to be some advantage to using mixed methods rather than only one method.(5,11)

In the affective domain, the dietetics professional seeks to influence the learner's interests, attitudes, beliefs, and values. This cannot be accomplished in an hour or a day, but requires ongoing contacts. At the lowest level in the affective domain, receiving and awareness, the professional may gain the learner's attention through the use of audiovisual materials or guided discussion, such as about the relationship of food choices and obesity. At higher levels, where the adoption of new attitudes and values is important, the individual must participate more fully in discussion. Attitudes are acquired through interpersonal influences, and commitments that are made public are more likely to be adopted than those that are kept private.

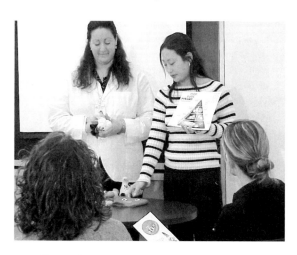

Discussion with visuals helps the learner.

Discussion in a group or where experiences are shared, discussion of case studies or critical incidents, and role playing may be effective. These methods may lead to higher self-awareness and public commitment to values. People may perceive that all members of the group support the new attitudes and behaviors. Active oral summarization after discussion is recommended because it leads to more elaborate thinking and integration into the person's conceptual framework.

Effective instructional strategies that influence deeper-level learning of nutrition and the modification of attitudes and dietary behaviors are recommended. Promoting the active involvement of participants and interpersonal interaction in a group can help.

Inquiry learning requires the use of the problem-solving process, in which the dietetics professional presents a puzzling situation or problem. The practitioner may ask people, for example, to calculate their daily fat or sodium allowance from food labels. Individuals identify and clarify the problem, form hypotheses, gather data, analyze and interpret data, select possible solutions, test solutions, and finally draw conclusions and select the best solution to the problem. People learn how to solve problems, evaluate possible solutions, and think critically. Clients can be guided through this process so that they learn to solve their own nutrition problems.

Experiments, such as with modifying recipes for fat or sodium, and hands-on activities, such as planning nutritious menus for a week or preparing varieties of new foods for a diet, are another approach. An example is to require clients to shop for and evaluate certain foods at the grocery store.

Modeling is also a method of influencing a person's behavior.(12) People learn by observing others and then imitating them in unfamiliar or new situations. The dietetics professional should behave as the client or employee is expected to behave, modeling the desirable attitude or behavior. People are more likely to accept new behaviors, such as healthful food choices, when they meet and have discussions with people who have successfully adopted them. This technique is appropriate for nutrition education.

Focus group research was used to plan diabetes nutrition education for a hard-to-reach, low-income, African-American community. Members wanted positive sessions rather than "don'ts," the demonstration of alternatives in preparing food, and not too many words. The resulting program "Learn, Taste, and Share" de-emphasized lecture in favor of more participatory methods—games, food prizes, a cooking demonstration, and cooking participation. Activities included ranking boxes of cereal from low to high fiber, guessing the amount of fat in foods, finding whole-grain crackers at a grocery store, experimenting with recipes, and preparing a dinner.(13)

Skills in the psychomotor domain are learned with direct experience and practice over time. The professional may begin with a demonstration, but then the learner needs to practice the skill under supervision. Coaching is a term that describes the assistance given to someone learning a new skill; it can apply to an educational experience as well as a sport. Coaching suggests a one-on-one, continuous, supportive relationship from which a person learns over time. It is perhaps the best method for on-the-job training of employees. After the demonstration, the trainer can give encouragement, confidence, and guidance as the trainee performs the task.(9) Coaching takes into consideration different learning abilities and needs, allows actual practice, and provides people with immediate feedback regarding their performance.

TASK ANALYSIS

A task analysis is a written sequential list of the steps involved in performing any task from beginning to end and including the knowledge, skills, and abilities needed as well as the conditions under which it is performed and the proper method of performance. Usually, the major steps are numbered, and each step describes what to do. Many job-related tasks involve the psychomotor domain; thus, actions are listed in the analysis. It is often necessary, however, to have some background knowledge from the cognitive domain in performing the task. Balancing a checkbook, for example, is both a manual and an intellectual skill, as is operating a cash register.

After the sequential steps are listed, each one should be examined to see whether there are explanations from the cognitive domain that need to be added. If step one, for example, is to plug in the meat slicer, a key point is to have dry hands to avoid the danger of electrical shock. If a final step in the wait staff's task analysis for bussing dirty dishes includes washing hands, an explanation may be added regarding the transfer of microorganisms to clean food and utensils. In food service, sanitation and safety statements are frequently needed. Other explanations of reasons why a step is necessary or notes on materials or equipment may be important to add. There are many ways to complete a task analysis.(9,14,15)

Employees need to learn the skills related to their jobs, and clients may need to develop skills in menu planning and food preparation using a new dietary regimen, such as sodium restriction. Regardless of the kind of skill involved, the learner needs to be able to perform the skill initially and then to improve the skill through continued practice. After grasping the basics of tennis, driving a car, or baking a cake, for example, a person requires repeated experience to develop a skill.

If available, a job description may be used as a starting point in determining job content, but job descriptions do not give information that is specific enough for determining the content of training.(9) All the tasks included in a job should be listed individually. If the job description is unavailable, it may be necessary to interview employees or observe their work to determine the job content. Wait staff, for example, complete a number of tasks during the day, such as greeting customers, taking their orders, placing orders in the kitchen, serving the courses of the meal, bussing dishes, setting tables, receiving payment for services, and maintaining good public relations. Each is a separate task making up the total job, and each task or set of actions can be defined in task analyses.

Once it is written, the task analysis should be used by both the professional and the trainee. The trainer may examine the task analysis to construct learning objectives, which describe the behavior expected at the end of training. In assessing the person's need for instruction, the professional should consider the difference between the skill described in the task analysis and the individual's current skill to define the gap in knowledge or skill that must be addressed. The practitioner should use demonstration to show what to do, and then allow the person to perform the task. The individual may use the task analysis as a reference, since it describes what to do in sequence. Using the task analysis in coaching or in supervised on-the-job training facilitates the learning of skills.

After mastering the basic skill involved and being able to recognize the correct sequence of procedures, the individual needs repeated practice to improve the skill. With time and practice, improvements in speed and quality of work should develop.

JOB INSTRUCTION TRAINING

A great deal of employee training takes place not in the classroom, but on the job. New employees require orientation and training with either an experienced worker or a supervisor. Current employees may need retraining periodically, may be assigned new tasks, or may receive promotions that require the development of new skills and abilities.

A four-step process entitled Job Instruction Training (JIT) was delineated for rapid training of new employees. It may be used to teach skills and is based on performance rather than subject matter. The four steps are (1) preparation, (2) presentation, (3) learner performance, and (4) follow-up. This is similar to Tell/Show/Do/Review. Before instruction, a task analysis should be completed, and the work area arranged with the necessary supplies and materials that the employee is expected to maintain.(9,16,17) Table 12-2 summarizes the main points.

Preparation

Part I of JIT prepares the employee psychologically and intellectually for learning. Since a superior may be the trainer, any tension, nervousness, or apprehension in the subordinate employee must be overcome because it may interfere with learning. A friendly, smiling trainer puts the person at ease by creating an informal atmosphere for learning, where mistakes are expected and tolerated. The trainer states the job to be learned and asks specific questions to determine what the individual already knows about it. When employees become interested in their jobs, their motivation for learning increases.

TABLE 12-2 How to Instruct

Part I: Prepare the learner.

Put the learner at ease.
State the job.
Find out what the individual knows about the job.
Develop interest.
Correct the person's position.

Part II: Present the operation.

Tell, show, and illustrate.
Explain one important step at a time.
Stress key points.
Instruct clearly, completely, and patiently, but no more than the learner can master.
Summarize the operation in a second run-through.

Part III: Try out performance.

Have the learner do the job.
Have the learner explain key points while performing the job again.
Make sure that the learner understands.
Continue until you know that the learner knows the job.

Part IV: Follow-up.

Put the learner on his or her own.
Designate where to obtain help.
Encourage questions.
Taper off.
Continue with normal supervision.

Finally, the trainer should be sure that the employee can physically see what is being demonstrated.

Presentation

In Part II, the trainer presents and explains the operation as the employee is expected to perform it. The trainer shows, tells, and illustrates the operation one step at a time using a prepared task analysis. Key points should be stressed. The instruction should be carried out clearly, completely, and patiently, with the trainer remembering the employee's abilities and attitudes.

Since the ability to absorb new information is limited, the trainer needs to determine how much the learner can master at a time. It may be five to 10 steps with key points, or it may be more. It may be 15 minutes or 1 hour of instruction. Overloading anyone with information is ineffectual, since the information will be forgotten. After this initial instruction, the operation or task should be summarized and performed a second time.

Performance

Part III tests how much the employee has retained as he or she tries out the operation using the written task analysis as a reference. The employee does the job while the trainer or coach stands by to assist. This is a form of behavior modeling. Accuracy, not speed, is stressed initially. As the employee completes the task a second time, the trainer should ask the employee to state the key points. To be sure of understanding, the trainer should ask such questions as "What would happen if...?" "What else do you do...?" and "What next...?" Employees may need to repeat the operation five times, 10 times, or however many times are needed until they know what to do. The trainer continues coaching and giving positive feedback, encouragement, and reassurance until the employee learns the operation.

Follow-up

Follow-up occurs in Part IV as supervision tapers off. At first, the employee is left alone to complete the task. The individual should always know, however, where to obtain assistance if it is needed. Any additional questions ought to be encouraged in case problems arise. Normal supervision continues to ensure that the task is done as instructed, since fellow workers may suggest undesirable short cuts.

Mager pointed out that when the learner's experience is followed by positive consequences, the learner will be stimulated to approach the situation, but that when adverse consequences follow, the learner will avoid the situation.[12] A positive consequence may be any pleasant event, praise, a successful experience, an increase in self-esteem, improvement in self-image, or an increase in confidence. Adverse conditions are events or emotions that cause physical or mental discomfort or that lead to loss of self-respect. They include fear, anxiety, frustration, humiliation, embarrassment, and boredom. In influencing learners in the affective domain, as well as the other domains, the dietetics professional should positively reinforce learner responses.

SEQUENCE OF INSTRUCTION

Since there is a great deal to learn, instruction requires some type of organized sequence. Sequence of instruction is characterized by the progressive development of knowledge, attitudes, and skills. Learning takes place over time, and the process should be organized into smaller units. Since the ultimate outcome is able performance or behavioral change, it is important to consider how meaningful the sequence is to the individual, not the teacher or trainer, and whether or not it promotes learning. Mager provides several recommendations for sequencing. Instruction may be arranged from the general to the specific, from the specific to the general, from the simple to the complex, or according to interest, logic, or frequency of use of the knowledge or skill.[2,15]

In moving from the general to the specific, an overview or large picture should be presented first, and then the details and specifics are presented. For example, present an overview of the reasons for the diabetic diet and the general principles of the diet before presenting the details. With a new employee, a general explanation of the job should precede the specifics. After the individual has digested some information, it is possible to consider a specific to general sequence.

Material may be organized from the simple (terms, facts, procedures) to the complex (concepts, processes, theories, analyses, applications) so that the individual handles increasingly difficult material. If the taxonomies are used in writing objectives for learning, the hierarchy of the taxonomies provides a simple-to-complex sequence.

Another possibility is sequencing according to interest, or from the familiar to the unfamiliar. One may begin instruction with whatever is of most interest or concern to the individual. Initial questions from patients, clients, employees, or other audiences suggest such interest and should be dealt with immediately so that they are free to concentrate on later information. "How long will I have to stay on this diet?" "Can I eat my favorite foods?" The information that the person desires is a good starting point for discussion.

Similarly, if the person perceives a problem, the dietetics professional can start with that problem rather than with a preset agenda. As learning proceeds, the individual may develop additional needs for information or goals for learning that may be addressed. Generally, people who have assisted in directing their own learning tend to feel more committed to it.

Logic may suggest the sequence. Certain things may need to be said before others. Safety precautions may need to be introduced early, for example, when discussing kitchen equipment. Sanitary utensil handling may be important to discuss with wait staff before discussing how to set a table.

Frequency of use of the knowledge or skill may also dictate sequence. The skill used most frequently should be taught first, followed by the next most frequently used skill. If training time runs out, at least the learner has learned all except the least frequently used skills. The dietetics professional should teach first what people need to know rather than the "nice to know" information.

Finally, the practitioner should provide learners with total practice. Even though learners may have been practicing individual elements of the job, they need practice on the total job. This practice may be provided in the actual job situation or through simulation.

EVALUATION OF RESULTS

The step often overlooked is probably that of evaluation. Evaluation is key to successful nutrition interventions, and a current demand in health care is to measure effectiveness in terms of outcomes. The wise professional defines outcomes expected before starting the intervention rather than later. Nutrition education that does not show improvement in client status cannot be considered effective. Thus, evaluation is important for accountability and for continuous improvement and refinement of education.

Evaluation connotes judgments about the value or worth of something compared with a standard. Everyone makes these judgments daily, both consciously and unconsciously. "The food tastes good." "The television show is worth watching." "She is not motivated." Our thoughts turn to evaluation automatically as we compare something with some standard and pass judgment.

Educational evaluation consists of a systematic appraisal of the quality, effectiveness, and worth of an educational endeavor, such as instruction, programs, or goals based on information or data.(18) That it is systematic suggests that advance planning has taken place and that the process will provide data on the quality or worth of the educational endeavor.

Consider not only what to evaluate, but also when to evaluate and how the evaluation will be done. An evaluation plan involves a number of steps: defining objectives or outcomes; designing the evaluation based on objectives; choosing what to evaluate; deciding how and when to collect data to obtain timely feedback; constructing a data collection instrument or method; implementing the data collection; analyzing results; reporting them; and setting a course of action.(19)

Although the terms "measurement" and "evaluation" are sometimes interchanged, their meanings are not equivalent. Measurement or "educational assessment" is the process of collecting and quantifying data in terms of numbers on the extent, degree, or capacity of people's learning in knowledge, attitudes, skills, performance, and behavioral change. Testing is one kind of measurement. Measurement involves determining the degree to which a person possesses a certain attribute, as when one receives a score of 85 on a test. However, such a measurement does not determine quality or worth. These systems require experimental designs, data collection, and statistical analysis of the data.(18,21) The term "assessment" can also mean estimating or judging the value of the data collected, as in nutrition assessment.

Evaluation, on the other hand, is based on the measurement of what people know, think, feel, and do.(20) Evaluation compares the observed value or quality with a standard or criterion of comparison. Evaluation is the process of forming value judgments about the quality of programs, products, goals, and the like from the data. One may evaluate the success of an educational program, for example, by measuring the degree to which goals or objectives were achieved. Evaluation goes beyond measurement to the formation of value judgments about the data. To be effective, evaluation designs should specify not only what will be evaluated, but also when it will be evaluated. Sometimes, several measurements are needed, as in pretesting and posttesting.

Purpose of Evaluation

Careful evaluation should be an integral part of all nutrition education programs and employee training programs.(5) There are several purposes of evaluation. One cannot make judgments about effectiveness without it.(22) Program evaluation may be used for planning, improvement, and justification. As a system of quality control, it can determine whether the process of education is effective, identify its strengths and weaknesses, and determine what changes should be made. To determine accountability, one needs to know whether people are learning, whether dietetics professionals are teaching effectively, whether programs accomplish the desired outcomes, and whether money is well spent. In times of limited financial resources, accountability requires an examination of cost/benefit ratios. Is the program useful and valuable enough to justify the cost?(23) Is there evidence that training is changing employee behavior on the job and contributing to the bottom line? It is important to determine whether the learning objectives were accomplished and whether the individual learned what was intended or developed in desired ways.

Evaluation helps dietetics professionals make better decisions and improve education. It is helpful in making decisions concerning teaching, learning, program effectiveness, and the necessity of making modifications in current efforts or even of terminating them. Evaluation provides evidence that what you are doing is worthwhile. Plans for evaluation should be made early, in the planning stages of an educational endeavor and not after it has begun or is completed.

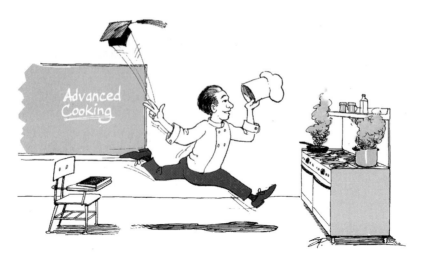

Does the training transfer from the classroom to the workplace?

With employees, training evaluation should show improved job performance and financial results. Another question often asked is: "Does training transfer?" One needs to determine whether the skills and knowledge taught in training are applied on the job. If they are, this demonstrates the value of the training to the organization, and the effectiveness of the method of training, If not, change is needed.(24)

As with other parts of his adult education model, Malcolm Knowles suggested that evaluation should be a mutual undertaking between the educator and the learner.(25) He recommends less emphasis on the evaluation of learning and more on the rediagnosis of learning needs, which suggests immediate or future steps to be taken jointly by the dietetics professional and the client or employee. This type of feedback from evaluation becomes more constructive and acceptable to adults. Thus, evaluation may be considered something you should do with people, not to people. If problems are apparent, then solutions may be found jointly by the professional and the individual.

Formative and Summative Evaluations

Formative and summative evaluations are two types of evaluations used to improve any of three processes—program planning, teaching, or learning. Formative evaluation refers to that made early or during the course of education, with the feedback of results modifying the rest of the educational endeavor. Summative evaluation refers to an endpoint assessment of quality at the conclusion of learning.(18)

Formative

Formative evaluation is a systematic appraisal that occurs before or during the implementation of a learning activity for the purpose of modifying or improving teaching, learning, program design, or educational materials. It is often qualitative in nature with data collection by observation, interviewing, and surveys.(21) It can help to diagnose problems in student learning and in teaching effectiveness. It pinpoints parts mastered and parts not mastered and allows for revision of plans, methods, techniques, or materials.

Formative evaluation may be performed at frequent intervals. If the learner appears bored, unsure, anxious, quizzical, or lost, or if you are unsure of the person's abilities, for example, it is appropriate to stop teaching and start the evaluation process. Ask the person to repeat what he or she has learned. In diabetic education, if formative evaluation shows that the person does not understand the concept of carbohydrate counting, he or she will not be able to master more complex behaviors such as menu planning. Having located the problem that carbohydrate counting is not comprehended, the dietetics educator can change approaches to try to overcome the problem. Perhaps an alternative explanation that is clearer or simpler or a concrete illustration is indicated. Sometimes in group education, a group member is able to provide an explanation that an individual understands better than the explanation of the professional.

Before nutrition messages and educational materials are designed and implemented, formative evaluation or market research activities, such as focus group interviews and structured discussions with members of the target audience, are designed and implemented. This type of qualitative evaluation helps the educator to learn about individuals' thoughts, ideas, and opinions and tells whether message recipients are likely to ignore, reject, or misunderstand the message or accept it and act on it.(5,26,27)

Formative research is essential for tailoring intervention strategies. The moderator of a focus group uses open-ended interviewing strategies with groups of eight to 15 people. The focus group approach has been used to assess consumer preferences, to plan and evaluate nutrition education interventions, and to pretest print materials. It can answer questions about readability, content, and applicability. Formative methods, including peer-led individual interviews, focus groups, and trips to Hispanic food markets, for example, were used to adapt nutrition education materials for four Hispanic subgroups.(28) In other research, data from student focus groups indicated that the barriers to eating healthfully were time and money; this knowledge resulted in interventions that focused on these issues.(29) Qualitative evaluation may be audiotaped or videotaped for later review and reference.

Failure to learn may not always be related to instructional methods or materials per se, but may derive from problems that are physical, emotional, cultural, or environmental in nature. By performing an evaluation after smaller units of instruction, the educator can determine whether the pacing of instruction is appropriate for the patient, client, or employee. Frequent feedback is necessary to facilitate learning. It is especially important when a great deal has to be learned.

Mastery of smaller units can be a powerful positive reinforcement for the learner, and verbal praise may increase motivation to continue learning. When mistakes are made, they should be corrected quickly by giving the correct information. Avoid saying such things as: "No, that's wrong." "Can't you ever get things right?" "Won't you ever learn?" Positive, not negative, feedback should be given. Approach the problem specifically by saying, for example, "You identified some of the foods that are high in sodium, which is very good. Now let's look a second time for others."

Summative

Summative evaluation has a different purpose and time frame from that of formative evaluation. Summative evaluation is considered final, and it is used at the end of a term, course, or learning activity. The purpose of summative evaluation is to appraise results, quality, outcomes, or worth using quantitative approaches. It may include grading, certification, or evaluation of progress, and the evaluation distinguishes those who excel from those who do not. Judgment is made about the learner, teacher, program, or curriculum with regard to the effectiveness of learning or instruction for the target population. This judgment aspect creates the anxiety and defensiveness often associated with evaluation.

Evaluation should be a continual process that is preplanned along with educational sessions. Evaluation preassessment determines the individual's abilities before the educational program, and progress should be evaluated continually during and immediately after the educational program. Follow-up evaluation at 3 to 6 months may measure the degree to which the person has forgotten information or has fallen back to previous behaviors.

Norm- and Criterion-Referenced Methods

Norm-Referenced Interpretations

Besides formative and summative evaluation, there are norm- and criterion-referenced interpretations. In norm-referenced results, the group who has taken a test provides the norms for determining the meaning of each person's score.(18,30) A norm is like the typical performance of a group. One can then see how the individual compares with the results of the group, whether above or below the norm.

Some instructors may believe that a test should not be too easy, but the degree of difficulty of a test may not be as important as whether a person can perform. The instructor may believe that some of the questions have to be difficult so that a spread of scores is produced to separate the brightest from the rest, the A's from the B's and C's. Some tests are purposely developed so that not everyone is successful, and variation in individual scores is expected. Students are graded in a norm-referenced manner by comparison with other individuals on the same measuring device or with the norm of the group. A norm-referenced instrument indicates, for example, whether the individual's performance falls into the 50th percentile or the 90th percentile in relation to the group norm.(18) This method is not as appropriate for affective and psychomotor objectives.(30)

Criterion-Referenced Interpretations

A more important question is whether or not the learner can perform what is stated in the objectives. This approach to evaluation is criterion-referenced. Instead of comparing learners with each other, the instructor compares each individual with a predefined, objective standard of performance of what the learner is expected to know or to be able to do after instruction is complete. A criterion-referenced measurement ascertains the person's status in respect to a defined objective or standard, and test items, if tests are used, correspond to the objectives. If the learner can perform what is called for in the objective, he or she has been successful. If not, criterion-referenced testing, which tends to be more diagnostic, indicates what the learner can and cannot do, and more learning can be planned.(18)

What is important should be made known to the learners so that their time and effort are not wasted. Well-written performance objectives accomplish this. These objectives should be the basis for assessing the results of instruction. If everyone does well, the instruction has been successful.(31) The Registration Examinations for Dietitians and for Dietetic Technicians are examples of criterion-referenced tests.

Formative evaluation is almost always criterion-referenced. The practitioner wants to know who is having trouble learning, not where they rank compared with others. Summative evaluation may be either norm- or criterion-referenced.

Types of Evaluation and Outcomes

After considering the purpose (why) and timing (when) of evaluation, the educator should resolve the question of what to evaluate. Several types of evaluation can be used in measuring effectiveness. These are (1) measurement of participant (client, employee) reactions to programs, (2) measurement of behavioral change, (3) measurement of results in an organization, (4) evaluation of learning in the cognitive, affective, and psychomotor domains, and (5) evaluation of other outcomes.(9,23,32) The evaluation of health education is usually focused on one or more types: knowledge, attitudes or beliefs, change in behavior, and other measures.(33)

Participant Reaction to Programs

The first type of evaluation deals with participant (employee, client) reactions to educational programs and whether or not they are favorable. Preferences may vary by age of the participants, cultural or ethnic group, gender, socioeconomic status, and other variables. You need to decide what should be evaluated. Were participants pleased and satisfied with the program, subject matter, content, materials, speakers, room arrangements, physical facilities, and learning activities? When a program, meeting, or class is evaluated, the purpose is to improve decisions concerning its various aspects, to see how the parts fit the whole, or to make program changes.

The quality of learning elements, such as objectives, techniques, materials, and learning outcomes may be included also. One study, for example, evaluated participants' perceptions of a weight-loss intervention in a hypertension prevention clinical trial as a basis for designing future programs.(34) Hedonistic scales or happiness indexes, such as smiley faces or numerical scales, have been used to determine the degree to which participants "liked" various aspects. Although these judgments are subjective, they are not useless, since learners who dislike elements of a program may not be learning.(35)

Behavioral Change

A second type of evaluation is the measurement of behavior. Did employee or client behavior or habits change based on the learning? In measuring behavior, the focus is on what the person does. In employee training, for example, you may assess changes in job behaviors to see whether transfer of training to the job has occurred. Continual quality improvement has influenced the need for this type of evaluation.(35) It is necessary to know what the job performance was before training and to decide who will observe or assess changed performance—the supervisor, peers, or the individual. This type of assessment is more difficult to measure and can be done selectively.

The ultimate criterion for effectiveness of nutrition education is not merely the improvement in knowledge of what to eat, but also changes in dietary behaviors and practices as the individual develops better food habits.(5,22) Is the person consuming more fruits and vegetables, for example? These changes are difficult to confirm and often depend on direct observation, which is time-consuming, on self-reports, and on indirect outcome measures, such as weight gained or lost in a person on a weight reduction diet, reduction in blood pressure in hypertensive persons, or better control of blood sugars in diabetes mellitus.(33)

Organizational Results

Professionals involved with employee training gather a third type of evaluative data to justify the time and expense to the organization. Management may want to know how training will positively benefit the organization in relation to the cost. Results in terms of the following aspects may be attributed, at least in part, to training: improved morale, improved efficiency or productivity, improved quality of work, better customer satisfaction, less employee turnover, fewer accidents or worker's compensation claims, better attendance, dollar savings, number of employee errors, number of grievances, amount of overtime, and the like. Did changing employee's behavior on the job improve business results? If not, it is not useful.

Learning

Whether learning has taken place is a separate question, even if the program rated highly on entertainment value. The learning of principles, facts, attitudes, values, and skills should be evaluated on an objective basis, and this task is more complex. If the learning objectives are written in terms of measurable performance, they serve as the source of the evaluation. To what degree were the objectives achieved by the learner?

Whether one has succeeded in learning can be determined by developing situations, or test items, based on the objectives of instruction. A program is ineffective if it has not achieved its objectives. It is important for the test items to match the objectives in performance and conditions discussed in Chapter 11. If they do not match the objectives, it is not possible to assess whether instruction was successful, that is, whether the learner learned what was intended.

Mager pointed out that several obstacles must be overcome to assess the results of instruction successfully. Some obstacles are caused by poorly written objectives, whereas others result from attitudes and beliefs on the part of instructors who use inappropriate test items.(31)

One of the problems in evaluation results from inadequately written objectives. If the performance is not stated, if conditions are omitted, and if the criterion is missing, it will be difficult to create a test situation. If these deficiencies are discovered, the first step is to rewrite the objective.

Mager suggested a series of steps to select appropriate test items:(31)

1. Note the performance (what the person will be able to say or do) stated in the objective. Match the performance and conditions of the test item to those of the objective.
2. Check whether the performance is a main intent or an indicator. If the performance is the main intent, note whether it is covert (invisible) or overt (visible, audible).
3. If the performance is covert, such as solving a problem, check for an indicator behavior, a visible or audible activity by which the performance can be inferred.

4. Test for the overt indicator in objectives containing one rather than the main performance.

The first step is to see whether the performance specified in the test item is the same as that specified in the objective. If they do not match, the test item must be revised, since it will not indicate whether the objective has been accomplished. If the objective states that the performance is "to plan low-fat menus," or "to operate the dish machine," for example, the test should involve planning menus or operating the dish machine. It would be inappropriate to ask the learner to discuss the principles of writing menus or to label the parts of the dish machine on a diagram.

In addition to matching performance, the test should use the same specific circumstances or conditions that are specified in the objective.

E X A M P L E : *(Given the disassembled parts of the meat slicer) is able to reassemble the parts in correct sequence.*

The conditions are "given the disassembled parts of the meat slicer." The practitioner should provide a disassembled machine and ask the employee to reassemble it. An inappropriate test would be to ask the learner to list the steps in reassembling the meat slicer or to discuss the safety precautions to be taken.

If the learner must perform under a range of conditions, you may need to test performance using the entire range. If a client eats at home and in restaurants, the dietetics professional must determine whether the person is capable of following the dietary changes in both environments. If students are learning to take a diet history, they should be taught to handle the range of conditions, including people of different ages, socioeconomic, and cultural groups. Not every condition will be taught and tested, but the common conditions that the individual will encounter should be included in the objectives and in testing.

The main intent of an objective may be stated clearly, or it may be implied. The main intent is the performance, whereas an indicator is an activity (visible, audible) through which the main intent is inferred.

E X A M P L E : *(Given a copy of a sodium-restricted diet) is able to plan a menu for a complete day.*

In the above example, the main intent is to discriminate between foods permitted and omitted on the diet, and the indicator is the ability to plan menus. You can infer that the client knows what is permitted and what is not if accurate sodium-restricted menus are planned. Test for the indicator in objectives that contain one. This, of course, does not prove that the person will change eating behaviors.

Covert actions are not visible, but are internal or mental activities, such as solving problems or identifying. If the performance is covert, an indicator should have been added to the objective, as explained in Chapter 11, and the indicator should be tested.

E X A M P L E : *Is able to identify the parts of the slicer (on a diagram or verbally).*

For this example, the employee should be provided with the indicator, a diagram of a meat slicer, and asked to identify the parts.

Although some performances are covert, others are overt. Overt actions are visible or audible, such as writing, verbally describing, and assembling. If the performance is overt, determine whether the test item matches the objective.

EXAMPLE: *Is able to reassemble the parts of the meat slicer.*

The employee should be provided with the parts of the meat slicer and asked to reassemble them. Performance tests are appropriate when skills are taught. If the employee is being taught to use equipment, the evaluation should be to have him or her demonstrate its operation. If a student is learning interviewing skills, an interview session is indicated as the evaluation.

The discussion so far has used examples of objectives in the cognitive and psychomotor domains. Affective objectives describe values, interests, and attitudes that are thought to predispose dietary changes. While the cognitive and psychomotor domains are concerned with what individuals can do, the affective domain deals with what they are willing to do. These changes are covert or internal and develop more slowly over a period of time. Evaluation of their achievement is more difficult and needs to take different forms.

Attitudes are inferred based on the evidence of what people say or do. To assess whether the individual has been influenced by education, the professional may conduct a discussion and listen to what the individual says or observe what he or she does, since both saying and doing are overt behaviors. In measuring attitudes and values, the person needs the opportunity to express agreement rather than deciding on right or wrong answers. A self-reported attitude survey may be used, for example. Statements can be given to which the person responds on a 5-point scale from "strongly agree" to "strongly disagree." To evaluate change in the person's behavior, the practitioner attempts to secure data that permit an inference to be made regarding the person's future disposition in similar situations. In the affective domain, this is a more difficult task.

It is conceivable that the individual may display a desirable overt behavior only in the presence of the practitioner. The attitude toward following a diabetic diet or an employee work procedure may differ depending on the dietetics professional's presence or absence. Since time is required for change in attitudes and values, evaluation may have to be repeated at designated intervals. To determine realistically how the person is disposed to act, the measurement approach needs to evaluate volitional rather than coerced responses.

SELF-ASSESSMENT

You have just discussed sodium restriction with a man with hypertension. How can you assess what he has learned?

Other Outcomes

An outcome is a result and can be defined as "what does or does not happen after an intervention."(36) The criterion of nutrition education program effectiveness has generally been improvement in knowledge, awareness, and in dietary behaviors and/or physiologic parameters.(5,22)

Outcomes should have clear interpretations related to the dietitian's intervention in improving nutrition and health status. They may be of several types: (1) physiological or biological measures; (2) behavioral change based on self-report; (3) diet-related psychosocial measures; and (4) environmental or other measures of dietary behavior. Biological indicators are changes in clinical or biochemical indices, such as serum lipid levels in cardiovascular disease, hemoglobin or serum albumen level in pregnancy, and glycosylated hemoglobin level in diabetes. Eating behavior changes such as decreasing fat intake or increasing fiber intake are based on self-reports, which can be subject to bias. Psychosocial outcomes include increased nutrition knowledge, attitude change, or self-efficacy for behavior but do not prove the change in food choices.(19) Other changes are in body mass index or weight, increases in the level of physical activity, decreased blood pressure, or reduction in risk factors for disease and improved health, both long-term goals. Care must be taken in interpreting some of these results, since they may reflect variables other than education. Stress, for example, can affect a person's blood sugar even when the diabetic diet is followed.

In nutrition education interventions, behavior has been measured in different ways ranging from observable food choices to dietary intakes.(22) Children's behaviors were measured by teachers and by parental reports of food preferences, such as refusing a food, willingness to taste a new food, and selecting a more nutritious food when other choices were available. In older children at school lunch programs, actual food choices and consumption, plate waste, and self-reported intake were used. Changes in adult food intake were measured by 24-hour dietary recall, food records and food frequency questionnaires, and changing food preparation practices and recipes. Older adults were observed in a residential dining room. Interventions to promote breastfeeding measured the percent of mothers still breastfeeding at specific times.

Physical measures included iron deficiency anemia in children, serum lipids, blood pressure, weight indices, urinary sodium, and physical activity status. In pregnancy, mean maternal weight gain, infant's birth weight, and Apgar scores at birth were measured to determine pregnancy outcomes and the health of newborn infants.(22,37)

Organizational changes included changes in school lunch menus, such as to lower fat and sodium, and food choices and nutrition information offered at the worksite have been assessed.

Attitudes and values correlate with food choices and preferences. Attitudes related to health and nutrition were noted by a willingness to eat new foods, a belief that "nutrition affects health," concerns about nutrition, and beliefs about the benefits of better food choices. Dietary self-efficacy scales asked whether respondents were "not sure," "sure," or "very sure" that they could choose healthful foods most of the time.(22)

A wide variety of approaches can be used to evaluate the effectiveness of nutrition education. Changes in dietary behavior should be the primary outcome of nutrition education, and interventions should be directed at behavior change in food choices and practices. The knowledge and skills needed to change behaviors are important to all age groups and are another type of outcome. The correlation between knowledge and behavior is low, however, and psychosocial, cultural, and other mediating variables need to be considered.

Data Collection Techniques

There are many techniques for collecting evaluation data: paper-and-pencil tests, questionnaires, interviews, visual observation, job sample or performance tests, simulation, rating forms or checklists, individual and group performance measures, individual and group behavior measures, and self-reports.(23,32) As measurement devices that will be analyzed statistically, they require the use of specific experimental designs. Regardless of the particular instrument or technique used, it should be pretested with a smaller group before actual use. Since comparisons are desired, it is usually necessary to collect preliminary data on current performance or behaviors.

Tests

Tests, especially written tests, are probably the most common devices for measuring learning. Tests sample what one knows, and schools depend heavily on them. Multiple-choice, true-false, short answer, completion, matching, and essay questions are used to measure learning in the cognitive domain. These tests are appropriate when several people are expected to learn the same content or material. Sometimes, both a pretest and a post-test are used to measure learning. This method assists in controlling variables, but be careful not to attribute all the changes noted on the post-test to the learning experiences, since other factors may have been involved.

Although tests are appropriate with school-age children, adults may respond less favorably. The dietetics practitioner should avoid evoking childhood memories associated with the authoritarian teacher, the dependent child, or the assigned degree of success and failure based on right or wrong answers. In one-on-one situations, the practitioner could ask the individual to state verbally what he or she learned as though telling it to a spouse or friend. Or, a self-assessment instrument may be used.

Questionnaires

Questionnaires may be preplanned and are often used to assess attitudes and values that do not involve correct answers. Questions may be open-ended, multiple choice, ranking, checklist, or alternate response, such as yes/no or agree/disagree. In evaluating behavioral change on the job, trainees and supervisors can both complete a questionnaire.

Interviews

Interviews conducted on a one-to-one basis are another form of evaluation. They are the oral equivalent to written questionnaires used to measure cognitive and affective objectives. Before the interview, the dietetics professional should preplan and draw up a list of questions that will indicate whether learning has taken place. After instruction, evaluation may consist of asking the client or employee to repeat important facts. An advantage of an interview is that the evaluator can put the person at ease and immediately correct any errors. Another advantage is that the interviewer can probe for additional information. Although this method is time consuming, it is appropriate for people with low literacy or those less educated. Focus group interviews, mentioned earlier, are an example of a qualitative, formative evaluation.

Observation

In many cases, visual observation is an appropriate method of evaluating learning. The behaviors to be observed should be defined, and an observation checklist may be helpful. When employees are under direct supervision, systematic ongoing observation over a period of time is a basis for evaluating learning. The supervisor can observe and report whether the employee is operating equipment correctly or following established procedures properly. If the employee has been taught sanitary procedures, for example, the professional can see whether or not they are incorporated into the employee's work. Evaluate the performance, using what was taught as a standard. If discrepancies are found, further learning may be indicated.

Performance Tests

When direct observation is not possible or would be too time-consuming and costly, a simulated situation or performance test can be observed. Performance tests are appropriate in the cognitive and psychomotor domains. You can ask a wait staff member to set a table, a cook to demonstrate the meat slicer, or a client to indicate what to select from a restaurant menu. The patient could be given a list of foods, some of which are permitted on the diet and some of which are not, and asked to differentiate them. With permission from the learner, audiotape or videotape may be used to record the simulation, so that the instructor and learner may discuss the results together and plan further learning to correct any deficiencies. The observer needs to delineate which behaviors are being observed and what is to be acceptable behavior.

Rating Scales/Checklists

Rating scales or checklists have been used to evaluate learner performance and teacher effectiveness. Categories or attributes such as knowledge level or dependability are listed and should be defined in detail to avoid ambiguity. Emphasis should be placed on attributes that can be confirmed objectively rather than judged subjectively. A 5- or 7-point scale is used, allowing a midpoint, and the ratings should be defined, for example, from "excellent" to "poor" or from "extremely acceptable" to "very unacceptable." The list should include as a possible response, "No opportunity to observe."

Rating scales are subject to a number of errors. Two evaluators may judge the same individual differently. To avoid error, definition of the terms and training of evaluators are essential. The ratings may suffer from personal biases. In addition, some raters have the tendency to be too lenient. Error may result if the rater is a perfectionist. Some evaluators tend to rate most people as average, believing that few people rank at the highest levels. Another possible error is the "halo" error, in which an evaluator is so positively or negatively impressed with one aspect of a person that he or she judges all other qualities according to this one impressive aspect.

Performance Measures

In employee training programs, individual and group performance measures, such as work quality and quantity, and number of errors, may be assessed. Individual and group behavioral measures, such as amount of absenteeism, number of grievances, and other types of problems that affect work performance, may be noted.

Self-Reports

Self-reports, self-evaluation, and self-monitoring are another approach to evaluation. In the affective domain, written questions or statements are presented, and the individual supplies responses. The dietetics professional may ask: "What changes, if any, have you made in your food choices?" "What are you doing differently?" Self-reports, such as a 3-day food record have been used to measure behavioral change. Responses may be distorted if the individual can ascertain the acceptable answer.

In one study, a food score was developed, permitting participants to score their own food choices.(38) A cholesterol-saturated fat index (CSI) scorecard was developed for self-monitoring to facilitate the adoption and maintenance of a cholesterol-lowering dietary pattern.(39) Studies have shown that self-evaluation or self-assessment of dietary status and behaviors enhanced motivation in older children, adults, pregnant women, and older adults.(5)

All methods of evaluation have advantages and limitations, which need to be considered. Although evaluation may not provide proof that an intervention and education worked, it does produce a great deal of evidence.(35) Evaluation of nutrition education programs is complex, and federal food assistance programs often have limited budgets to undertake evaluation.(40) In assessing adult learning, the dietetics professional should be careful to protect the individual's self-concept and to treat errors as indicators for additional instruction.

RELIABILITY AND VALIDITY

Validity

The concepts of reliability and validity are essential to the measurement of the effectiveness of nutrition education outcomes and employee learning. Validity indicates whether we are measuring what we intend to measure.(19,41,42) There are different types of validity, such as content-related, construct-related, and criterion-related (concurrent and predictive) validity, all of which help to "defend" the validity of the instrument. Content-related validity, which is the simplest and perhaps the most important, refers to whether the test items or questions correspond to the subject matter or purpose of instruction or to the knowledge, skills, or objectives they are supposed to measure for a specific audience by culture, age, literacy level, and the like. If interested in knowledge of dietary fiber, for example, are the questions appropriate in content.

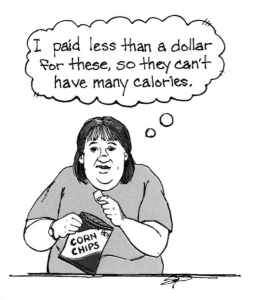

We need to evaluate what people learn.

Reliability

Reliability refers to the consistency and accuracy with which a test or device measures something in the same way in each situation or over time.(41) For example, if a test is given twice to the same students to sample the same abilities, the students should place in the same relative position to others each time if the test is reliable. Methods for determining the reliability and validity of tests may be found in the educational literature.(18,22) In all cases, keep in mind that the measuring device should assess whether the learner has attained the requisite knowledge, skill, or competence needed and whether behavior has changed. Pretesting evaluation instruments with the intended audience is essential. If the learner has not attained the intended knowledge or skill, additional learning may be indicated.

After the data from evaluation are collected, they should be compiled and analyzed. The statistical analysis of data is a lengthy subject of its own beyond the scope of this book. Future plans or programs may be modified based on the results of the evaluation. Results should be communicated through evaluation reports to others such as participants, management staff, decision makers, and future learners.

LESSON PLANS/PROGRAM PLANS

A lesson plan is a written summary of information about a unit of instruction. It is prepared and used by the instructor and may be submitted to an administrator. Various formats for lesson plans are available, but the content is essentially the same. A lesson plan is a blueprint that describes all aspects of instruction. It includes the following:(15)

- Preassessment of the participants or needs assessment
- The performance objectives identified
- The content outline (introduction, body, conclusions)
- How the content will be sequenced
- A description of the activities participants will engage in to reach the objectives
- Instructional procedures (lecture, discussion, and the like)
- Educational materials, visual aids, media, handouts, and equipment
- Amount of time allotted or scheduled
- Facilities to be used
- Method of evaluating whether the learner reached the objectives, outcomes, or other results
- References

Once written, a lesson plan is a flexible guide to instruction that can be used with many different individuals or groups.

A series of lesson plans or activities may be grouped into a larger unit of instruction covering a longer time frame, such as a whole day or several days. The term program planning is also used. A plan for a longer program would include essentially the same components as a lesson plan with the addition of the names of speakers or others responsible, and cost considerations. Sample lesson plans are found in Tables 12-3 and 12-4.

TABLE 12-3 Sample Lesson Plan on Sanitary Dish Handling

I. Target audience: New wait staff
II. Objective: When setting tables, wait staff will be able to handle dishes and utensils in a sanitary manner.
III. Time allotted: 15 minutes
IV. Preassessment: Question new employees to determine what they already know about sanitary dish and utensil handling.
V. Content and sequence:
1. Wash hands. Handling of flatware by the handles.
2. Handling of cups by the base or handle and glassware by the base.
3. Handling plates and bowls on the edge without touching the food.
4. Use a tray.
5. The hands and skin as major sources of disease causing bacteria and their transmission to food and utensils.
6. Proper bussing of dishes to avoid contamination of the hands.
7. Hand washing.
VI. Learning activities:
Demonstration and discussion of proper handling of dishes and utensils when setting tables, serving food, and bussing tables.
Discussion of hand washing.
Actual practice by new wait staff.
VII. Materials: Dishes, utensils, tray, handout of important points to remember.
VIII. Evaluation: Whether or not dishes and utensils were handled properly during the actual practice; continued observation of the employee's performance on the job.

DOCUMENTATION

Dietetics professionals are accountable for the nutrition care they provide in all settings, including in consulting and private practice and at the worksite. Accepted standards of practice for quality control and accreditation agencies, such as the Joint Commission on Accreditation of Healthcare Organizations (JCAHO), mandate that dietetic services be documented and communicated to other health professionals providing care.(43–45) Patient records also provide evidence in malpractice suits and are important to the denial of legal liability. This is increasingly important when transferring information to others over the internet.(46)

Documentation provides a developmental history of nutrition services to clients. Measurement and documentation of desired outcomes—medical, clinical, educational, and psychosocial—are essential. Documentation provides the information needed to evaluate how well medical nutrition therapy strategies have worked. What takes place between the dietetics professional and the patient or client should be recorded, including such data as nutrition screening, assessment, and reassessment as needed, nutrition care interventions planned and provided with timetables, measurable goals, plans for achieving goals and their outcomes, meal intakes and tolerance problems, nutrition counseling and education provided to the patient and/or significant other, patient's or client's reactions or responses, monitoring of progress including adherence to recom-

TABLE 12-4	Sample Lesson Plan on Calcium in Pregnancy

I. Target audience: Pregnant women

II. Objective: To be able to identify foods and quantities of foods that will meet the daily calcium needs for pregnancy and plan menus using these foods.

III. Time Allotted: 30 minutes

IV. Preassessment: Question audience about which foods contain calcium and how much of these foods should be eaten daily during pregnancy. Determine any previous pregnancies and what was eaten.

V. Content and sequence:
1. Total daily calcium needs with the important functions of calcium during pregnancy.
2. Dairy foods as a source of calcium with quantities of calcium in each.
3. Other foods as good sources of calcium with quantities of calcium.
4. Calcium sources for lactose-intolerant individuals.
5. Have audience suggest a breakfast, lunch, dinner, and snacks that meet the need for calcium.
6. Questions from the audience.
7. Have each person plan her own menu for tomorrow.

VI. Learning activities: Group discussion of food sources of calcium. Show actual foods and food models for portion sizes. Group planning of a day's menu followed by each individual planning something appropriate for herself for the next day's menu.

VII. Materials: Actual food samples, food models, paper and pencils for menu planning, chalkboard or flip chart for writing menus, handout with good sources of calcium and the amount of calcium in each including the DRI for pregnancy, and a sample menu.

VIII. Evaluation: The menu planned by each individual. Discussion with individuals during their follow-up prenatal visits.

mendations, actual outcomes and behavioral changes, as well as where efforts ought to be directed in the future.(44,47) The information communicated demonstrates what the dietetics professionals contribute to health care delivery and that their services provide the patient or client with a specific benefit that will offset the cost of the service.

The usual place for documentation is in the medical or client's record. Although several formats are available, traditionally the professional makes notes on the patient's medical record using the SOAP procedure.(43) The acronym SOAP stands for Subjective data, Objective data, Assessment, and Plan. Subjective data, obtained primarily through an interview, includes the patient's or client's perception and thoughts about the nutrition problem and his or her food intake. Objective data are the results of laboratory tests, such as serum albumin, or physical findings, such as weight, height, ideal weight, and diet orders. Assessment is the practitioner's analysis of the person's problem based on the subjective and objective data. The plan tells what the professional recommends or intends to do to solve the identified problem, such as plans for dietary alterations, patient counseling, education, referral, or other follow-up practices.

Documentation of employee education and training programs is also essential. Records should be kept of all information included in employee orientation. The use of

CASE STUDY 1

Susan Grey has decided that there is a need for prenatal nutrition classes in the outpatient clinic. Many of the patients are teenagers with limited incomes who are on suboptimum diets. The nurse is also interested in cooperating to reduce the time she spends in individual counseling with patients.

1. Develop a lesson plan for a prenatal nutrition class.
2. What audiovisual materials would you suggest?
3. What handout materials would you recommend?
4. How long should the presentation be?

CASE STUDY 2

Susan manages the kitchen at a major medical center with 600 beds. In the past month, there has been some employee turnover, and three new employees are involved in the preparation of hot foods. Susan is unsure of their knowledge of sanitation and knows that it is past time to be sure that they know the standards and the HACCP (Hazard Analysis Critical Control Points) procedures.

Susan decides to get the three employees together to assess their knowledge and discuss standards for personal hygiene and time-temperature standards for cooking and holding hot foods.

1. What are some ways to determine what the new employees know already, that is, their current level of knowledge?
2. What are possible ways to approach and fill any gaps in their knowledge?
3. What ways can Susan follow up and evaluate the results of her discussions?

an orientation checklist is helpful in ensuring that everything the employee needs to know has been communicated to him or her. Records should be kept on file showing the date and content of ongoing training sessions such as inservice programs, and off-the-job experiences such as continuing education.

This chapter has examined the selection and implementation of learning activities in the cognitive, affective, and psychomotor domains. The use of task analysis and job instruction training has been explained. The final step in planning learning is evaluation, in which assessment data are collected and analyzed to determine the success of educational endeavors.

The dietetics professional seeks to change people's eating practices, and in training employees, seeks to change the employee's job performance. Techniques and strategies that influence the acquisition of knowledge, the development of appropriate attitudes, and behavioral change were discussed. The relationship of knowledge and attitudes to behaviors is complex, however, since behavior is subject to many motivations all operating at the same time. The fact that clients and employees are informed does not mean that they will always act appropriately. Motives may be conflicting, and information may be disregarded or altered to serve one's own purposes. If time is limited, for example, little thought may be given to food choices. Instructional techniques that reflect the cultural and social context are important influences in nutrition education.

REVIEW AND DISCUSSION QUESTIONS

1. What are the advantages and disadvantages of the educational methods and techniques?
2. What methods and techniques are appropriate for objectives in the cognitive domain? The affective domain? The psychomotor domain?
3. Explain how a task analysis would be used with Job Instruction Training (JIT).
4. In what ways may educational instruction be organized or sequenced?
5. What are the purposes of evaluation?
6. Differentiate the following: formative and summative evaluation; reliability and validity; criterion-referenced and norm-referenced evaluation.
7. What are the major types or levels of evaluation? If you had to describe each to someone desiring to evaluate employee training, what major elements of each would you emphasize?
8. If you had to evaluate a diabetes education program, what would you do? How would you go about it?
9. What are the parts of a lesson plan or program plan?
10. What should be documented in the medical record?

SUGGESTED ACTIVITIES

1. Complete a task analysis for using a procedure or a piece of equipment (coffee urn, meat slicer, dish machine, mixer, oven, grille, broiler, etc.), listing the sequential steps and key points.
2. Using the JIT sequence and a task analysis, teach someone to use an unfamiliar piece of equipment.
3. Plan learning using one of the techniques in the chapter (other than lecture), such as discussion, simulation, or a demonstration. Carry out the plan.
4. Develop one or two performance objectives on a topic of interest for a target audience defined by age, sex, socioeconomic status, and educational level. The audience may be pregnant women, mothers, schoolchildren, adolescents, adult men or women, elderly, employees, executives, sports figures, or a person with a chronic disease. Plan the preassessment, content, techniques for presentation, teaching aids and handouts, and evaluation methods. Carry out the educational plan.
5. Develop one or two visual aids to use in teaching.
6. Give a pretest of knowledge on a subject. Instruct the learner on the subject. Follow up with a post-test to examine results.
7. List three ways in which you might evaluate whether an employee learned from a training program. List three ways in which you might evaluate whether a patient comprehended instruction regarding a diabetic diet.

WEB SITES

Patient education materials can be obtained free from government sites and some other sites as well. Also, see the web addresses in Chapters 5 and 8.

www.aboutproduce.com / Produce Marketing Association
www.aicr.org / American Institute for Cancer Research
www.Americanheart.org / American Heart Association
www.arches.uga.edu/~noahnet / University of Georgia free lesson plans
www.hrsa.gov / Health Resources and Services Administration
www.cancer.org / American Cancer Society
www.cnpp.usda.gov / USDA Center for Nutrition Policy and Promotion
www.cspinet.org / Center for Science in the Public Interest
www.diabetes.org / American Diabetes Association
http://exhibits.pacsci.org/nutrition / nutrition games
http://familydoctor.com / American Academy of Family Practice
www.fightbac.org / partnership for food safety
www.foodsafety.gov / food safety information
www.4women.gov / site for women
www.healthanswers.com / streaming video
www.healthAtoZ.com / health information from health professionals
www.healthfinder.gov / fact sheets, games, Spanish site
www.healthtouch.com / patient educational materials
www.ific.org / International Food Information Council
www.ifst.org / Institute of Food Science and Technology
www.intelihealth.com / affiliated with Harvard University
www.medicinenet.com / doctor produced information
www.kidney.org / National Kidney Foundation
www.niddk.nih.gov/health/health.htm / National Institutes of Health (NIH) fact sheets
www.nal.usda.gov/fnic / USDA Food Nutrition Information Center
http://nccam.nih.gov / National Center for Complementary and Alternative Medicine at the NIH
www.nutrition.gov / links to government resources
http://ods.od.nih.gov / NIH Office of Dietary Supplements
www.quackwatch.com / guide to health fraud
http://vm.cfsan.fda.gov/list.html / Food and Drug Administration
www.vrg.org / Vegetarian Resource Group
www.webmd.com / consumer health information
www.wheatfoods.org / Wheat Foods Council

REFERENCES

1. Gagne RM, Briggs LJ, Wager WW. Principles of instructional design, 4th ed. Fort Worth: Harcourt Brace Jovanovich, 1992.
2. Tracey WR. Selecting a delivery system. In: WR Tracey, ed. Human resources management & development handbook, 2nd ed. New York: American Management Association, 1994.

3. Wlodkowski RJ. Enhancing adult motivation to learn, rev ed. San Francisco: Jossey-Bass, 1999.

4. Farrah SJ. Lecture. In: Galbraith MW, ed. Adult learning methods: a guide for effective instruction, 2nd ed. Malabar, FL: Krieger, 1998.

5. Contento I, Balch GI, Bronner YL, et al. Executive summary. J Nutr Ed 1995;27:279.

6. Hartman TJ, McCarthy PR, Park RJ, et al. Focus group responses of potential participants in a nutrition education program for individuals with limited literacy skills. J Am Diet Assoc 1994;94:744.

7. Abusabha R, Peacock J, Achterberg C. How to make nutrition education more meaningful through facilitated group discussion. J Am Diet Assoc 1999;99:72.

8. Gilley JW. Demonstration and simulation. In: Galbraith MW, ed. Adult learning methods: a guide for effective instruction, 2nd ed. Malabar, FL: Krieger, 1998.

9. Wexley KN, Latham GP. Developing and training human resources in organizations, 3rd ed. Englewood Cliffs, NJ: Prentice Hall, 2002.

10. Carroll JM, Stein C, Byron M, Dutram K. Using interactive multimedia to deliver nutrition education to Maine's WIC clients. J Nutr Ed 1996;28:19.

11. Contento I, Balch GI, Bronner YL, et al. Nutrition education for adults. J Nutr Ed 1995;27:312.

12. Mager RF. How to turn learners on . . . without turning them off, 3rd ed. Atlanta: CEP, 1997.

13. Hahn J. How do you provide diabetes education to hard-to-reach, at-risk populations. J Am Diet Assoc 1996;96:1136.

14. Nolan M. Job training. In: RL Craig, ed. The ASTD training and development handbook, 4th ed. New York: McGraw-Hill, 1996.

15. Mager RF, Beach KM. Developing vocational instruction. Belmont, CA: Fearon Publishers, 1967.

16. Brinbrauer H. Skills/technical training. In: WR Tracey, ed. Human resources management & development handbook, 2nd ed. New York: American Management Association, 1994.

17. Leatherman RW. Conducting one-on-one training. In: WR Tracey, ed. Human resources management & development handbook, 2nd ed. New York: American Management Association, 1994.

18. Popham WJ. Modern educational measurement: practical guidelines for educational leaders, 3rd ed. Boston: Allyn & Bacon, 2000.

19. Kristal AR, Satia JA. Evaluation of nutrition interventions. In: Coulston AM, Rock CL, Monsen ER, eds. Nutrition in the prevention and treatment of disease. San Diego: Academic Press, 2001.

20. Dignan MB. Evaluation of health education, 3rd ed. Springfield, IL: Charles C Thomas, 1995.

21. McDermott RJ, Sarvela PD. Health education: evaluation and measurement. A practitioner's perspective, 2nd ed. New York: WCB/McGraw Hill, 1999.

22. Contento IR, Randell JS, Basch CE. Review and analysis of evaluation measures used in nutrition education intervention research. J Nutr Ed Behav 2002;34:2.

23. Phillips JJ. Handbook of training evaluation and measurement methods, 3rd ed. Houston: Gulf Publishing, 1997.

24. Garavaglia PL. How to ensure transfer of training. Training & Development 1993;47:63.

25. Knowles MS. The adult learner: a neglected species, 4th ed. Houston: Gulf Publishing, 1990.

26. DiLima SN, Schust CS. Community health: education and promotion manual. Gaithersburg, MD: Aspen Publishers, 1996.

27. Betts NM, Baranowski T, Hoerr S. Recommendations for planning and reporting focus group research. J Nutr Ed 1996;28:279.

28. Gans KM, Lovell HJ, Fortunet R, et al. Implications of qualitative research for nutrition education geared to selected Hispanic audiences. J Nutr Ed 1999;31:331.

29. Evans AE, Sawyer-Morse MK. The right bite program: a theory-based nutrition intervention at a minority college campus. J Am Diet Assoc 2002;102:S89.
30. Woolfolk AE. Educational psychology, 8th ed. Boston: Allyn & Bacon, 2001.
31. Mager RF. Measuring instructional results or got a match? 3rd ed. Atlanta: CEP, 1997.
32. Kirkpatrick DL. Evaluating training programs. The four levels. In: Piskurich GM, Beckschi P, Hall B, eds. The ASTD handbook of training design and delivery. New York: McGraw-Hill, 2000.
33. Dignan MB. Measurement and evaluation of health education, 3rd ed. Springfield, IL: Charles C Thomas, 1995.
34. Mattfeldt-Beman MK, Corrigan SA, Stevens VJ, et al. Participants' evaluation of a weight-loss program. J Am Diet Assoc 1999;99:66.
35. Gerber B. Does training make a difference? Prove it. Training 1995;32:27.
36. Schiller MR. Practical approaches to outcome evaluation. Top Clin Nutr 1999;14:1.
37. Long VA, Martin T, Manson-Sand C. The great beginnings program: impact of a nutrition curriculum on nutrition knowledge, diet quality, and birth outcomes in pregnant and parenting teens. J Am Diet Assoc 2002;102:S86.
38. Remmell PS, Gorder DD, Hall Y, Tillotson JL. Assessing dietary adherence in the Multiple Risk Factor Intervention Trial (MRFIT). J Am Diet Assoc 1980;76:351.
39. Mitchell DT, Korslund MK, Brewer BK, Novascone MA. Development and validation of the cholesterol-saturated fat index (CSI) scorecard: a dietary self-monitoring tool. J Am Diet Assoc 1996;96:132.
40. Sims LS, Volchick J. Our perspective: nutrition education enhances food assistance programs. J Nutr Ed 1996;28:83.
41. Monsen E. Research: successful approaches. Chicago: The American Dietetic Association, 1992.
42. Cheney C. Eight faces of validity. J Am Diet Assoc 2000;100:256.
43. Grace-Fargaglia P, Rosow P. Automating clinical dietetics documentation. J Am Diet Assoc 1995;95:687.
44. Krasker GD, Balogun, LB. 1995 JCAHO standards: development and relevance to dietetics practice. J Am Diet Assoc 1995;95:240.
45. Rankin SH, Stallings KD. Patient education: principles & practice, 4th ed. Philadelphia: Lippincott Williams & Wilkins, 2001.
46. Ashley RC. Telemedicine: legal, ethical, and liability considerations. J Am Diet Assoc 2002;102:267.
47. The ADA Standards of Practice for Dietetics Professionals. J Am Diet Assoc 1998;98:83.

13 Group Facilitation and Dynamics

After reading this chapter, you will be able to

1. list the factors increasing group cohesiveness.
2. discuss the suggestions for promoting group change.
3. explain the informal work group.
4. identify the group facilitation skills.
5. list and explain facilitator and participant functions in groups.
6. differentiate between formal and informal groups.
7. develop skill by leading a small group discussion.
8. identify the benefits and limitations of cohesive groups.
9. list the strengths and weaknesses of group decision making.
10. discuss the advantages and disadvantages of group counseling.

Never doubt that a small group of thoughtful, committed citizens can change the world. Indeed, it is the only thing that ever had.

Margaret Meade

As you peruse the list of objectives for this chapter, you may be surprised at the range of communication behaviors related to groups that the professional in health care is expected to develop. We humans, as social animals, spend most of our lives working, living, and playing among groups, but too few of us actually understand group dynamics and the accompanying behaviors that allow for us to be influential, persuasive, and a group asset. Activities such as conducting performance appraisals, counseling, disciplining staff, facilitating group meetings, team building, enhancing morale through the building of group cohesiveness among staff, initiating change and managing the resulting resistance all require well-honed communication skills.

When people are advanced into management without adequate training in these areas, the chances of their succeeding are hindered. During the twenty-first century, dietetics practitioners who manage need not only an extensive understanding of the applications of computer science and technology to assist them in decision making but also the knowledge and ability of how to harness the power of their employee and client groups.(1,2)

This chapter provides the practitioner with a general overview of the dynamics inherent in groups, including how the group functions internally, how the members relate to one another, how they communicate among themselves, and how they do their work as a group. The following topics are discussed: team building and management, change in groups, cohesiveness in groups, informal work groups, facilitator preparation, group facilitation skills, facilitator/participant functions, synergy, and groups as a supplement to individual nutrition counseling.

Much of this chapter is devoted to exploring skills required of the group facilitator and participants. The reader is cautioned, however, that one cannot develop these skills simply from reading a chapter, or even from reading it again and again. To develop these skills, you must make a personal commitment to risk feeling unsure and awkward as you attempt to practice them, and you need not wait until you are in management positions. In fact, the time to develop group skills is while you are still a student or staff member. You can practice these skills with friends, with family, and in the community. In this way, when you advance to a position of authority, you will have refined your skills from the earlier practice and experience.

Although interpersonal and group interaction skills can be taught, the most effective way for people to learn them is through experiencing, observing, and modeling others whom they admire and view as effective communicators. Communication skills often are more effectively "caught" than taught, and professionals need to be conscious of their opportunity to develop these skills among staff and clients through their own modeling of appropriate behaviors. Whether or not you intend it and whether your behavior is optimal or not, the professional is a role model for staff and clients. By learning interpersonal and group skills and then consciously applying them, dietetics practitioners constructively and proactively enhance the development of these skills among staff and clients.

A committee is a group that keeps minutes and loses hours.

Milton Berle

CHARACTERISTICS OF AN EFFECTIVELY OPERATING TEAM

Political, economic, and social change is pressuring health-care organizations to reinvent themselves. Staff and directors alike live with the anxiety arising from the question of whether or not the belt-tightening efforts, combined with structural changes and strategic alliances, will achieve the necessary improvements in efficiency and help to secure an adequate patient base.

It is reasonable to expect that health care institutions can realize the major gains in quality, productivity, efficiency, and competitive edge that organizations in service industries have enjoyed for the past several years by using proven methods, such as work redesign, team-based structures, and an empowered workforce, which have helped to restore competitiveness to many firms.

Spates of studies in health care generally and dietetics specifically examine the value of the team approach. Furthermore, the studies are being done not only within separate disciplines but also across disciplines and among the multidisciplines that are included in health care. Topics such as the efficiency of service and total quality of delivery, overcoming resistance to change within the work units, understanding the team's dynamics and the effects of team approaches on stress and burnout of staff all are being considered.(3–14)

By and large the studies confirm the superiority of the team approach, albeit directed by an enlightened director/facilitator, over the traditional authoritative style. The studies cited confirm that the team approach is more cost-effective and efficient and promotes more harmony and less resistance among staff and between the team leader and the work team. The contemporary dietetics professional therefore needs to be skilled in the practices of team leadership and development. The most critical of these skills is the operational knowledge of how to create the appropriate atmosphere among the team members, a climate that is comfortable, informal, and relaxed and yet encourages the team to perform optimally, free from obvious tensions, and to work together while involved and interested.

The contemporary team leader recognizes that his or her role is not to dominate or unduly defer to the group. The leader understands that leadership often shifts, depending on the circumstances. Different members, because of their special knowledge or experience, may be in positions at various times to act as resources for the group. In such teams, there is generally little evidence of a struggle for power; the issue is not who controls but how to get the job done.

The team leader also has the responsibility for motivating team members to stay focused on the team's goals and objectives. For example, if two team members are not getting along, the team leader is responsible for bringing the discussion back to the team's goals and off individual personalities.

The team leader reinforces member behavior that promotes healthy team dynamics. One of the key functions is to teach team members to monitor themselves and their work-related responsibilities independently. A well-functioning team processes their progress and attempts to discern what may be interfering with the operation. Whether

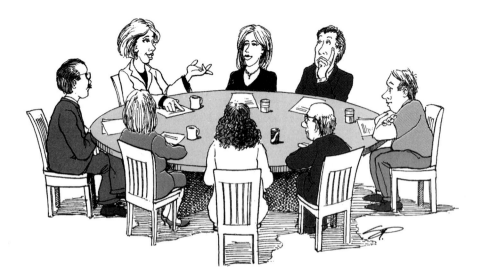

Groups should be seated in a circle so that everyone can see one another.

the problem is that of an individual whose behavior is interfering with the accomplishment of the group's objectives or whether it is a matter of procedure, the preferred method of resolution for today's workforce is open discussion until a solution is found.(15,16)

Another of the team leader's responsibilities is to stimulate a climate in which the members communicate openly and frankly. Although they are cohesive, they are not afraid to disagree or be rejected by teammates for sharing a contrary view. Conflict is regarded as healthy, and members understand that "managed" disagreement often leads to synergetic solutions. Members expect to voice their alternative opinions so that mutually satisfying solutions may be found. Criticism is frequent and frank and given with a minimum of anxiety. When members feel invested in one another, they feel freer to express their feelings authentically. When all members of the team participate in the problem-solving and decision-making processes, team members feel responsible and committed to the successful implementation of the team's decisions and objectives.

STIMULATING CHANGE IN TEAMS/GROUPS

Groups and teams are similar but not the same. All teams are groups, but not all groups are teams. A group is a collection of people who are together because of a common cause, goal, or purpose; they are not just a collection of people. The word "team" implies all of what constitutes a group, plus more. Teams ordinarily have structure imposed to facilitate the accomplishment of their agenda, and a team has a director, a coach, and a facilitator whose task it is to act as their catalyst. To be such a catalyst, team leaders or facilitators require group skills to manage change with both staff teams and client groups.

Ongoing change in organizations is inevitable. When changes are minor, the administrator can simply announce the changes and expect others to follow without resistance; however, other changes may be perceived as threatening by the staff. When changes arouse a sense of fear, ambiguity, and uncertainty, they are resisted. One of the first steps in overcoming this resistance is to facilitate the overt expression of concerns, even when such disclosures may provoke conflict. The professional needs to learn how to process the conflict that arises in the group so that it can be managed constructively.

A direct correlation exists among the amount of time, consideration, and participation in the proposed change allotted to those affected by the change and the amount of resistance likely to occur. When people are given consideration and an opportunity to voice their anxieties and questions, with their recommendations being incorporated whenever possible, they are less likely to resist the changes and more likely to assist in upholding them among others who may resist. When an entire work group is involved in discussion of problems and potential changes, with their supervisor acting as facilitator, agreement can be reached to use new methods, procedures, or solutions. The members of the group who later object are reminded by the others that they had adequate opportunity to make suggestions and express their concerns and that objecting now is inappropriate.(17–21) Subsequent discussion examines the group phenomena of change and cohesiveness and their effect on one another.

Communication among work groups is affected by a constellation of variables, each of which is related to every other. Currently, no theoretical model takes into account all the elaborate networks of sender, receiver, and message variables in small groups. In this section the two most salient variables, "change" and "cohesiveness," are explored. It is to the practitioner's advantage not only to understand the power and influence of the two phenomena on organizational life, but also to understand and apply appropriate strategies to use the change and cohesiveness variables for the good of the organization, department, and staff.

COHESIVENESS IN GROUPS

Cohesiveness is an elusive concept; there is no single definition that completely defines it. An eclectic definition is perhaps the best way to discuss the concept. A cohesive group has strong feelings of "we-ness," that is, members talking more in terms of "we" than "I"; displaying loyalty and congeniality to fellow members; working together for a common goal with everyone ready to take responsibility for group tasks; possibly enduring pain and frustration for the group; and defending against criticism and attack. A summary of factors influencing group cohesiveness is found in Table 13-1.

TABLE 13-1   Factors Increasing Group Cohesiveness

1. All members perform worthwhile tasks and feel they are appreciated by the group.
2. Members clearly perceive the group's goals and consider them to be realistic.
3. Members perceive the group as an entity in its own right and refer to it as such, calling it "the group" or "our group."
4. The group develops a history and tradition. All cohesive groups (church, state family, work, etc) perform traditional rites and rituals, passing on to new members the "secrets" of the past and strengthening the existing ties among the group's veterans.
5. The group has prestige.
6. Members possess knowledge or material needed by the group.
7. Member participation in the determination of the group's standards is full and direct.
8. Members perceive the issues at hand to be of importance.
9. Personal interaction among members is based on equality, with no one exercising much authority over anyone else.
10. Members share ideals and interests, a common enemy outside the group, or a common satisfaction of individual needs for protection, security, and affection.
11. Members are not jealous and competitive with one another.
12. Group size is small rather than large.
13. The group is more homogeneous than heterogeneous.

Because employee turnover is constant in most organizations, intense cohesiveness in work groups is rare; however, a knowledgeable manager can enhance the group's level of attraction and support toward one another through an understanding and application of what behavioral scientists have learned regarding group cohesiveness.

The specific reasons why cohesion thrives in some groups, dissipates in others, and fails to emerge at all in still others are as elusive as its definition. The most fundamental reason for groups tending to gravitate toward cohesive units stems from a basic tenet of human nature: people like to be liked. This desire to be accepted and liked leads people to engage in actions that will maintain or increase the esteem they receive from those around them. There is, therefore, a tendency to go along with the group. After a group feels cohesive, it attempts to preserve the state. Cohesiveness, however, is not static. Even highly cohesive organizations change employees, altering the nature of the internal structure and the interaction patterns of members. Over a period of time, therefore, a group may lose its cohesiveness.

Not all teams are cohesive, and those that are may not remain so indefinitely. Cohesiveness relates to the feelings of belonging and acceptance that each member feels in the group. Unless the norms of authenticity, openness, and nonjudgmental acceptance of differences are regularly reinforced among the members, the level of cohesiveness will diminish.

In addition to the increase in self-esteem that generally accompanies members' participation in a cohesive group, other benefits emerge as well: members or individuals can be honest in their dialogue with other members, and they can relax and not be continually on their guard. Because members feel a stake in the group, they are more likely to disagree and argue about decisions affecting it. When a decision is made, each member feels committed to it and takes responsibility for it. Even if meetings are uninhibited and less structured, the topic is more likely to be fully explored, errors are more likely to be pointed out, and poor reasoning or attempts at manipulation on the part of various individuals are more likely to be exposed in the cohesive group than in the more self-conscious and cautious noncohesive group. From the dietitian's perspective, maintaining high cohesiveness provides a highly desirable work climate, especially when the manager uses participative decision-making and group problem-solving strategies.

People in noncohesive groups are likely to argue less, to be more polite, and to be more easily bored. When members disagree, they feel less secure in expressing themselves and often give no overt signs; instead, they may frown, look away, or plead ignorance. Members who are worried about their own security hesitate to challenge others; therefore, noncohesive groups frequently stick to irrelevancies or safe topics or procedures rather than become involved in discussing the real issues. Unlike members of cohesive groups, members of noncohesive groups generally do not fully explore the topic, expose manipulation or poor reasoning, argue for what they believe, or take full responsibility for the group's decision. Agreement may be only for the sake of apparent cohesion (external), in which case the individual does not feel bound to the group's goals or decisions. Clearly, the quality of any group decisions or solutions to work-related problems made in these groups is poorer than those made in more cohesive work groups. It is the manager's responsibility to create a climate in which individuals dare to differ from the group without fear of expulsion.

Generally, the newer members of a group are the most easily intimidated because they are more likely to feel inferior to the established members of the work group. The individual's sense of acceptance in the work group is a highly prized possession, and anything that produces disharmony or conflict of views is likely to disturb it. New members are the most likely to accept and adopt the group's norms because of the pressures of being in a group in which everyone else is acting, talking, or thinking in a certain way. This can occur even without any overt or conscious pressure by group veterans.

In summary, the major advantage of the cohesive group is its tendency toward a greater quality of communication, with the interaction more equally distributed than in the noncohesive group. Members feel freer to disagree and challenge one another, provided that they do not perceive the message as a threat to their own status or security. Messages are usually more fully explored in the cohesive group, and the communicator has a better chance of achieving a shared understanding of the message, which could lead to a favorable attitude change in the entire group. If, however, the group interprets a message as a threat to its cohesiveness, it will reject it more hastily than the noncohesive group will.

Conforming to norms may stifle the person's identity and creativity and may restrict, inhibit, and change the values of individual members. It is paradoxical that cohesive teams or groups also provide individuals with opportunities for need fulfillment and personal growth through work satisfaction and camaraderie and are the most likely to achieve synergy. Developing cohesiveness within the team and then using it to produce superior problem-solving and decision-making can only be achieved consistently through the enlightened facilitator's careful monitoring and "fine-tuning" of the group's dynamics. The manager needs to solicit and reinforce authentic reactions from individuals within the group while at the same time safeguarding the sense of unconditional acceptance among the other team members.

THE RELATIONSHIP OF COHESIVENESS TO CHANGE IN GROUPS

Group change can be fostered through coercion and intimidation, but permanent change promoted in this way is rare. Group change is most easily and optimally developed in meetings and workshops, where trust, team building, and open communication are facilitated among members. Change has the best chance for acceptance and permanence when the need for and value of the change arise from within the group. Change occurring under these conditions receives mutual support and reinforcement from the entire group. After all channels of communication are opened and the needs for change explored, the members may experience a short-lived increase in hostility, but eventually after all have shared perceptions and arrived at mutual agreement or compromise, the new norms are enforced.

Although some group members may disagree with the change and revert to the old behavior, frequently group pressures and the persons' perceptions of their own dissonance cause them to abide by the group-accepted behavior. Suggestions for promoting group change are summarized in Table 13-2.

TABLE 13-2 Suggestions for Promoting Group Change

1. If attitude change is desired, small open-ended, off-the-record discussion groups in which the person feels secure are most effective.
2. When people need to change behaviors, participation in group discussions is 2 to 10 times more effective than a lecture that presents the reasons for and pleas for change.
3. Active discussion by a small group to determine its goals, methods, work, and new operations, or to solve other problems is more effective in changing group practices than separate instructions, supervisor's requests, or the imposition of new practices by an authority. Group involvement brings about better motivation and support for the change and better implementation and productivity of the new practice.
4. Group change is easier to bring about and more permanent than change in the individual members of the group. The supposed greater permanence stems from the individual's assumed desire to live up to group norms. It follows that the stronger the group bonds, the more deeply based are the individual's attitudes. Another explanation suggests that the public commitment to carry through the behavior decided on by group members creates an awareness of the expectations that members have for each other, thus creating forces on each member to comply.
5. The best way for a manager to initiate change is to create an atmosphere that leads to a shared perception by the entire group of the need for change. Then the members will call for the change themselves and enforce it. After all facts have been shared with all members and all channels of communication have been opened, there is frequently a sudden but short-lived increase in hostility; however, without this complete sharing among all group members, there can be no real change, only mistrust and subtle hostility.
6. High-status persons have more freedom from group control than do other members. The greater the prestige of individual group members, the greater the influence for change they can exert on the others.
7. The "buddy system" of change, in which the change is suggested by a peer, is better than having it demanded by an authority figure.

Modified from Breuer J. Orchestrating culture shock: what happens when companies must change. Inform 1989;3:46. Modified from Brilhart JK, Galanes GJ. Effective group discussion, 8th ed. Dubuque, IA: Wm C Brown, 1995.

In summary, people's attitudes, beliefs, and values all are rooted in the various groups to which they belong. The more genuinely attached people are to their groups and the more attractive these groups become in fulfilling the various needs of group members, the more likely these members are to be in close and constant contact with their group. Under these conditions group-anchored behaviors and beliefs are extremely resistant to change, with the group being able to exercise firm control over its members. The more attractive a group is to its members, the greater its power to change them. For the group itself to be used most effectively as an agent of change, it must first be cohesive with a strong sense of oneness existing between those who are to be changed and those who desire change. Attempts at changing group members must be aimed at either countering the influence of the group or encompassing it in the change. Either way, all attempts at changing individuals must also consider the dynamics of their groups.(22–25)

INFORMAL WORK GROUPS

Dietetics professionals need to be aware of the inherent power and influence of the informal work group. Since the 1920s, when the Hawthorne studies were carried out at the Western Electric plant near Chicago, social scientists have been studying the Hawthorne Effect. The Hawthorne Effect refers to the theory and its corollaries that employees perform more efficiently when they believe that they are being given special attention. The theory suggests that the major influences affecting efficiency and production are group social structures, group norms, and group pressures.

Professionals need to be sensitive to the dynamics and influences of the informal work group. They must learn ways to provide a forum in which social, task-related, and organizational concerns can be expressed, responses can be offered, and any resistance to change can be overcome. To become conscious of the influence inherent in the informal work group and to tap into the grapevine of informal communication, the manager needs to be aware of the networks of communication that exist within the department as well as the networks within the organization.

Communication networks are the patterns of message flow or linkages of who actually speaks to whom. In all organizations, there are distinctions between the "permissible" structured or organizational and the actual channels of communication and network linkages. The permissible channels are the linkages dictated by the organization's structure, which determines the hierarchy of power and influence; the actual channels are the patterns that do, in fact, occur. Often, administrative assistants are ultimately more influential, because of their connections within the network, than others who are considerably higher on the organization chart.

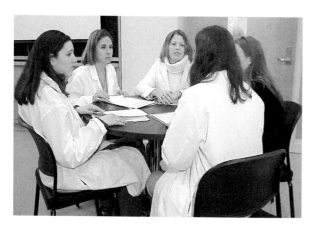

Groups can provide solutions superior to those of one individual.

Although they constitute a minority, some people perform best when under the direction of an authoritarian leader. When persons come from backgrounds in which they have not been encouraged to think and have been punished for initiating ideas, predictably in a work situation they will lack the self-confidence to offer suggestions within a group. If treated with patience, however, and given continued positive reinforcement each time they risk contributing an idea, they may gradually gain the confidence to become valuable group members. In general, however, members of today's work force have grown up with a preference for egalitarian treatment and perform best in groups with a leader who can act as a facilitator, involving employees rather than prescribing to them. Facilitators are those who understand the value of group decision-making and see their function as helping the group to get started, to establish a climate of work, to give support to others, to guide the group, and to keep the group on track so that its objectives are achieved. The group's activities and the facilitator's attitude toward the group are based on respect for what can be accomplished through group discussion and on the fostering of a group climate in which people feel comfortable and secure enough to contribute their ideas.

FACILITATOR PREPARATION

Facilitators' responsibilities begin before the discussion in their preparation of the appropriate meeting environment. They must make sure that the room itself is comfortable, with adequate ventilation and lighting and with a consciously arranged seating pattern. Sitting in a circle, for example, allows group members to see one another's faces, which tends to increase interaction among them. When people are arranged at long rectangular tables, they tend to interact most with those in direct view and little with those on either side of them.

When meetings involve persons who do not know one another, the facilitator should supply nametags or cards for everyone in the group. A sense of group spirit develops more quickly when people use one another's names as they interact. Allowing members time to introduce themselves is time well spent toward developing a comfortable climate. "Small talk" in groups in not a small matter. Just hearing one another allows the members to make some assumptions that help them to reduce anxiety. The individuals' tone of voice, dress, diction, and manner provide valuable clues to their character. Often, negative inferences disappear after the other's voice is heard and some information regarding the person's background is gathered.

Facilitating is like driving—you've got to pay attention a lot.

Kevin Elkenberry

GROUP FACILITATION SKILLS

Nutrition counselors and managers need to assist in group problem-solving by developing their roles as expert information disseminators, diagnosticians, team members, empathizers, and group facilitators. Most practitioners eventually need to direct in groups and facilitate interaction among them. Effective facilitation requires training and discipline to stay in the role of guide and not become a participant. Described in the following paragraphs are specific skills that need to be practiced as you train to develop group facilitation skills.(25–28)

Relieving Social Concerns

A tenet of group dynamics suggests that social concerns take precedence over task- or work-related concerns. In other words, a person's first concern is with being accepted and acknowledged as worthy. If people feel anxiety about being with unknown others or others who may bear them ill will, they generally do not participate. One way in which a facilitator can attend to social concerns is to spend a few minutes at the beginning of each meeting allowing people to interact socially, providing "open-time" to reestablish positive regard for one another. If ill will does exist among some of the participants and the facilitator is aware of it, he or she can attempt to have the members resolve their conflict before the meeting, or, if they are willing, the conflict can be resolved at the meeting. Only after the members have had their social concerns met can they wholeheartedly participate in task concerns.

Tolerating Silence

After facilitators have made opening remarks, have made sure that everyone knows everyone else, have articulated the desire for everyone's participation, and have stated the reasons or purpose for the meeting, they might rephrase the topic in the form of a question and then invite someone to comment. Because members frequently hesitate to express opinions with which their superior might disagree, they often wait to hear the supervisor's opinion first. At times no one may want to initiate discussion and reduce the tension. Silence is likely to occur most during the early stages of an ongoing group. After the group comes to understand that the facilitator truly does not intend to dominate, lead, or force opinions, members begin to use the meeting time to interact with one another. For those first few meetings, however, the facilitator should repeat the intention not to participate, should encourage others to participate, and then should just sit patiently. Ordinarily, if the silence is tolerated long enough, someone eventually takes the responsibility for directing the discussion.

Guiding Unobtrusively and Encouraging Interaction

The facilitator guides indirectly, helping the members to relate better to one another and to complete the task. Facilitators ought not allow themselves to become the focus. The facilitator can encourage interaction among the group members by looking away from speakers in the group as they attempt to harness his or her eyes. Although this behavior may seem rude, the speaker quickly gets the idea and looks to the other group members for feedback and response as the talk continues. The facilitator should resist the temptation to make a reply after others talk, but needs to wait for someone else to reply. If no one else makes a comment, however, the facilitator can ask for reactions. A question such as "Any reaction to that, Mary?" is preferred to "my reaction is. . . ."

Because facilitators wish to keep the focus on the group, they should remind group members during the first few minutes of the meeting that their purpose primarily is to get things started and then simply to serve as a guide. This assertion will eventually be tested. Most people have heard the same sentiment expressed by teachers and others and have learned that while some do mean it, the majority are paying it lip service only, want things done their way, and expect ultimately to be followed.

Knowing When and How to Resume Control

Just as a facilitator who rules and dominates in an authoritarian manner can stifle the group's creativity, facilitators who are too timid, uncertain, or frightened and who let the group wander can hinder the group's potential for synergy, that is, for finding superior solutions. Facilitators need to determine whether the group is capable of facilitating for itself. When it is, the facilitator's function is to remain on the sidelines. Only when no competent participant is available to perform the necessary functions does the facilitator become an active member of the group.

Reinforcing the Multisided Nature of Discussion

The facilitator can reinforce the nondogmatic, multisided nature of discussion by phrasing questions so that they are open-ended. Examples are: "How do you feel about that, Helen?" "Who in you opinion. . .?" and "What would be some way to. . .?" Facilitators need to think before asking questions to avoid closed and leading questions, questions that can be answered by only one or two words, and questions that suggest a limited number of alternative responses.

Exercising Control Over Loquacious Participants

The most common problem that facilitators have is knowing what to say to someone who is overly talkative. There are many appropriate ways of handling this participant, and individual facilitators need to decide which techniques they feel most comfortable using, keeping in mind that when they interact with any single member of the group, all other participants experience the interaction vicariously. If the facilitator treats individual participants without respect or humiliates or embarrasses them, all members are affected by the experience.

Several techniques may be effective in dealing with the loquacious participant. The facilitator may interrupt the participant, commenting that the point has been understood, and begin immediately to paraphrase concisely so that the participant knows that he or she has been understood. Although some group members talk excessively because they enjoy talking and because they believe that they are raising their status within the group through the quantity of their interaction, other talkative members often repeat themselves because of insecurity. They are not convinced that they have been understood. Usually, this kind of participant stops talking after being paraphrased. Of course, this process may need to be repeated several times during the course of the discussion.

A second problem arises with the participants who simply enjoy talking and do perceive increased status from it. These people do not stop talking after being paraphrased. They may need to be told that short concise statements are easier to follow, that they need to limit the length and number of comments, and/or that the group is losing the point from their extensive commentary. If that does not work, the facilitator may need to talk with the participant privately. Often, talkative group members are unaware that others are offended by their domination. The facilitator can point out to them that he or she has noticed others stirring and wanting to enter the discussion. It needs to be stressed to these participants that being long-winded cuts down on the time allowed for others to contribute to the discussion.

Establishing additional meeting guidelines on an ad hoc basis can also control "time-wasters." The facilitator, for example, may say, "Because of the brief time remaining, we will no longer be able to permit interruptions."

Encouraging Silent Members

For various reasons, including boredom, indifference, felt superiority, timidity, and insecurity, there are usually some members who refuse to participate. The facilitator's action toward them depends on what is causing them to be silent. The facilitator can arouse interest by asking for their opinions of what a colleague has said. If the silence stems from insecurity, the best method is to reinforce positively each attempt at interjection. A smile, a nod, or a comment of appreciation for any expressed opinion is sufficient. Sometimes silent members "shout out" nonverbal signals. An overt frown, nod, and pounding fingers all are signals that should be interpreted as the silent member's willingness to be called on to elaborate; however, if silent members have their heads down and blank facial expressions, it would be a mistake to force them into the discussion.

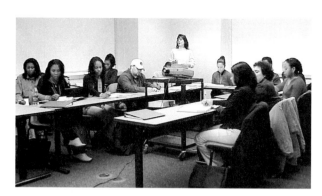

Meetings should have an agenda.

Halting Side Conversation

Generally, the facilitator should not embarrass members who are engaged in private conversations by drawing attention to them in the presence of the group. If the side conversation becomes distracting to other members of the group, those engaged in the conversation might be called by name and asked an easy question.

Discouraging Wisecracks

If someone in the group disrupts with too much humor or too many wisecracks, the facilitator needs to determine at what point the humor stops being a device to relieve tension in the group and starts to interfere with the group's interests. When facilitators believe that the humor is taking the focus off group issues and onto the joker, they need to interrupt, preferably smiling, with a comment such as "Now let's get down to business." If the comment needs to be made a second time, intense eye contact with the joker and no smile as the same remark is repeated usually halts the disruption.

Helping the Group to Stay on the Topic

When the group itself seems unable to stick to the agenda and wanders, a device under-used by facilitators is a flip chart to jot down points that have been agreed on as a way to chart the group's progress. With a minimum of interaction, the facilitator can prod the group on by simply summarizing and writing down the points. Generally, the group's reaction is to go on to the next item on the agenda.

Avoiding Acknowledgment of the Facilitator's Preferences

Facilitators hinder the group when they praise the ideas they like and belittle those they dislike. It is particularly important that they avoid making comments that may be taken as disapproval, condescension, sarcasm, personal cross-examination, or self-approval. Once the group members know the facilitator's preferences, they will tend to incorporate these preferences in their own comments. Because the professionals are in a position to reward or punish subordinates, the group members quickly learn that if what the supervisors want is to be followed and not disagreed with, that is how they will behave toward them.

FACILITATOR/PARTICIPANT FUNCTIONS

In addition to the specific skills required of facilitators, there are numerous group skills that both participants and facilitators should possess. There is a mistaken notion that it is the facilitator's responsibility alone to see that the group's tasks are accomplished and that a healthy group spirit is maintained. In reality, these responsibilities belong to anyone who has the training and insight to diagnose the group's weaknesses and who has the skills to correct them. Because most people are used to being "led" in groups, the facilitator may need to reinforce verbally the functions that all participants are expected to perform. The following paragraphs describe some of these skills and functions that both facilitators and participants have a mutual obligation to develop in themselves.

1. Groups need members to propose new ideas, goals, and procedures. Individual members are expected to accept the responsibility of **initiating.** Any member who has the insight into what should be initiated and waits for someone else to do it is ignoring an obligation. The facilitator might also remind participants of the spate of behavioral literature that verifies the correlations between employee-participant involvement and superior decisions.(29–33)
2. Everyone shares the responsibility of **seeking information and opinions**. You do not need to have vast knowledge of the topic being discussed to be a valuable member. Asking the right questions and seeking information from others in the group who have knowledge are valuable functions.
3. **Clarifying** what others have said by adding examples, illustrations, or explanations is a major contribution. People are not all on the same wavelength. Because of background, life experiences, education, natural intelligence, and environment, some people tend to understand one another more easily than do others. Two people who have grown up under similar conditions, for example, have an easier time commu-

nicating than two people from different backgrounds. People who understand what someone else in the group is struggling to make clear and add examples and explanations to clarify the thoughts for the others have made significant contributions. Simply nodding in agreement and saying nothing is a disservice to the others.

4. Another function related to clarifying is **coordinating** relationships among facts, ideas, and suggestions. If one member has the insight to understand how the ideas and activities of two or more group members are related and how they can be coordinated, that member serves a valuable function in expressing this relationship to the others.

5. **Orienting** is a term given to the function of processing for the group the pattern of its interaction and progress. The orienter clarifies the group's purpose or goal, defines the position of the group, and summarizes or suggests the direction of the discussion. Orienting by providing frequent internal summaries, for example, allows the group an opportunity to verify whether everyone is understanding the direction in which the group is going and provides those who disagree or who have misunderstood with the opportunity to speak.

6. Perhaps the least understood and most valuable function a person can perform for a group is being a **supporter**. Supporters are those who praise, agree, indicate warmth and solidarity, and verbally indicate to the others that they are in agreement with what is being proposed. It is a valuable function because without verbal support from others, good ideas and suggestions are often disregarded. If one person expresses an idea that the majority dislikes and that no one supports, the idea is quickly dismissed. Generally, if only one person supports the idea, the group will seriously consider the proposal. Frequently, a minority opinion can gain majority support because a single supporter agrees, causing the group to consider seriously the possible merits of the proposal. Support can be given by briefly remarking, "I agree," "Well said," "I wish I had said that," or "Those are my sentiments, too." Generally, one person alone cannot influence a group: one person with a supporter, however, has an excellent chance of doing so.(34) This topic is developed further in the final section of this chapter.

7. **Harmonizing** is also a valuable contribution to the group. It includes mediating differences between others, reconciling disagreement, and bringing about collaboration from conflict. It is common for group members to sit silently as they hear the valid arguments on both sides of an issue. One of the ways in which discussion differs from debate, however, is that discussion assumes that most issues are multisided, whereas debate tends to lend itself to two-sided issues only. The group member who verbally reinforces the positive aspects of the various factions and helps to suggest new and alternative solutions that include the best points of all sides is harmonizing.

8. Conflict, stress, and tension in groups are inevitable. When the stress or the tension mounts, it can enhance the conflict and the disagreement. People who can find humor in the situation, reduce the formality or status differences among group members, and relax the others are called **tension relievers**. A problem can occur when the tension reliever seeks recognition for him- or herself and continues to joke, drawing the attention away from the issues. Relieving tension is valuable up to a point, after which it can be disruptive.

9. The final function in this discussion is **gatekeeping**. In gatekeeping, one notices which members have been sending out signals that they want to speak but have not

had the courage or opportunity to enter the discussion. Gatekeeping ensures that all have an equal chance to be heard. As pointed out in the discussion of the facilitator's functions, there is a difference between people who are nonverbally signaling that they have strong feelings—by raising their eyebrows, tapping loudly, or grunting—and people who are silent. Group members become uncomfortable when they sense that other members might force them to talk. All members share the responsibility to protect others from being coerced into sharing opinions. Gatekeepers tend to say things such as "You look like you have strong feelings," or "I can tell by your face that you disapprove." Such comments are generally all the prodding the silent participant needs to enter the discussion.

Too often individuals believe that in the ideal group, a single leader is responsible for each of the functions just discussed. In fact, all members—participants as well as facilitators—are responsible, and they need to be alert to perform as many of the functions as they see a need for. Some people may be natural harmonizers or natural orienters or may be able to effortlessly perform some other valuable function. However, if the group needs a gatekeeper and none is present, the natural harmonizer who sees the need must exercise the gatekeeping function. One of the ways in which people familiar with group dynamics and with the skills needed to enhance the working of groups can detect members who have had training in the same area is by their willingness to act on their insight to correct a weakness in the group. The mind operates several times faster than the speed of human speech. While members of the group are talking, other sophisticated group members need to be reflecting on the dynamics of the group and on the needs at the moment. This process leads to an understanding of which functions need to be performed to help the group accomplish its task and maintain its healthy spirit.

PARADOX OF GROUP DYNAMICS

There is a paradox inherent in groups. They possess the potential, on the one hand, to stimulate creative thinking and to promote a decision or solution that is superior to what any individual working alone could accomplish. On the other hand, groups possess the potential to stifle creative thinking and thus promote a quality of outcome inferior to what individuals working alone might accomplish. Ordinarily, no one person is solely responsible for what happens in any given session; however, whether a group becomes a force to promote creative thinking and problem solving or a force that inhibits these functions depends primarily on the skills of its leader and, to a lesser degree, on the skills of the participants. Specific behavior patterns help a group to function effectively; others hinder the progress. Knowing how to facilitate positive behavior in groups and how to inhibit the negative behavior is an asset to dietetics practitioners.

SYNERGY

Professionals need to appreciate "group process" and to discover what can be done to stimulate their staff and/or client groups so that they become a creative force that promotes synergy. Synergy refers to the phenomenon in which the group's product (i.e.,

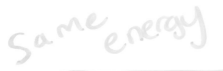

conclusion, solution, or decision) is qualitatively and/or quantitatively superior to what the most resourceful individual within the group could have produced by working alone.(35) Today, much is understood about the phenomenon; however, it has not yet filtered into management practice. Although greatly influenced by the style of their facilitators, all groups possess the potential to be either a force for creative innovative thinking or a force that works to preserve the status quo and stifle new ideas.(16) The purpose of this section is to offer suggestions on how to promote the former. The major variables that affect the group's potential for synergy are the availability of a single expert within the group, the heterogeneity or homogeneity of the group, and the existence of training of the group and its facilitator in the consensus-seeking process.

Facilitators should begin each meeting by stating their desire to promote a climate of acceptance and freedom of expression. Hearing the facilitator express this desire helps to set a group "norm" whereby everyone has a responsibility to participate. A norm is an unwritten rule to which the group adheres. Members pick up the code of appropriate behavior by noticing what the facilitator reinforces positively, ignores, tolerates, or rejects. Eventually, the facilitators' expressions of their desire for everyone to participate and the rights of each member to express subjective opinions without being abused by others will be tested. It is not enough to articulate norms; they must be enforced. If people are abused by others, told to be silent, embarrassed, humiliated, or insulted, for example, and the facilitator does not intervene to protect them, his or her articulated norm will be discounted and the actual behavior that has been tolerated will be considered the "real" norm. For that reason, it is critical that group facilitators realize the importance of their function to stimulate group interaction while protecting group members from being verbally abused or stifled. Realizing that synergy is most likely to occur in groups in which people can react authentically and are free to challenge the facilitator and the other participants, the dietetics practitioner needs to convince the group that they need to listen and respond honestly to one another's ideas.

As a rule, if a single expert is available and the rest of the group members are relatively ignorant of the matter being discussed, the expert should make the decision. In practice, however, there is usually no single expert available, and some group members are more informed than others, with a wide range of opinions being represented in the group. Under these conditions, the potential for synergy exists.

The variable of a heterogeneous versus homogeneous group of participants is more complicated. When group members are untrained in the consensus-seeking process and form a homogeneous group, they have less conflict and generally produce superior decisions to those produced by an untrained heterogeneous group. It is understandable that people who are similar in age, background, culture, life experiences, values, and the like have an easier time agreeing than with those with whom they have little in common.

The heterogeneous group that is untrained is likely to respond in one of the following ways. If the members of the group do not know one another, they will probably remain silent. Most people become anxious in the presence of strangers, whose response to them is unpredictable. Rather than risk sharing a contrary opinion and being insulted, humiliated, or embarrassed, they tend to go along with the opinions expressed by other members of the group. Decisions in such groups may appear to be produced by consensus, because there is no apparent disagreement, but in fact consensus may not be present. Because there is no group commitment and cohesion, conflict presents a threat to the group's interpersonal structure. Members try to smooth conflicts rather than resolve them. When disagreement arises, the members make quick compromises to get along. They resort to conflict-reducing techniques, such as majority rule and trade-offs. The quality of decisions made in these groups tends to be low.

The other possibility is that a great deal of verbal conflict will occur among the untrained members in a heterogeneous group, with each member insisting on his or her own point of view, so that the group never arrives at a decision with which everyone can be satisfied. This tends to occur most often in ad hoc groups with high-power personalities.

The variable of training in the consensus-seeking process is the most critical of all for producing synergy. In studies conducted by Dr. Jay Hall, a social scientist, trained and untrained groups were measured; both types of groups produced synergy. In the trained groups, however, synergy occurred 75% of the time, whereas in the untrained groups, synergy occurred only 25% of the time.(35) The implications are obvious: group leaders, facilitators, managers, supervisors, and all those who try to work with others in a participative manner need to understand the principles of training and instruct their groups in the process. A second conclusion was that under conditions of training, heterogeneous groups performed better than homogeneous groups. In fact, the broader the range of opinions presented, the better the group's chances of arriving at superior decisions. The implication here is that a group of "lemons," group members who fight and cannot agree, can be turned into lemonade, if the facilitator trains them in the consensus-seeking process.

GUIDELINES FOR SEEKING CONSENSUS

The training required to move a group from 25% to 75% efficiency in achieving consensus is based on a set of guidelines for group behavior; it is simple and not time-consuming. Professionals who decide to use this method with staff need to understand, however, that it may take several weeks of regularly reminding the group of the guidelines and interrupting each time the guidelines are not followed, before the process becomes natural to the group. The following are guidelines for achieving consensus in groups:

1. All group members have the responsibility and obligation to share opinions.
2. After group members have expressed opinions on a particular issue, they have the right to ask others to paraphrase these comments to their satisfaction.
3. After being paraphrased, they may not bring up their perspective again unless asked to do so by another group member. Insisting on one's own point of view or blocking discussion is not acceptable.
4. Everyone has the responsibility to understand the arguments and opinions of the other members and may ask questions for clarification.
5. After all perspectives are understood, the group needs to arrive at a solution or decision that can satisfy everyone. In accomplishing this task, the group may not immediately resort to the stress-reducing techniques of majority rule, trade-offs, averaging, coin-flipping, and bargaining.
6. Differences of opinion should be viewed as natural and expected.

Members need to be encouraged to seek them out so that everyone is involved in the decision process. Disagreements can help the group's decision because with a wider range of information and opinions, there is a greater chance that the group will develop superior solutions. Frequently, when the group members suspend their own judgment, new solutions emerge that no single individual would have been able to develop alone. These solutions tend to incorporate the best points of all views—of both the majority and the minority. Such solutions tend to be synergistic. At times, however, after considerable discussion, no new solution emerges. In these instances, alternative problem-solving techniques can be applied.(36)

Alternative Problem-Solving Techniques

When a group is unable to agree on a solution, several other methods—each with its advantages and disadvantages—can be used. One method is for the leader to make the decision. The advantage is that the decision is arrived at quickly; the disadvantage is that those who dislike it may not support it. Leaders may feel that they have "won," but others who feel that they have "lost" may attempt to subvert the decision or solution. Another possibility is for some members to accommodate others by no longer insisting on their preferred solution. This method immediately relieves the group of conflict, but those who accommodated may later resent having done so and may not feel obliged to uphold the solution. Perhaps the most common method is compromise, each side giving in a little until both can agree. The problem with compromise is that often what is given up is sought back eventually. Compromise solutions tend to be short-lived. Other conflict-reducing techniques such as majority rule, trade-offs, and coin-flipping also tend to be short-lived because the members who gave up something to satisfy the immediate need for a solution feel no obligation to support the solution.

GROUP PARTICIPATION IN DECISION-MAKING

There are both advantages and disadvantages to participative decision-making. The practitioner needs to be aware of them to decide, on a contingency basis, when this method is appropriate.

Advantages

1. When managers meet their team members one at a time, problems of communication and perceptual distortion may occur. Each time the manager discusses the issues on a one-to-one basis, the superior's manner and language vary, with each subordinate asking questions from a different perspective. Meeting together to discuss such matters as operational activities and politics provides an opportunity for everyone to hear the same descriptions at the same time and to ask questions, which may clarify perceptions, so that everyone shares a common understanding.
2. Interpersonal relationship problems can be resolved, particularly when the staff is aware of the need for teamwork.
3. Motivation can be enhanced, since the individuals involved in the decision may become more committed to it and may better understand how it is to be carried out. Resistance to change is reduced when individuals consider the alternative actions

together and decide together on the goals and objectives for achieving change. They experience a greater commitment to changes that they themselves have either initiated or participated in developing.

4. The synergy of problem-solving can occur, allowing the group to arrive at solutions that are qualitatively superior to any that a single individual could arrive at alone.

Disadvantages

1. Group participation in decision-making can be time consuming; however, the time spent in goal setting, problem definition, and planning can result in more rapid implementation of the solution and less resistance to change.
2. Cohesive groups can become autonomous and work against management's preferences.
3. Groups can sometimes become a way for everyone to escape the responsibility for taking action, since each person may assume that someone else is ultimately responsible.
4. The goals and interests of employees and those of management may not be compatible.
5. Employees may not be qualified to participate. Participation requires not only a desire to be involved, but also knowledge and/or experience in the problem area, as well as an ability to communicate insights, reactions, and desires. Not everyone possesses these skills to the same degree, and some who have the desire, but not the ability, may need to be trained.
6. People whose ideas are continuously rejected can become alienated.
7. Managers may use groups as a way to manipulate employees into making the decision that they, the managers, have already decided on.
8. Work group involvement may raise employees' expectations that cannot always be met or that the manager did not intend; once started, employees may want to be included in all decision-making, whether or not their participation is appropriate.
9. The hazards of "groupthink" refer to the phenomenon of a group stifling individual creativity to preserve the status quo. It is the mode of thinking that persons engage in when seeking concurrences becomes more important in a cohesive group than a realistic appraisal of the alternative courses of action. The symptoms of groupthink arise when group members avoid being too harsh in their judgments of their leaders' or their colleagues' ideas for the sake of preserving harmony. All members are amiable and seek complete concurrence on every important issue to avoid conflict that might spoil the cozy, group atmosphere.(36,37)

Dr. Irving Janis, social psychologist and pioneer researcher in this area, is the leading expert on the groupthink phenomenon. Below are some of the remedies he suggests to prevent its occurrence. Dietetics practitioners need to consider ways of adapting these practices to their own style of group facilitation with staff.(36)

1. At each meeting, the facilitator should verbalize the desire that all participants assume the role of "critical evaluator." Members need to be encouraged to look for the weaknesses in one another's arguments. The facilitator's acceptance of criticism from others is critical if the others are to continue the practice with them and with one another.

2. The facilitator should adopt from the start an impartial stance rather than stating preferences and expectations. Such a stance encourages open inquiry and impartial probing of a wide range of policy alternatives.

3. The organization should routinely or periodically set up several alternative policy planning and evaluation groups to work on the same policy question, with each group deliberating under a different leader. This practice can prevent the insulation of an in-group.

4. Before reaching a final consensus, the group members should discuss the issues with qualified associates who are not part of the decision-making group and should then report back to the others the results of their informal surveys.

5. The group should invite one or more outside experts to some meetings on a staggered basis and encourage the experts to challenge the views of the dominant group members.

6. At every meeting of the group, whenever the agenda calls for an evaluation of policy alternatives, at least one member should be assigned to play the "devil's advocate," challenging the testimony of those who advocate the majority position.

7. After reaching a preliminary consensus about what seems to be the best policy, the group should hold a "second-chance" meeting, during which members express all their residual doubts as vividly as they can. This meeting gives everyone a last opportunity to rethink the entire issue before making a definitive choice.(37–41)

GROUPS AS SUPPLEMENT TO INDIVIDUAL COUNSELING

Group and individualized counseling may be used together. Even those who require intensive counseling can benefit by the examples, support, and ideas available in

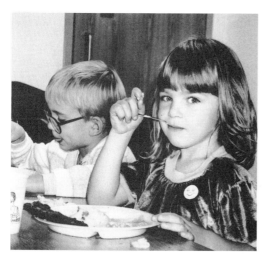

Peer groups may influence children's food habits.

groups. When specialized and intense one-on-one nutrition counseling does not produce the desired results, group counseling may be advantageous. When problems are mutual, the group can provide support, reinforcement, and all the advantages of synergy in solving problems. Groups also provide the resources for conducting role plays and rehearsing actions for the real world.

As used in nutrition counseling, groups differ from group therapy. Group counseling is intended to be not a form of therapy, but a format to help people find solutions to dietary problems. These solutions can then be demonstrated, attempted, and evaluated with group support. A primary goal in nutrition counseling is to promote self-sufficiency in clients. In groups in which people learn basic change strategies by helping other group members design personal dietary change programs and by encouraging mutual follow-through, this self-sufficiency goal is enhanced. Once the group understands the basic strategies, the practitioner can facilitate nondirectively, allowing the members to consult with one another.

Some consider group counseling impractical when it is limited to a single session. One-on-one counseling, however, is time consuming. With the limits on staff at some hospitals, any time saver, such as the use of groups, is helpful. Behavior change requires more than one session, but a single group session may be an efficient and time-saving way of giving information to a group of patients or clients with similar problems. The practitioner is saved from having to explain basic concepts over and over. Being with others who share similar problems often encourages participants to change more than if they were counseled individually.

When the group is designed primarily for the professional to convey nutrition and dietary information, to teach principles of dietary change, and to encourage group members to use them, several principles should be incorporated into the teaching aspects of the group sessions.

CASE STUDY 1

Betty Smith, RD, is planning a series of group meetings for her clients who are parents of children who have type I diabetes mellitus. Her concern today is planning for optimum group participation in the first session, which will be 1 hour long. She also wants to be sure to meet the needs of the group so that they will return for future sessions.

1. What suggestions do you have for the first session?

CASE STUDY 2

Doris Johnson, RD, has worked for the past 5 years in a school lunch program at an elementary school. In the past year, there has been 35% turnover of employees. Although all new employees have received training, Doris has noticed that sanitation has slipped considerably. It is not as sharp as in the past.

Doris has decided to bring together a group of employees at the end of the lunch service for a discussion of the problem. About 10 employees will be present.

1. How should Doris introduce the problem?
2. What role should Doris take in the discussion?
3. What should she do to facilitate discussion?
4. How would Doris go about promoting a synergistic solution?

1. The number of major points covered per meeting should be limited. The dietetics practitioner should focus all efforts toward motivating the group to understand and use the main principles.
2. Since learning is a gradual process, teaching time in groups should be devoted to essential and necessary information. The intricate technicalities can be taught later.
3. The principles of education covered in other places in this book should be used: the goal of the session should be stated, examples should be given, and group discussion and problem solving should be stimulated. Participants should be encouraged to summarize the points learned and their intended applications of them.
4. The content should be presented and reinforced through a variety of means: written handouts, presentations, audiovisual media, role-playing, and demonstrations.
5. Group members should be required to write down or publicly verbalize short-term goals that are specific and "doable," so that they can be reviewed in the group the following week.

This chapter has stressed the necessity for practitioners to study group process and internalize the behaviors needed to participate in, facilitate, and model group interaction skills. With proper facilitation, groups can stimulate solutions and insights the individual might not experience otherwise. Once dietetics professionals develop the skills needed to diagnose group needs and the ability to correct them by focusing on the group's resources, they can function as change agents and as communication models for the other group members, while at the same time becoming more effective mangers.

REVIEW AND DISCUSSION QUESTIONS

1. What is the role of the team leader?
2. What distinguishes autocratic from participative leadership?
3. Why is a team approach superior?
4. How should a facilitator halt a side conversation?
5. Discuss the significance of the informal work group.
6. What is "synergy" and how can it be stimulated in groups?
7. Discuss several of the participant functions and how they generally either aid in promoting the group's effectiveness or assist in accomplishing the group's task.
8. Discuss the suggestions for promoting group change.

SUGGESTED ACTIVITIES

1. In groups of three, discuss the best small group experiences you have ever had. What occurred that qualifies them as superior? Describe specific behaviors of both the group's leader/facilitator and the participants that seem to have made a difference. Time should be allotted for each group to share its insights with the others.
2. In groups of three, plan to meet in three different settings over the next 2 days, with different seating, room size, lighting, etc. Report your observations on the effects of

the environment to the entire class. Notice whether different groups had simpler reactions and were influenced by the same factors. A simpler variation on this activity would be to hold a discussion for 10 minutes with the group arranged in a circle and then to continue the discussion with the group sitting in a straight row.

3. Make a list of at least three small groups in which you have been active, and describe the functions you performed in each. Compare your perceptions of yourself as a contributing group member with the perceptions that your friends or classmates had of you. Do you notice that you performed different functions in different groups? Do some functions overlap from group to group? Are your classmates in agreement with you regarding your functions within their group?

4. Thinking back to some recent experiences in group discussions, complete each of the following statements:

    A. My strengths as a group participant are....
    B. My strengths as a group facilitator are....
    C. What is keeping me from being more effective both as a participant and facilitator is....
    D. My plans for improvement are....

5. How do you determine whether needed leadership and facilitative services are being provided during a discussion? Compare your observations with those of your classmates.

6. Write a question or description of a food or nutrition problem or issue, preferably from your own personal or professional experience, for which you do not have a solution. Present it to a small group and facilitate their discussion. Possible questions might include "What populations need to take vitamin supplements?" "What are the best food choices when eating at a fast food outlet?" and "What recommendations should one give to someone who desires to reduce calories or exercise more?"

7. Group together four to five people who have a common problem such as (1) wanting to lose weight, (2) to start eating breakfast, (3) to control excess consumption of snacks, (4) to select nutritious meals, (5) to increase the fiber content of their diets, or (6) to exercise more often. State the problem, and have the group attempt to solve it.

WEB SITES

Change in teams/groups:
> http://www.users.csbsju.edu/~aimmelma/text0024.htm
> http://www.vcu.edu/hasweb/psy/psy633/change.htm

Cohesiveness in groups:
> http://www.mapnp.org/library/grp_skll/theory/theory.htm
> http://www.accel-team.com/work_groups/informal_grps_04.html
> http://www.brookes.ac.uk/services/ocsd/2_learntch/small-group/sgt1.7.html
> http://interzone.com/~cheung/SUM.dir/humcohesive.html

Team management:
> http://www.workteams.unt.edu
> http://management.bus.okstate.edu/faculty/eastman/mgmt5113/teams/

Self-management in teams:

http://www.russellconsultinginc.com/docs/white/tdosmwt.html

http://www.clanwilliam.ie/selfmgt.html

Developing group leadership skills:

http://www.consultskills.com/leadasse.htm

http://www.consultskills.com/getpart.htm

http://www.healthcaredynamics.com/hcd-pas.html / **group dynamics in healthcare**

http://crs.uvm.edu/gopher/nerl/group/a/h.html / **developing group facilitator skills**

http://adrenaline.ucsd.edu/onr/disaster/summary.htm / **consensus in groups**

REFERENCES

1. The American Dietetic Association Standards of Professional Practice for Dietetics Professionals. J Am Diet Assoc 1998;98:83.
2. Scope of practice for qualified dietetics professional in diabetes care and education. J Am Diet Assoc 2000;100:1205.
3. McGuinness M. Team management in community mental health. Prof Nurse 2000;5:312.
4. Finn S. President's page: partnerships forge opportunity, innovation, and action. J Am Diet Assoc 1993;93:195.
5. Eagleson G, Waldersee R, Simmons R. Leadership behavior similarity as a basis of selection into a management team. Br J Soc Psychol 2000;39:301.
6. Parcellis B. The tough work of turning around a team. Harv Bus Rev 2000;78:179.
7. Cuny F. Fred Cuny memorial continuing educations series lesson 10: group dynamics in disasters: managing work groups. Prehospital Disaster Med 2000;15:215.
8. Winship G, Hardy S. Disentangling dynamics: group sensitivity and supervision. J Psyciatr Ment Health Nurs 1999;6:307.
9. Kanas N, Caldwell B. Summary of research issues in personal, interpersonal, and group dynamics. Aviat Space Environ Med 2000;71:26.
10. Fox L, Rejeski W, Gauvin L. Effects of leadership style and group dynamics on enjoyment of physical activity. Am J Health Promot 2000;14:277.
11. McKendall M. Teaching groups to become teams. J Ed Bus 2000;75:277.
12. Dreachslin J, Hunt P, Sprainer E, Snook D. Communication patterns and group composition: implications for patient-centered care team effectiveness. J Healthcare Mgt 1999;44:252.
13. Carless S, DePaola C. The measurement of cohesion in work teams. Small Group Research 2000;31:71.
14. Terry K. Should doctors see patients in group sessions? Medical Economics 1997;74:70.
15. Robbins S. Organizational behavior. Upper Saddle River, NJ: Prentice Hall, 2000.
16. Frey L. Innovations in group facilitation. Cresskill, NJ: Hampton Press, 1995.
17. Weber V, Joshi M. Effecting and leading change in health care organizations. Jt Comm J Qual Improv 2000;26:388.
18. Horak B. Dealing with human factors and managing change in knowledge management. Top Health Mgt 2001;21:8.
19. Gareau B. Driving change: up the organization. Hosp Mater Mgt Q 1999 21:59.
20. Lesic S. Using instrumental leadership to manage change. Radio Mgt 1999;21:44.
21. Dupre B, Mritton L, Catlin R, Milam S, Miranda A. Riding the waves of change in health system material management: team building in times of uncertainty. Health Care Super 1999;17:49.
22. Galanter M, Brook D. Network therapy for addiction: bringing family and peer support into office practice. Int J Group Psychother 2001;51:101.

23. Dreachslin J, Hunt P, Sprainer E. Communication patterns and group composition: implications for patient-centered care team effectiveness. J Health Mgt 1999;44:252.
24. Dasgupta N, Banaji M, Abelson R. Group entitativity and group perception: associations between physical features and psychological judgment. J Pers Soc Psychol 1999;77:991.
25. Schulte T. Facilitating skills: the art of helping teams succeed. Hosp Mater Manage Q 1999;21:13.
26. Schwartz C. Teaching coping skills enhances quality of life more than peer support. Health Psychol 1999;18:211.
27. Rosner B. Facilitation takes real pluck. Workforce 2000;79:104.
28. Anonymous. The art of facilitation. Women in Business 1999;5:38.
29. Weber V, Joshi M. Organizational change and learning. Jt Comm J Qual Mgt 2000;26:388.
30. Kolodziel J. The lean team. Mich Health Hosp 2001;37:24.
31. Doyle B. It takes teamwork to produce big savings. Hosp Mater Mgt Q 2000;25:14.
32. Sager K, Gastil J. Reaching consensus on consensus: a study of the relationship between individual decision-making styles and use of the consensus decision rule. Comm Q 1999;47:67.
33. Tracey A. Conflict and consensus: a general theory of collective decisions. J Occ Organ Psyc 2000;8:131.
34. Brilhart JK, Galanes GJ. Effective group discussion, 8th ed. Dubuque, IA: Wm C Brown, 1995.
35. Hall J. Decisions, decisions, decisions. Psychol Today 1971;6:61.
36. Janis I. Groupthink. Psychol Today 1971;6:43.
37. Choi J, Kim M. The organizational application of groupthink and its limitations in organizations. J Applied Psychol 1999;84:297.
38. Druskat V, Wolff S. Building the emotional intelligence of groups. Harv Bus Rev 2001;79:80.
39. Hinojosa J, Bedell G. Team collaboration. Q Health Res 2001;11:206.
40. Soloman C. Team spirit. Health Facil Mgt 2001;14:41.
41. Bliese P, Britt T. Social support, group consensus and stressor-strain relationships. J Organ Behav Special Issue 2001;22:425.

CHAPTER 14

Delivering Oral Presentations and Conducting Workshops

After reading this chapter, you will be able to

1. list the three parts of a presentation and what each should provide.
2. explain how the credibility of the speaker can be established.
3. discuss how to overcome stage fright and enhance communication with an audience.
4. identify how to conduct a workshop.
5. list suggestions for working with the media.
6. give a presentation for classmates or others.

Whether you think you can or whether you think you can't, you're right.

Henry Ford

Dietetics professionals are expected to be good communicators. Working knowledge of public speaking is a competency required for professional practice according to the Commission on Accreditation/Approval for Dietetics Education of the American Dietetic Association. Eventually, the dietetics practitioner will be asked to give an oral presentation or public speech in his or her area of expertise.(1–5) Information on planning the visuals to go with the speech can be found in Chapter 15. The presentation skills discussed in this chapter will serve the dietetics practitioner equally well in teaching—to students, patients, and employees. Like so many of the other skills discussed in this book, the skills needed to deliver a message orally and articulately cannot be learned by reading alone; you must be prepared to digest the information and then have the courage to RISK.

Although entire books are written on the broad and general subject of giving oral presentations, the purpose here is to develop and discuss concisely the most salient principles occurring in the process of preparing and delivering oral presentations and workshops and dealing with the media.

Following are suggestions for advance planning and organizing of a presentation, advance physical arrangements of the room, delivering the presentation, and post-presentation actions.

When you have nothing to say, say nothing . . .

Charles Caleb Colton

ADVANCE PLANNING AND ORGANIZATION
FOR THE PRESENTATION

The key to holding the attention of an audience, particularly an audience with limited time to absorb the speaker's ideas, is for the speaker to be coherent and to communicate simply; otherwise, listeners' minds will wander. The secret of conciseness and simplicity is for speakers to know their objectives before planning their talk. What do they want to accomplish? What changes do they want to take place in the attitude or behavior of the audience? Do they want them to perform a task or recall some information? A common mistake made among untrained presenters is to attempt to cover too much in the time allotted. Inexperienced speakers often feel the need to parade their expertise and overload the audience with information.

Unlike with reading in which one can go back and reconsider an idea, listening requires ongoing concentration. When the brain begins to feel overloaded and saturation sets in, it protects itself by shutting down. Hasn't everyone had the experience of pretending to be listening to an overly meticulous speaker, while the mind was wandering elsewhere? Oral presentations need to be limited to a few major points, generally 5 to 10, which can be clearly explained and reinforced through details, examples, and a variety of media. Too much information and too many different points defeat the purpose. When listeners know where the presentation is going and are able to follow the presenter's reasoning, grasping examples with ease, they are much more likely to give their full attention.

Although presentations are often as brief as 10 minutes or as long as 90 minutes, presenters should remember when adapting their goals to their group what the

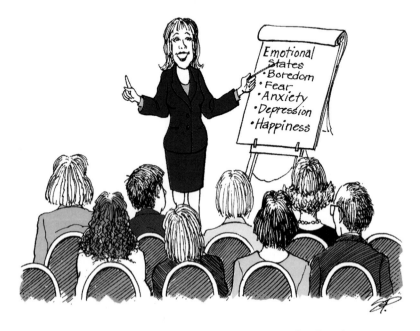

*In discussing emotional eating, the professional
enhances her presentation with visuals.*

Reverend William Sloane Coffin said about the length of an effective sermon, "No souls are saved after 20 minutes." Once presenters have their general and specific goals tailored to their group, the next task is to organize them.

INTRODUCTION
CRITICAL TO SPEAKER CREDIBILITY

Each of the three generally accepted divisions of a presentation (introduction, body, and conclusion) requires its own internal organization and serves a specific function. The introduction serves speakers by providing them the opportunity to establish credibility, to link themselves in some way to their audience, to let them know in what ways they will be better off as a result of having attended, and to describe for the audience in some serial fashion the points they intend to cover.

Often when speakers are introduced, their credentials are presented in advance; however, at times no one is present to introduce the speaker or the "introducer" may neglect to mention important items related to enhancing the speaker's credibility. Although self-serving comments delivered in a braggadocio manner may have a negative effect on audiences, audiences do nevertheless want to know that the person talking to them is worthy and knowledgeable. Practitioners, therefore, should subtly let listeners know during the introduction that they are qualified. For example, one might say, ". . . in an article I wrote last year for the *Journal of the American Dietetic Association . . .*," or "of the several hundred patients I have worked with in the past. . . ."

Audiences tend to be more attentive when they believe that the person speaking to them is able to relate to their circumstances. During the introduction, whenever it is possible, speakers would do well to underscore any connection they may have with a particular group. For example, you might say, "I have lived in this community for 15 years . . . ," or "I was once 25 pounds overweight myself . . . ," or "I see we are all baby boomers and share many of the same sentiments about wellness." If one gives it some thought, almost all audiences have some traits with which the speaker can identify.

During the introduction, speakers need to let the audience know how the topic relates to their needs; in other words, presenters should answer the unasked question in everyone's mind, "What is in this for me?" Abraham Maslow has synthesized the basic human needs into five areas: physiological, safety and security, belonging and social activity, esteem and status, and self-realization and fulfillment. When the professional announces that after listening to the speech, the listeners will in some way be better able to control their health, provide more nutritious meals to their families, be more secure, be in a position in which others think better of them or respect them more, think more of themselves, or feel they have the knowledge to develop latent potential in themselves, the audience perks up and prepares to be attentive to the forthcoming message. Not every human need can be related to every topic, but as many as possible and as appropriate should be suggested during the introduction. During the body and conclusions of the speech as well, the speaker should remind the audience how what is being discussed can be related to fulfilling their own needs.

Finally, the last critical component to be included in the introduction is a list of the topics that will be discussed. It might be presented something like this: "Today I intend to discuss three specific points. Number one, I will discuss the relationship of diet to heart disease; number two, I will discuss how to read food labels for the fat and cho-lesterol content of foods, and third, I will model how to order at a restaurant." Not only does this help the audience to listen to the talk with an expectation of what is to come, but also the organization itself adds to the "halo effect" and increases the audience's per-ceptions of the speaker's credibility.

KEY OBJECTIVES OF THE BODY OF THE PRESENTATION

The body of the presentation is the second major division and the place where the points mentioned in the introduction are actually developed. Presenters need to have a rationale for the way they decide to organize this major section. The overall objectives generally are threefold: that the audience fully understands the message, that the audience believes the speaker, and that they are comfortable enough with the speaker to share their objections in the event that they are confused or wish to challenge the presenter. One other possible objective is for the audience members to do something differently after the presentation. Examples are to start reading food labels, to try a new recipe, to purchase a different food at the store, to eat breakfast, to change the choice of snack food, and the like.

To safeguard the first objective, understanding the message of the presenter, the speaker needs not only to construct the message clearly and concisely, but also to design visual aids, handouts, and/or participative experiences to enhance the audience's understanding. The second objective, content and speaker credibility, needs to be con-tinually reinforced throughout the presentation. The third objective, to develop a rap-port with the audience to the extent that they are comfortable enough to challenge or question, is critical. When objections are unexpressed, presenters may infer falsely that the audience agrees and understands, causing the speaker to move too quickly from one point to another, leaving confused members behind.

CONCLUDING A PRESENTATION

Like the first two, the third division of the presentation, the conclusion, may be han-dled successfully in many ways. The key is that all the ingredients be included some-where. The first ingredient is for the audience to feel that the presentation is "winding down" and about to end. This needs to be done gradually and smoothly. It sounds non-professional and haphazard to end with remarks like "any questions," "that's all folks," or "thank you for your attention." Remember that the presenter's credibility is influ-enced by the audience's perceptions of how well he or she is organized. Clues such as "in conclusion . . . ," "to summarize," "before concluding, I want to leave you with one more thought" are helpful in letting the audience know that the presentation is about to terminate. If a summary is warranted, it should be given; if a final plea or pitch is warranted, that should be given; if a final quote, anecdote, or joke makes the point one more time, then that is appropriate.

One last word about conclusions is to be proactive in asking if your listeners have any questions. Of course, people are often hesitant to ask questions. The speaker should prepare a few for the audience, and then ask for a reaction from a participant who has been paying attention. You might say, "I noticed that you looked confused when I was discussing the fatty acid content of foods. What is it you would like further discussion of?" After responding to the first question, which was generated by the presenter, it is often simpler to get others to respond when the question is asked, "Are there any *other* questions or comments?"

CORRELATION BETWEEN FORM AND SPEAKER CREDIBILITY

Although the discussion of the presentation's design is generally divided into the three areas of introduction, body, and conclusion, there is no single perfect way to organize. Speakers with varied styles can be successful. However, you should consider several points when deciding on a presentation's specific format.

Most people are not aware that the presentation's organization is critical, primarily because it relates to the presenter's credibility. For example, if a speaker were to deliver the same talk to two different audiences, giving one audience 10 bits of information in an organized way and giving the second audience the same 10 bits of information in a disorganized way, both audiences would retain about the same amount of information after hearing the talk, but only one audience would consider it seriously or possibly change their attitude toward the subject matter.

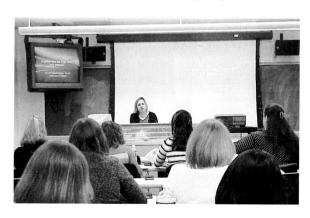

A presenter should be familiar with the site and equipment.

When an audience hears an organized speaker who gives the audience a sense that he or she knows exactly where the talk is going, with a defined beginning, middle, and end, they are more likely to infer that the speaker is competent in the area. Many brilliant and qualified professionals, however, are not taken seriously when giving presentations because they sound too "loose," too unprepared, too disorganized.

If you refuse to accept anything but the best, you very often get it.

W. Clement Stone

MEDIA AS RELATED TO PRESENTER'S CREDIBILITY

All media, the way they are designed, presented, and used, are an extension of the speaker and consequently reflect directly on the speaker's credibility. Media include such things as Power Point slides, handouts, blackboard, flip chart, pad/mock-ups, and even actual foods. A superior standard is inferred from media supplements that are obviously carefully put together. For example, a presenter whose Power Point slides are designed with large print and attractive clip art, rather than a black-and-white transparency with small print, allows for the inference of an experienced and considerate presenter. Other signs include using stenciled letters in bold colors on posters rather than sloppy printing or cursive writing. The condition of the poster itself leads to either positive or negative impressions of the speaker. Posters that are discolored, bent, and old looking suggest that the presenter does not care enough to add fresh visual aids for the group. Even the quality and color of the paper used in handouts can add or detract from the overall impression.

If it is possible, the presenter is wise to try to coordinate all aids in colors that may be symbolic or meaningful. For example, a presenter giving a talk to an Italian-American Club could be done in red, white, and green. This may sound superficial, but audiences do respond on an unconscious level to the extra care and preparation the speaker has made in tailoring a presentation on their behalf.

ORAL PRESENTATIONS

In Contrast to Written Presentations

The written text and the oral presentation are entirely different. There is no objection to a presenter writing out the entire talk, carefully organizing it according to topics, causes and effects, chronology, or whatever else seems appropriate. However, once the talk is written, the speaker needs to recognize that the written manuscript represents the "science" of a presentation; the actual delivery represents the "art." Each time it is delivered, the presentation should be somewhat different, with different words, different examples, different anecdotes, and so forth, to suit particular audiences and situations. The word choice in the spoken language also tends to be different from the word choice used in the written language. Sentences in oral speech tend to be simpler, shorter, and more conversational, including common words and contractions, whereas the written manuscript may be more erudite and academic. The only way for speakers to develop this art is to rehearse from a simple outline and not a manuscript and to rehearse in front of real people who will react and comment, rather than in front of mirrors, walls, or car windshields.

Never to Read or Memorize

There are other good reasons for not rehearsing from a manuscript. The speech tends eventually to become memorized and that can be deadly. Once a speech is memorized, speakers tend to become more speech-centered than audience-centered, which means that they tend to become more concerned about whether they can remember each line exactly as it is written on the manuscript and less concerned about whether the audience is enjoying, learning, listening, and understanding. Another problem that arises from manuscript speaking is that it is *dull*! Because the speaker's facial expressions and vocal intonations are not spontaneous, the monologue tends to sound memorized and can easily become boring to listeners.

Advance Arrangements

Take control of seating the listeners before everyone settles down. It may be their boardroom, gymnasium, or meeting hall, but it is the presenter's "show." Conscious decisions should be made about whether or not to pull the group into a circle, half-circle, rows; sitting around tables; and so forth. When it is possible to know beforehand which persons are the most influential, their seats should be reserved and placed in the best position to see, hear, and appreciate visual aids as well as the speaker. A final checklist for presentations is found in Table 14-1.

Creating Positive Impressions

Presenters are being sized up and are adding to the presentation's ambiance from the moment they enter the room. Whenever possible, they should arrive early and make an effort to meet people. Their own self-confidence, whether real or feigned, will relax the audience and increase their perceptions of the speaker's desire to share information. Presenters should never volunteer any negative information regarding their own stress or fear of speaking. The audience wants to learn and enjoy, and when they are aware of the speaker's fragility or stage fright, they tend to become nervous themselves in sympathy.

If the presenters are waiting to be introduced and are seated among the audience or on a stage, they should be aware that audience members who know they are the guest speakers, will be watching their every move. That means that even before begin-

---

TABLE 14-1 **Checklist for Oral Presentations**

Attend to details and prepare a checklist. Listed below are a few questions that the presenter might consider to avoid last-minute problems.

Do I have my presentation notes?
Do I have all my supporting materials?
Have I enough copies for each of the attendees?
Will the facility be unlocked and open?
Are the tables and chairs arranged to suit my design?
Do I understand how to operate the lighting system?
Do I understand how to operate the ventilation system?
Do I know the location and operating condition of the electrical circuits?
Do I know how to work the projector?
Do I have an extra bulb, cassette, video, extension cord, etc.?
Will the projection screen be in place and adequate for this size group?
Do I have the type of sound system I require? Is it working?
Have arrangements been made to handle messages during the presentation?
Are there arrangements for hats and coats?
Will there be a sign to announce the place of the presentation?
Will someone be introducing me, and have I given all the information I want
  shared with the group?

ning the presentation, speakers must be careful to smile, look confident, and extend themselves to others. After the speaker is introduced, the way he or she walks up to the dais is critical. During those first moments an initial impression is being created. The speaker should consciously walk confidently, looking and smiling toward the audience. Before uttering the first words to the audience, it is a good technique to spend a long 3 seconds just looking out at the audience, smiling and establishing eye contact with several people. This allows them to infer poise, confidence, and the speaker's desire to connect with them.

DELIVERING THE PRESENTATION

Internal Feelings of Fright or Anxiety

One of the worst things that presenters can do is to admit to an audience that they are scared, ill prepared, missing material, sick with a cold, or have done the presentation better in the past for other groups. The audience does not know what it may be missing and is generally much less critical of speakers than speakers are of themselves. The speaker must act confident, even when he or she does not feel it internally. Speakers experience themselves in the situation from the inside out; the audience experiences them from the outside in. This means that if asked whether they are nervous or anxious, speakers should always answer "no!" The audience picks up the tip of the iceberg from their observations of the speaker, but they do not feel the intensity of the speaker's anxiety and are probably totally unaware of it unless it is brought to their attention through the speaker's own confession.

Stage Fright

The feelings commonly referred to as stage fright may date back to the dawn of the human race, when our prehistoric ancestors had to survive by living in caves and sharing the food supply with other beasts. Faced by a predator, our ancestors had a genuine use for a sudden jolt of energy, which gave them the power to do battle or run (i.e., fight or flight response). The vestiges of this power, stemming from the secretions of the adrenal gland, still manifest themselves today when people sense danger. Who hasn't felt that ice block in the stomach while being reprimanded by the boss or experienced sweaty palms and racing heart while walking into a room full of strangers? Occasionally, one still reads newspaper accounts of a person exhibiting superhuman strength under conditions of fear or danger, as in the father who lifts a car off his child who has been pinned under the wheels. This is an example of the power that comes with the adrenaline jolt; however, when a person is unable to fight, run, or in some other way utilize this surge, he or she may become overwhelmed by the internal feelings themselves. This feeling before and during a presentation is commonly labeled "stage fright."

The best safeguard against stage fright is adequate preparation and rehearsal. The more you practice in front of *live others,* the less nervousness you will have. Other ways of dealing with these feelings include being active during the presentation and "acting" calm and confident. If presenters know they are going to be full of extra energy because of their excess adrenaline secretions, they could plan on engaging in demonstrations during the presentation, passing handouts, using a pointer, or any other activity that involves motion. Motion is a release for the tension and anxiety and allows the audience to infer enthusiasm from the speaker's movement rather than fright, nervousness, or tension. It may not work for everyone, but many people can learn to control their public behavior if they visualize themselves as acting.

All movement should be meaningful. Do not pace. Presenters ought to look for opportunities to break the invisible barrier between themselves and their audience.

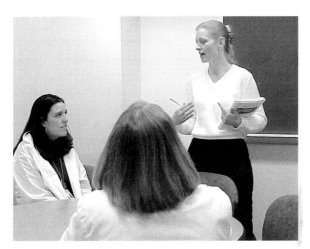

Walking toward the audience, walking around the audience, walking in and out of the audience and walking among the audience all are acceptable ways of delivering a presentation. What is not acceptable is pacing back and forth, particularly with eyes down, as the speaker pulls his or her thoughts together before uttering them. Movement into an audience is a communication vehicle in itself. When presenters penetrate that invisible barrier between themselves and the audience, they are nonverbally indicating their desire to connect, to be close,

Barriers between the presenter and audience should be omitted.

to better sense what it is the audience is feeling about the speakers and the content. In fact, as speakers walk among the audience, the audience can begin to be seen from a different perspective and the speaker may gain new insights into how better to clarify particular points and issues from this experience.

Omitting Unnecessary Barriers

Presenters do best when they omit all barriers between themselves and their audience. Avoid using a podium or lectern, even when one is provided by the sponsoring organization. Of course, there may be times when because of the quantity of material, a place to store things may be required. Even under this condition, using a table on which to set handouts and other materials is preferred to a podium. A lectern should be used only when the speaker does not intend to move about but intends to lecture and needs a stand to rest against and place notes on. Adults generally do not learn optimally through the lecture method. Unless the speaker is extraordinarily good, straight lecture behind a podium should be avoided. When delivering a message while standing in front of a group without a barrier, the speaker is more disposed to stop the talk to respond to the verbal or nonverbal feedback of listeners. Gestures and movement, too, can be expansive and visible without the lectern barrier.

Verbal Behavior

Vocal inflection and variation add interest and the impression of speaker enthusiasm. For some people, controlling this variation is simple and natural; for others, it is a challenge. Nevertheless, the presenter needs to attend to voice modulation. The goal when speaking in front of a group is to sound natural and conversational. However, what sounds natural and conversational when standing in front of a large group is not the same as what sounds conversational in a small face-to-face group. "Natural and conversational" from the presenter's point of view is exaggerated. The highs need to be a bit higher and the lows need to be a bit lower. What may sound to the presenter's ear as phony and theatrical generally sounds far less so to the listener. The good news is that this trait can be fairly easily and quickly developed, even in those who recognize a problem in this area. It requires risking sounding foolish and exaggerated in front of trusting others, until adequate reinforcement has convinced the presenter that the increase in vocal variation is really an advantage and allows him or her to be attended to more easily. In any case, a delivery that is of narrow range or monotone is difficult to attend to for more than a few minutes.

When talking in front of a group, the speaker should generally attempt to speak more slowly than in ordinary conversation. What is an appropriate rate in a small face-to-face discussion is probably too fast for a group presentation. For some reason, there seems to be a correlation between the speech rate of the speaker and the size of the audience. What might be easily grasped at a more rapid rate in face-to-face conversation, is not understood as quickly in large groups. Also the speaker's slower rate allows him or her to scan the audience better while speaking to see if he/she is being understood, to see if some people need an opportunity to disagree, to see if he/she needs to talk louder, or to increase the variation because some listeners look bored.

Professional speakers attend to their diction, particularly when pronouncing words such as "for," "can," "with," "picture," "going to," and "want to." In ordinary conversation one is not likely to judge negatively a speaker who mispronounces common words and engages in sloppy diction saying, for example, words like "fer," "ken," "wit," "pitcher," "gunna," and "wanna," for the words listed above. However, when that speaker is in front of an audience, these mispronounced words often stand out and lead to negative inferences regarding the speaker. Professionals who present themselves in front of groups must attend to their diction because they risk losing credibility if it is poor. Logical? No! True? Yes!

When speakers have decided to become conscious of their diction and decide to improve it, several steps are required. Step one is to inform trusted others who are often around them to listen critically and to stop them each time a diction error occurs. Only after people are made aware of their common errors can they begin to train themselves to hear the errors. That is step two. Because the human mind operates generally at five times the rate of human speech, it is possible to listen critically to ourselves as we speak. People attempting to rid themselves of poor diction or some other vocalized interference (e.g., "um," "ah," "and a") can train themselves to listen for the error and to correct themselves. Like learning to ride a bicycle or use a computer, this learning and training task is uncomfortable at first, but improvement comes quickly. Working on diction is an ongoing task. Professional speakers never stop listening to the way their words are coming out and planning ahead to pronounce them correctly.

Nonverbal Behavior

It is good practice to keep your hands away from your body and from one another. Allow them to be free to gesture, and avoid holding anything in them while talking unless it is a useful prop like a pointer or a visual aid. After 35 years of teaching presentational speaking to college undergraduates, this writer (RJC) knows empirically that once speakers allow their hands to mesh together or to grasp one another behind the back, there is only a slight chance of their being released to gesture. People often feel awkward with their hands hanging loosely at their sides. Perhaps if they could see themselves on videotape in this posture, they would realize that it is natural looking, but even more important, they would probably see that one tends not to stay in that position. If you talk with your hands hanging loosely at your sides, eventually your hands begin to rise and gesture spontaneously to emphasize points that are important.

It is dangerous to begin a presentation holding a pen, paperclip, rubber band, or other instrument not directly related to the presentation. Unconsciously, the fingers begin to play with the instrument, and the audience becomes fascinated with watching to see what the speaker will do. A former student actually straightened out a paper clip and began to stab herself while talking. Needless to say, for the remainder of her presentation the class could not take their eyes off the mutilation scene and missed the speaker's concluding points.

Presenters need to train themselves to keep their faces animated, using a variety of facial expressions. For many of the same reasons expressed earlier, it is important that speakers use all the communication vehicles available to them to maintain the audience's attention. Facial expression is itself a communication vehicle. When it is lively, animated, expressive, and changing regularly while the speaker reacts to the feedback coming toward him or her from the audience, it enhances the verbal message and allows the audience to go on unconsciously inferring the speaker's audience-centeredness. Because of natural dispositional personality, ethnic background, and so forth, this is easier for some people to do than for others; however, everyone can improve. Because it is not easy for a speaker to "act" expressive does not mean that this person cannot grow considerably in the ability to look expressive.

Eye contact is a vehicle of communication. It should be used to see everyone and respond to the nonverbal feedback. It is surprising how many people seem to remember having learned some rule about being able to fool the audience into thinking that the speaker is seeing them while actually looking over the heads of the people in the last row. The point is that when speakers have the opportunity to present themselves and their ideas to an audience, they want the audience to understand them, to believe them, and to follow their recommendations. A speaker has the best chance of being successful in achieving these goals when able to interpret the audience's ongoing reactions to what is being said. Even though presentational speaking is generally considered a one-way communication situation with the speaker talking at the audience as they listen, it is actually a two-way situation with audience and speaker communicating with one another constantly and simultaneously.

Trained speakers see almost everything from their position in front of the room. If they are alert, they may see people who are beginning to fidget, and they can interpret and act on this feedback. They might decide consequently to give the audience a short break; they might liven their own movements to regain attention; or they might engage in a new activity, perhaps one that involves audience participation. They might see some people coming in late, looking awkwardly for a seat. This gives them the opportunity to publicly welcome them and ask others to move over to provide seating. They might see people who look angry. This gives them the opportunity to say, "You look angry. What has been said to offend you?" In other words, speakers who use their eyes to connect with the audience make them a part of the presentation. The audience knows it and will begin to send signals when they realize the speaker is sensitive to them.

Facial expressions are important. Presenters must remember to smile and look as if they are enjoying the experience of sharing information. Smiling can be rehearsed and may feel phony, but it needs to be built into the design of the presentation. Speakers do not need to be constantly grinning, but they do need to maintain an expression of gentleness, approachableness, and nondefensiveness. The easiest way to convey these impressions is by smiling often. Unfortunately, it is not easy to smile when you are unsure of the material. All the above principles can be heeded only after the speaker has sufficiently mastered the content and has consciously, through rehearsal, developed skills.

Although individual situations may make this difficult, a general rule is that when speaking for an hour or less, always plan on at least 10 minutes for some audience interaction. In talks of more than 45 minutes, actual audience participation activities should be planned whenever possible and appropriate.

POST-PRESENTATION

Remember to bring business cards and to remain after the presentation for people who may want to talk. Speakers who have done a good job with eye contact and smiling and have prompted the inference of warmth almost always have some audience members who wish to engage them in some consultation. This is frequently a source of additional speaking engagements, and it is therefore an opportunity for the best kind of public relations, face-to-face. When there is a long line of people waiting to talk and time is limited, pass out business cards and tell everyone they are entitled to one call for free consultation. It is amazing how many people follow up on the offer.

WORKSHOPS

There are significant differences between a presentation and a workshop or training session. The differences are in the amount of time needed, the amount of audience participation recommended, and the goals of the leader. Presentations generally run no more than 90 minutes, whereas workshops may run from 90 minutes to several days. Audience participation and training are an integral part of workshop design, and the goals of workshops are generally to teach and train. A presentation's goal often is to persuade the audience to accept a specific proposal or behavior change. The following suggestions are particularly appropriate when designing workshops.

Workshop leaders should plan on using techniques that involve all participants and encourage open communication between themselves and the participants and among the participants. Ways to encourage participation include dividing the larger group into smaller groups, always giving them time in their small group to get to know one another, and then giving the small group activities related to the workshop topic. These small group activities may include such things as case studies, either real or hypothetical, role-playing, and questionnaire completion or discussion. Occasionally, a group may be given a pre-workshop assignment to complete a questionnaire, read material related to the workshop, or perform some other task. Reactions to these tasks can be processed among the participants in small groups.

Frequently, the most important point in determining the climate and direction of the workshop occurs during the first 20 minutes. Some suggestions for using the opening minutes to establish an open climate include using a group introductory activity to promote a relaxed and open atmosphere. When the group is small enough, generally 20 or less, spending time allowing participants to express themselves by identifying their major concerns and questions tends to promote this involvement. Workshop leaders can relieve participant anxiety by introducing themselves, sharing both personal and professional information, and giving a brief overview of their objectives for the workshop, the main topics to be covered, their sequence, and approximate time span. They should also reinforce that they do have expectations in terms of participants' cooperation and participation. Even when such introductory activities take as long as an hour, they are justifiable because of the importance in establishing a common frame of reference with shared goals in a relaxed and receptive setting.

The workshop leader should be aware of signals of fatigue or boredom from participants. These include identifying two or three participants whose behavior provides some type of clue to group climate, providing a variety of activities to break up the routine, and providing a change of pace. Most successful workshops are a blend of information-presenting activities with hands-on experiential type of activities. Another way to safeguard understanding and attention is regularly to summarize what has occurred, especially before moving on to a new topic. Continuity of training is promoted if there are purposeful and periodic reviews and summaries during the workshop. Leaders should note that it is not essential to do the summarizing; in fact, having the participants do it for themselves provides feedback as to whether or not the group has grasped the important points.

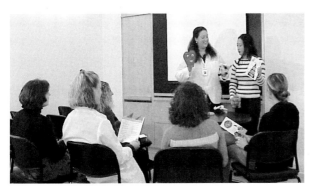

A presenter should arrange the seating area in advance.

Just as the introductory period to the workshop should not be rushed, so, too, should closure be carefully attended to. In a full day's workshop of 6 to 8 hours, allowing a full hour at the end for closure is appropriate. Of course, it depends on how much time is available for the entire workshop. During the closure, loose ends are tied and the presenter has a final opportunity to verify whether the group's original expectations have been met.

Requiring the group to complete an evaluation of the workshop during the time provided is the method most likely to get the largest return. These evaluations are most helpful to leaders who want to continue growing. They process the evaluations and make changes in subsequent workshops based on the responses. The emphasis in a workshop is always on quality, not quantity. It is not how much the audience has heard; it is how much they have learned, will remember, and will use in the future that is the final measure of the workshop's success.

COMMUNICATING THROUGH THE MASS MEDIA

Increasingly, public health and dietetic interventions depend on effective health communication. Numerous studies during the past few years have examined the influence of media politics, the accuracy of media reporting, the use of media for health education and advocacy, the availability of training in media relations for staff members, and whether media interaction facilitated or impeded achievement of public health objectives.(3–9) The data are clear that the organization's image and credibility are most certainly influenced by both the manner and content of the organization's spokespersons as presented by the media. This portion of the chapter on presentation skills deals specifically with tips for presenting oneself or one's organization in the media.

When given the opportunity to present information through the mass media, you need to understand the power of the media to influence and the inferences that listeners or viewers make based not only on the speaker's presentation and speaking skills but also on the speaker's manner. When you grasp the enormous persuasive power of mass media, you can train yourself to use it to your advantage. However, if you are unaware and make no special adaptations for the media, you may be unsuccessful— even though the content is excellent.

When communicating through the mass media, speakers need to remember that in more than 50% of the listeners' interpretation of the message is influenced not by the content, but by the form—the speaker's manner, energy, level of enthusiasm, vehicles and media used for transmission, and so forth. Listed in the text that follows are specific suggestions to assist the reader in preparing for media presentations. When you are given the choice of delivering a manuscript for someone else to read or showing up in person and presenting the information directly without a manuscript, the second choice is preferable. Other people who may paraphrase or quote ordinarily will not have the same tone of confidence, integrity, passion, sincerity, and so on, that the person, speaking for him- or herself, will be able to demonstrate. To demonstrate passion, for example, the speaker needs to know the material thoroughly, have strong feelings about it, and allow him- or herself to emote and not read.

The following paragraphs offer specific suggestions for working with the media.

Airtime is expensive and interviewers may interrupt or give signals to wind up the comments. When invited to be interviewed or share information through the mass media, speakers need to verify how much time they will be allotted and plan accordingly. When time is limited, the speaker needs to decide ahead of time what points are most essential, have these points highlighted, and express them first. If additional time is provided he or she can then elaborate or add additional information.

If there is an alternative possibility for time on a news show, you will increase your chances of being selected if you submit videotaped clips, slides, objects, pictures, and so on. Television is a visual medium, and producers favor opportunities to provide multiple images.

Try always to accept invitations to be on mass media, even when they are original-ly being produced for small audiences, esoteric cable programs, or minor rural stations. Once something is taped, there is no telling where else it may eventually be played or whom it will eventually reach.

Because time and talent are so expensive in the media, programs, even when being taped ahead of time, tend to run strictly on schedule. Guests should plan on arriving early, never late. This may mean verifying directions, bringing a cellular phone and the number of the station's direct line just in case, and reconfirming the time and place.

Often radio and television interviewers do not have time to become well informed regarding the specifics of their guest's causes. Don't become offended or defensive by their ignorance. Being polite and kind will be interpreted by listeners as genuine human warmth; being short with an interviewer may well be interpreted as arrogance and reflect negatively on the speaker's cause.

Keep the message simple, not complicated. It would be wise to rehearse and tape answers and then listen carefully. Is the language clear, concise without sounding too erudite, jargonized, or technical?

There will probably be commercial breaks, and this should be viewed as a positive. If there are questions that you as the interviewee want to be asked or suggestions you want to make, by all means, make them at this time.

Humor is a powerful communication vehicle, but not all people have the gift. Interviewees should be particularly careful about trying to be funny. It may make them look foolish unless they are confident they have the special gift. When, however, the material itself is genuinely funny and has been tried successfully in other audiences, the humor should be brought out.

Often television and radio programs conduct pre-interviews to determine whether the guest is articulate and interesting enough to hold the audience. This is the time to do your best. Really try here! Because the host is being kind and polite does not mean that he or she won't decide to omit the least interesting or articulate guests.

After you have seen or heard yourself on mass media several times, you will even-tually become adept at processing the experience while it is happening. Presenters need to develop a third eye to monitor themselves on the media and send back messages to themselves about how they are doing during the presentation or interview. Because the human mind whirls several times faster than speech speed, it is possible to see and hear yourself while talking and to modify accordingly. The rule generally is that on the mass media, natural behavior should be exaggerated somewhat bigger than life without being outrageous. Speakers need to behave in a way that generates inferences of self-confi-dence, sincerity, and even charisma.

Hand gestures on television should be carefully controlled; they tend to be dis-tracting on the screen. Speakers need to sustain interest through their dynamic voice, cadence, inflections, pauses, tone, and facial expression. Although large expansive ges-tures generally don't work well, variety and variation do work.

Very few nonprofessional presenters are able to improvise very long and come off looking professional. Answers to questions that the interviewee expects to be asked should be rehearsed and not read from notes. If you are asked a question you can't answer, the smartest thing to do is admit it and offer to locate the answer and forward it to the appropriate people.

Part of the self-monitoring process should include the interviewee judging the length of his or her own answers. Avoid long-winded answers or monologues. They tend to get boring to listeners and irritate the interviewer.

Dress is a communication vehicle itself and should be attended to carefully when on the visual media. The best advice is to dress conservatively and in good taste, without being flashy or drawing attention to yourself through clothes. Busy ties, socks, plaids, or large jewelry all are inappropriate.

If you are representing your organization, you may find yourself being asked the same questions over and over, day after day. Remember this is the first time this audience is hearing it; presentations need to sound fresh each time, even though it may be the speaker's twentieth time in 2 days answering the same questions.

Bored listeners and viewers change channels. Guest interviewees and presenters need to prepare themselves with interesting anecdotes and aphorisms. Personal experiences tend to hold attention. The deadliest mistake is to become too intellectual or abstract.

When several guests are on the same panel or are involved in a simultaneous interview, someone may attempt to dominate or interrupt . If this occurs, it is easiest to bite your lip and become angry but say nothing. If you do that, you will hate yourself later. You need to be prepared to assert yourself if this occurs. Push yourself back into the conversation and say something like, "please let me finish my point," or "I'm almost finished, and don't interrupt." This should be done with a smile and kind voice, but it should, by all means, be done. Listeners and viewers respect the person who stands up for him- or herself—politely. Never, never, never get defensive to a member of the audience or another panelist who takes the offensive angrily. The speaker should simply look to the moderator to move the program on.

If you are offended publicly or have your feelings hurt, you need to grin and bear it rather than react emotionally. You can say "I don't agree" or "that feels unkind," but if you snap back a retort, you risk being heard as weak or overly sensitive.

Because so much of what is produced for the media eventually gets repeated, speakers should avoid mentioning the time, place, or date of the live broadcast. If a piece isn't "dated," it has a better chance of being used at a later date by other affiliates who may need material.

There may be times when as the speaker you believe that you are being invited to talk about your cause and once you get there the interviewer steers you to other topics. When this happens, it is your responsibility to get your message across even if the host isn't considerate enough to afford the right opportunities. If questions become inappropriate or are about topics that you would rather not discuss, simply say, "I would rather not discuss that." Don't waffle or "double talk." Credibility is destroyed when listeners infer deception.

If a program is being pretaped, it would be a mistake to ask for a second chance. Generally, second chances cost too much money and annoy the director. The guideline is to come prepared to do it right the first time. That may mean taking in a sheet of notes of key points. Before the program's conclusion, you can glance at your notes and make sure you have said all that was critical.

Every show and moderator tend to have a unique style. Speakers should attempt to learn as much as they can about the format before their appearance. It will relieve their own anxiety and allow them to plan a strategy for ways to communicate their message best. They might also request to have 15 minutes alone with the interviewer before the broadcast to go over the questions. The interviewer may not get it, but if the speaker doesn't ask, they definitely won't get it.

Final impressions count, especially on the media. The speaker should use the final public moments to leave a positive impression of a composed, assertive, and controlled person. Privately, before leaving, the speaker should look for the producer and director and thank them personally as well. A firm handshake and looking people in the eye while talking is a separate nonverbal message itself apart from the verbal one being expressed.

CASE STUDY 1

Joan Stivers, RD, works in a corporate wellness program. She has noticed that some employees who eat in the employee cafeteria make less than optimum food choices for lunch. Others go out to a nearby fast-food restaurant. She was asked by management to give a 30-minute presentation on healthy, nutritious lunches.

1. What should she do in the introduction?
2. What are the objectives of the body of the presentation?
3. What approaches would you recommend with this audience?
4. How should she handle the conclusion?

CASE STUDY 2

The state university campus wellness center has assessed the need for nutrition education programs. One finding was that some of the athletes on campus do not seem to understand the importance of maintaining fluid intake and balance before, during, and after sports events. Coaches have asked the dietetics professional on campus to give a presentation on fluid balance to reinforce what they have told players. Joan Little, RD, has agreed to give the presentation and to be available for individual counseling sessions on nutrition as well.

1. What additional information should Joan gather before planning her presentation?
2. What major five to six points should Joan cover in her presentation?
3. How can Joan evaluate the outcome or success of her presentation?
4. What could Joan mention in her introduction to secure the audience's motivation to listen to her?

The suggestions provided in this chapter need to be practiced rather than memorized for an examination. Presenters need to understand, too, that when speaking with adults regarding possible changes in their eating habits, they need to be involved as much as possible in the discussion. Because people eat, they consider that they have some expertise on nutrition. Many do, in fact. Women, for example, who have been pregnant before have some knowledge of prenatal nutrition. Mothers feeding young children often have some knowledge of what is appropriate for them. People who have a medical problem, such as hypertension or heart disease, may have read articles or books or have visited the website of the American Heart Association. Presenters do have to recognize this. Straight lecture without interaction among participants who are informed to some degree is less effective in bringing about change than lecture with discussion.

Developing presentation skills and handling the myriad of problems that can occur with media or interviewers constitute a process that occurs over time. You will get better and better with each subsequent opportunity or practice. (Websites related to topics covered in this chapter are included with the endnotes.)

REVIEW AND DISCUSSION QUESTIONS

1. What are the three generally accepted divisions of a presentation?
2. What should an introduction provide?
3. What are the three key objectives of the body of the presentation?
4. Why is it important for a presenter to proofread all materials, including handouts, flip charts, posters, and transparencies?
5. What does it mean to be audience-centered?
6. How can presenters avoid stage fright?
7. Why are a presenter's facial expressions important?
8. What is the difference between a presentation and a workshop?

SUGGESTED ACTIVITIES

1. Presentation I: Design and deliver a 10-minute presentation on some issue related to foods, nutrition, or dietetics, such as safety of the food supply, a new food product, fiber in foods, reduced fat or calories in foods, snacks, restaurant meals, or sodium.

2. Presentation II: Design and deliver a presentation intended for a group of parents of obese children. A minimum of two visual aids are required, and transparencies and posters. Included with the 20-minute presentation should be 5 full minutes of audience/speaker interaction. "Are there any questions" at the conclusion is not acceptable.

3. Presentation III: Design and deliver a 30-minute presentation intended for a group of people who have recently learned they have diabetes. A minimum of three visual aids are required, including flip chart and handout material. Plan on at least 8 minutes of interaction with the audience; this should be prompted by the speaker's perceptions of the nonverbal feedback emanating from the audience.

4. Presentation IV: Design and deliver a 60-minute presentation intended for a group of people who have paid to be taught or trained by you in an area related to your specialty in the area of dietetics. Develop whatever aids seem appropriate.

If possible all presentations should be videotaped. Presenters should provide reaction sheets to the audience and later write a critique of the taped presentation responding to their own subjective reactions, the critique sheets of the audience, and the instructor's comments.

WEB SITES

http://www.allsands.com/HowTo/publicspeaking_zaf_gn.htm / public speaking tips
http://www.artofspeaking.com / public speaking
http://freenet.edmonton.ab.ca/toast/tips.html / public speaking tips
http://www.educationunlimited.com/Camps/youth/moderncomm/speaking/
    pubspeak.htm / public speaking
http://ok.essortment.com/publicspeaking_reod.htm / art of public speaking
http://www.mhhe.com/socscience/comm/pubspeak / public speaking
http://www.speakeeezi.com / fear of public speaking
http://www.speechtips.com / speech tips
www.stresscure.com/jobstress/speak.html / conquering fear of public speaking

REFERENCES

1. Naughton D. Make your words count. Washingtonian 1996;3:78.
2. Roach R, Pichert J, Stetson B, et al. Improving dietitians' teaching skills. J Am Diet Assoc 1992; 92:1466.
3. Schiller MR, Wolf KN. Preparing for practice in the 21st century. Top Clin Nutr 2000;16:1.
4. Johnson DB, Eaton DL, Wahl PW, Gleason C. Public health nutrition practice in the United States. J Am Diet Assoc 2001;101:529.
5. Ireton-Jones CS, Gottschlich MM, Bell SJ. Practice-oriented nutrition research. Gaithersburg, MD: Aspen Publications, 1998.
6. Kristi N. New technology is in the cards: wallet-size CD-Roms offer multimedia presentations, web links. Advertising Age's Business Marketing 1999;84:30.
7. Michas IC, Berry DC. Learning a procedural task: effectiveness of multimedia presentations. Applied Cogn Psychol 2000;14:555.
8. Nemec R. New media open new doors for communicators. Communication World 2000;17:33.
9. Perry P. Uncovering the top 10 secrets to a better show experience. Builder 1999;4:10.

ADDITIONAL SOURCES

Coughlin C. Overcoming the fear of public speaking. Today's Dietitian 2000;14:18.
Garmston RJ. Ouch! Journal of Staff Development 2000;21:76.
Horn P. So, you've been invited to speak? Rise to the occasion. Presentations 2000;14:92.
Kaye S. Its showtime! How to give effective presentations. Supervision 1999;60:8.
Messmer M. Building your presentation skills. Strategic Finance Magazine 2000;81:10.
Nowling B. Keep it short and simple. J Am Diet Assoc 1994;94:972.
Rosner B. What is the key to an effective business presentation? Workforce 1999;78:24.

Samson T. Master, but don't fear presentations. InfoWorld 2000;22:105.

Schmidt JJ, Miller JB. The five-minute rule for presentations. Training and Development 2000;54:16.

Small R. Having an impact: a model for improving instructional presentations. Teacher Librarian 2000;28:30.

Spaeth M. On presentations, risk managers making presentations at conferences. Risk Management 2000;48:9.

Steward B. Winning the engagement. CA Magazine 2000;133:53.

Wilma D, Kline S. Ace your presentations. J Accountancy 1999;187:61.

Wircenski JL, Sullivan RL. Winning presentations. Training and Development 2000;54:73.

Planning, Selecting, and Using Instructional Media

After reading this chapter, you will be able to

1. describe the key points for making visual materials.
2. identify when to best use various instructional media.
3. measure literacy level of educational materials.
4. have an awareness of the potential uses of asynchronous and synchronous education.
5. plan, use, and evaluate instructional media used in a presentation.

Instructional media are the teaching tools that enhance teaching through the use of various technologies. Using media correctly and effectively enhances your delivery of a message.(1) Whether making a presentation or working one on one with an individual, visual displays such as food models or attractive bulleted points, charts, and graphs make your message more understandable. Trainers who use visuals are "perceived as better prepared, more professional, more persuasive, more credible, and more interesting."(2) This chapter examines the types of instructional media most commonly available, offers suggestions for use, and discusses the advantages, limitations, and evaluation of various forms of media. In whatever aspect of dietetics you work, communication is a part of the business and media can help enhance communication.

BENEFITS OF VISUAL MEDIA

"A picture is worth a thousand words." How true. Four pictures, therefore, are worth 4,000 words. The more you want to get across, the more visual assistance is helpful. When people can see things rather than merely hear them or read about them, they remember more. Visual media are especially helpful to low-income groups with limited reading ability and ethnic groups who speak little English. All professionals should bear in mind that just because you are talking is no guarantee that anyone is listening. This fact has major implications for professionals who plan educational presentations for patients, clients, employees, other professionals, and the public.

How much do people learn from visual media? Following is an estimate on the amount of learning using the senses. We learn 10% from reading, 20% from listening,

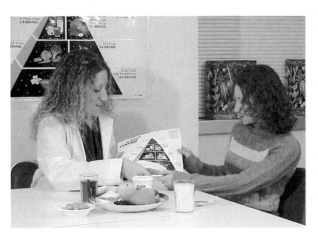

A picture is worth a thousand words.

and 80% from what we see.(3) What about recalling information 2 weeks later? We remember 20% of what we hear, but 50% of what we both see and hear and 90% of what we say and do.(4) It is obvious that giving the audience visuals helps in learning and remembering. Lecturing alone, such as about nutrition to a group of pregnant women, about low-fat diets to men with hyperlipidemia, or about sanitation to employees, is going to get only limited results. Visual methods are not the total answer to presenting information. Active participation is the key to learning.(4)

Visual media are part of the instructional input. Visuals enhance written and oral communication methods and make them more interesting. Pictures and sounds have the power to compel attention, to enhance understanding, and to promote learning in a shorter time frame than by using solely verbal explanations. A study of nutrition education focusing on a low-fat, low-cholesterol diet for patients in a clinical setting, for example, compared three methods: individualized instruction for 30 to 45 minutes, a slide/verbal classroom presentation for 45 minutes, and a videotape presentation with a 15-minute follow-up visit by a dietitian. The videotape method proved to be just as effective, as measured by a test of comprehension, and considerably more time-efficient.(5)

When media quality is high, your total presentation looks more professional, better prepared, more credible, interesting, and persuasive, because you appeal to individuals through their senses of sight, sound, touch, taste, and smell.(2) Of course, poor-quality materials produce the reverse results.

PLANNING VISUAL MEDIA

Planning what instructional media to use is part of the overall program planning for the learning situation. Answers to the following seven questions will help your thinking:

1. What are the objectives/aims of the session? What should audience members learn or be able to do?
2. What methods or activities (lecture, discussion, individual counseling, simulation and the like) will facilitate accomplishing the objectives? Where can media fit into these plans?

3. Who is the audience? What are the characteristics of the learner, such as age, gender, educational and literacy level, and cultural or ethnic group?
4. What is the learner's current level of knowledge of the topic? A presentation to a lay group, for example, would need different visuals than a presentation to a group of professionals. And new employee training may need a different approach from that for long-term employees.
5. What purpose(s) do the visuals serve? Is it to generate interest in the subject; to affect attitudes, emotions, or motivation; to entertain; to present information; to attract and hold attention; to involve the learner in mental activity promoting learning; or some combination of purposes?
6. How can you concisely organize and sequence the points to be made and emphasize them with visuals? How are the key messages being reinforced? Can you break down the learning into key steps and assess knowledge at each step?
6. How will you evaluate the effectiveness of the total presentation including visuals?(3, 6)

The instructional media that you select depends on the goals, the size of the audience, the physical facilities, equipment and time available, and the learning style of the audience. Before discussing types of visuals, let's identify key principles for all visuals.

ART AND DESIGN PRINCIPLES

The quality and effectiveness of media may depend to a great extent on art and design principles. You do not have to be a great artist, but some understanding of simple principles will improve results. First and foremost, the visual must be large enough for all participants to see. Know the size of the facility and the type of presentation before you create the visuals.

Simplicity/Unity

The presenter should try to convey only one idea at a time, since too many ideas confuse the audience. Decide what should be at the center of attention or interest and then build around it. This may need to be the largest-size item for the audience, so focus on it immediately.

Margins

To look professional, visuals need a margin in the same way that pictures need a frame. Overhead transparencies, for example, need an inch on all sides. Posters, charts, and bulletin boards also need margins. It is not advisable or attractive to write all the way to the edge or to crowd visuals.

Wording/Lettering

Be concise and use the fewest words possible. Working on conciseness of visuals should help to organize the thoughts that you as the presenter want to get across. Titles and labels are placed at various locations. Headings or headlines need to clarify the emphasis and should be in larger print.

Standardizing the size of the lettering and the kind of lettering or fonts makes a more professional appearance. Times Roman and Gothic are more readable than some stylized scripts. See Table 15-1 for examples of fonts.(6,7) The size must be large enough to be read by the reader who is sitting the farthest away. A rule of thumb on the size of lower-case letters projected on overhead transparencies, for example, is that they are ½ inch high for each 10 feet of viewer distance.(3) So, for someone standing 20 feet away, 1-inch letters should be readable. A study of 38 printed materials on cholesterol education found print size that was typically too small for many older adults.(8) For handouts, a minimum of 12-point font size is recommended.(6) For the elderly, 14- or 18-point and dark colors on light background work better.

For slides, the number of words should be limited to 20 to 36. Raines and Williamson recommend the "rule of six," which is to use not more than six lines and not more than six words per line.(7) Capital letters are appropriate for short titles of five to six words or less, but a combination of capital and lower case is

---

TABLE 15-1 Type Styles, Fonts, and Print Sizes

10 point type
12 point type
14 point type
18 point type
24 point type
36 point type
48 point type

Times Roman
Century
Courier
Helvetica
AvantGarde
Tekton
COPPERPLATE BOLD
Poetica Chancery

preferable for longer titles, allowing space for readability. A Combination of Upper and Lower Case Letters Is Preferable. ALL CAPS ARE MORE DIFFICULT TO READ. You may wish to number lists or use bullets (•), underline words for emphasis or add stars to key points.

Color

Color can enhance visuals and demand attention. You may combine colors that are pleasing aesthetically and not clashing. It is best to decide on the focus of the visual and select the color for that first. Colors have meanings to people. In most Western countries, red and orange are considered "hot," whereas green, blue, and violet are considered "cool" colors.(3) The presenter should start by considering the background color. If it is light, any bright colors may be used. With a dark background, lighter shades are needed and print has to be larger to be read.

Pictures, Artwork, Graphics, and Cartoons

Visuals can illustrate difficult concepts well. This includes proportions, relationships, similarities, and differences. An illustration evokes a visual picture of a procedure or technique. A cartoon can add fun to the presentation and increase the viewer's memory of a concept. As with the other principles, the dietetics professional should consider the layout of the illustration and its effect on the audience's understanding. Is it too crowded? Confusing? Pleasing? Is it serving its purpose? A complex table or chart may be better as a handout than as an overhead or slide.

Balance

There are two kinds of balance, formal and informal. Informal balance is asymmetrical and more attention getting and interesting than symmetrical balance. Formal balance occurs when one has the mirror image of the other half. Bear in mind that our society reads from left to right and top to bottom, so that is the way your audience will view any visual.(6)

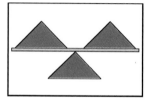 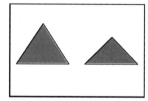

Formal balance   **Informal balance**

Formal and informal balance.

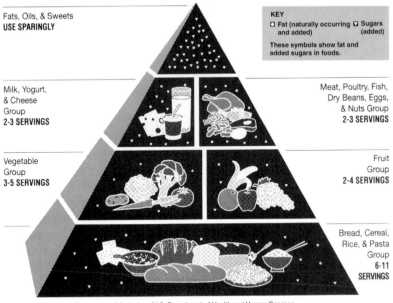

Food Guide Pyramid.

Emphasis

Try to create a "center of interest." This can be slightly above the center of the space or the intersection of two lines or by different size pictures.(6)

Back-ups

Have a plan to deal with media and equipment that does not work or that is too small for the space. Ask about back-up projector bulbs, have a back-up copy of a presentation, and have a printed-out copy. Be ready to do the presentation without the assistance of media.(9)

ASYNCHRONOUS OR SYNCHRONOUS LEARNING

Instructional information may be given in a synchronous or asynchronous manner. In synchronous learning, all the participants are learning at the same time. This may be one on one, as a small group, or as a large group. Traditionally, synchronous learning was done in one location in an office, classroom, or conference room. Today, synchronous learning can occur at two or multiple sites via videoconferencing and cable or tele-phone connections, compressed video connections, telephone or computer conference calls with materials distributed over the internet, or live chats on the internet, "Webinars." Asynchronous learning is "anytime learning." Reading a journal article or watching a videotape or CD-ROM or participating in an e-mail discussion based on your schedule are examples of asynchronous learning. Asynchronous learning gives learners much more freedom over their approach to learning. They can read, listen, or watch the material until they are comfortable with it; especially in distance education, the student must actively participate in the learning whether by participating with others or by completing tutorials and quizzes.

Computer-based instruction is becoming common in many worksites. Computer-based instruction can be used in various ways. It provides time flexibility and a consistent message.(10) The read/listen and do practice tests were the early computer-assisted learning. This is particularly good for learning facts, such as medical terminology, or calculations, such as designing a total parenteral nutrition (TPN) solution. The clients/employees are given rapid feedback on how well they comprehend the material. Tutorials, games, and simulations may augment the learning.

Today, the technology and teaching methods have advanced to the point that very interactive facilitated learning between teacher and student can occur via the computer. The addition of interaction between teacher and student, and student and student via the internet has allowed computer-based distance education to grow rapidly across the world. A computer-based distance education class generally has all the components of a traditional class: textbooks, readings, assignments, and tests. The class discussion is replaced by a web-based discussion facilitated by the teacher. The lecture is replaced by readings, websites, written lectures, and audio or video CD-ROMs. The students and faculty need internet connections via a modem or cable connection.

For "just-in-time" patient/client/employee education, many institutions are using stand-alone computer kiosks (terminals). A WIC (women, infants, and children) program used a multimedia nutrition education program for clients in a freestanding kiosk.(11) This allows clients to get information when they need it. It does not replace, but rather augments, the dietetics professional's message.

THE ENVIRONMENT FOR THE SYNCHRONOUS PRESENTATION

For synchronous learning, the type of visuals recommended depends on the environment. The decisions are based on the answers to the following questions.

1. What is the size of the audience and the room? Ten, fifty, one hundred, five hundred? What is the setting? How are the acoustics, lighting, and seats arranged?
2. What equipment is available in the room of the presentation, and what is the cost of use of the equipment, if any?
3. Is anyone available at the presentation to assist with setting up and using the media? Will the internet be available?
4. What is the preference of the audience for media: visual, auditory, reading material, or a combination?

5. What is the preference of the presenter for media? What are you comfortable using?
6. How much time will it take to prepare your own media? What people with technical expertise in design and production are available to assist? How many times will the material be used?
7. Would handouts work just as well as media? Would handouts augment the presentation?

Plan ahead for missing equipment and poor connections. Be prepared to have a back-up disk and be prepared to give the presentation without media. It is important to evaluate media as you use them. Eventually, you want to know what proves most effective in the shortest time frame in learning and retention, thus providing efficiency.

Assessing Knowledge

When giving a talk to a small lay group, you may give as a handout a short preassessment of multiple-choice and completion questions. This is a self-assessment or series of questions around which to frame the presentation. The questions elicit audience participation, discussion, and additional questions. This approach is valuable because it recognizes that adults come with many answers from their past experience. You need to find out what the audience already knows, compliment them on their knowledge, and present information at their level. The presenter can use the audience handout to write the additional points to be made, thus avoiding switching back and forth from the handout to notes for the presentation.

KINDS OF VISUAL MEDIA

After considering what needs to be communicated and thinking about the audience, the dietetics professional may select the appropriate media for the purpose. Any one or several may be applicable. Table 15-2 outlines the possibilities. This section discusses the types of media to consider—from real objects to multimedia presentations.

Real Objects

Nothing is more realistic than showing actual foods or food packages. A lesson on food labeling, for example, may include a variety of food packages so that the audience can participate hands-on with actual products in learning to read and understand the labels. To avoid audience distraction, keep items covered or out-of-sight when they are not being used. Passing items around may also be a major distraction. Photocopies of labels work well and reduce storage space or the amount to carry to an alternate site.

Making recipes to be tasted in group sessions when teaching about nutrition or modified diets is another suggestion. A person with heart disease, for example, who has seen the dietetics professional prepare a tasty recipe, sampled it, and received the recipe is more likely to try it at home. In a series of classes, audience members may assist and provide recipes.

TABLE 15-2 Types of Media

Real Objects/Presentations	Print Media
Foods	Handouts
Food demonstrations	Brochures/newsletters
Food packages/labels	
Food models	
Food service equipment	

Audio Formats	Projected Visuals
Audiotapes	Overhead transparencies
Compact discs	Slides/computer-based presentations
DVDs	VHS tapes
	CD-ROMs

Display Media	Graphics
Chalk or white board	Diagrams
Flip chart	Charts
Bulletin or display boards	Cartoons
Photographs	Clip art
Pictures	Menus
Magnets and pens	

Moving Images
Videos
CD-ROMs
Multimedia

A tour to the grocery store is another possibility. A nutrition intervention study based on the American Heart Association's grocery store tour taught adults to read food labels so they could decrease the risk of coronary heart disease by selecting foods lower in total fat, saturated fat, and cholesterol.(12) The tour was provided in three formats: an actual tour of a grocery store, an American Heart Association video, and a home study program. Results showed that those who took the actual tour reported that they learned an extreme amount, were likely to make at least one food purchasing change, and liked the delivery format more than those who participated in the other two formats. Even though the actual tour was more effective in promoting behavioral change, the educators preferred the video because it demanded less of their time and was the easiest format with which to recruit participants.

In training employees, it is preferable to train them using the real object, such as a meat slicer, dish machine, cash register, or other equipment. Actual hands-on experience is preferable. Breaking the learning into small segments is also preferable to facilitate learning.

Advantages

Realistic.

Hands-on learning and audience participation enhance motivation and retention.

Limitations

Some foods are perishable.

Cooking facilities may not be available.

Not suitable for large groups.

Food Models

Food models are representations of the real objects. Many professionals maintain an inventory of three-dimensional plastic food models. They are helpful in estimating client portion sizes, for example, during an assessment of food intake and in teaching portion sizes on controlled caloric intakes. Besides the visual stimulation, putting the model in the person's hands makes a more active experience using another of the senses—touch. Plastic, life-sized food models may be purchased from sources, such as Nasco Nutrition Teaching Aids in Fort Atkinson, Wisconsin.

When discussing portion control of beverages or foods, show the diversity of sizes available. You may need a variety of sizes and shapes as well as disposable cups when portion size is important. If you are going to suggest 4- and 8-ounce servings, you should encourage using a measuring cup at home to train the eye to portion correctly.

Advantages

Are realistic and colorful.

Are portable.

Show portion sizes.

Limitations

Cannot be seen in large groups.

May lose items.

Pictures/Packages/Menus

Pictures from magazines or catalogs or clip art may be displayed on posters or on computer screens. Sample packages and containers of recommended foods may be displayed. To discuss a "Nutrition Facts" label or ingredients labeling with a client, it is helpful and realistic to have actual labels available. Labels may be removed from packages and mounted on cardboard or into a book for display or as photocopies. You may want to have different collections, for example, when teaching about healthy snacks, low-fat food choices, sodium-controlled, low-calorie foods, and the like. One method of teaching about the values on the label and the ingredients is to have clients guess the product by the nutrient composition and ingredient list. Menus from local eating establishments are excellent for learning about eating out.

Advantages
May be colorful and eye catching.

Generally inexpensive.

Packages and pictures are portable.

Limitations
Lacks motion.

Can be overdone unless the message is focused.

Photographs/Drawings

The professional may take photographs or have them done professionally. Photos can be enlarged to any size. They may be used on bulletin boards and computer screens. If you are photographing people, such as employees and clients, a signed form releasing the use of the photos without limitation is advisable.

Advantages
Relatively inexpensive.

Reflects real situations.

Attracts interest.

Limitation
Distracting to pass around in groups.

Charts/Posters

Information may be presented in charts or on posters that you make or purchase. The US Department of Agriculture's graphic design of dietary recommendations in the Food Guide Pyramid is an example. Numerical data can be presented in bar charts, pie-shaped charts, or line graphs.

A table, easel, or tripod should securely hold the display. It is not necessary to read word for word from a visual. At most, you may tell why the visual is significant or paraphrase the content. If possible, remove it from audience view after discussing it.

Posters are also a medium for sharing research findings and other information at professional meetings. Often the posters are divided into specific segments that are prepared on separate sheets. They may be attached onto mounting boards at the meeting site or be free-standing tabletop posters.(13) Guidelines for poster sessions from the American Dietetic Association are in Figure 15-1.

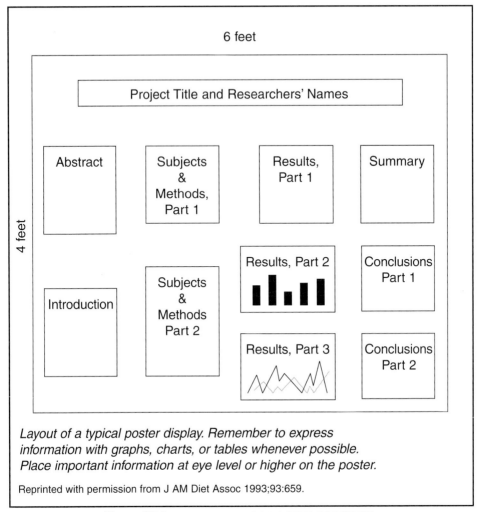

Layout of a typical poster display. Remember to express information with graphs, charts, or tables whenever possible. Place important information at eye level or higher on the poster.

Reprinted with permission from J AM Diet Assoc 1993;93:659.

Figure 15-1 GUIDELINES FOR POSTER SESSIONS.

Advantages

Inexpensive.

Portable for short distances.

Limitations

Cannot be seen except in very small (15–20) groups.

Homemade charts may be overcrowded with content.

Get worn with repeated use.

Bulletin or Display Boards

Bulletin boards or display boards can spark interest in a topic. They should be totally self-explanatory. The concept should be simple, and the display should visually attract attention.

Advantages

Inexpensive.

Limited preparation.

Limitations

Cannot be used with large groups.

Not generally portable.

Chalkboard or Whiteboard

Everyone has seen the chalkboard or whiteboard used and misused. If you write legibly and large enough to be seen, it is a good supplement to a presentation. Major pitfalls occur if you are a poor speller and if you turn your back to the audience and talk to the board while writing. You need to avoid standing with your back to the audience. If this is a problem for the presenter, overhead transparencies are preferable. Chalkboards, whiteboards, and flip charts all foster participation.

Advantages

Inexpensive.

Easy to use.

Allows audience opinions to be written down.

Spontaneous.

Limitations

Requires good timing so that one does not talk to the board.

Not good in large groups.

Poor spelling and handwriting are liabilities.

Flip Charts

If a chalkboard or whiteboard is unavailable, a flip chart with a display easel may substitute. Flip charts have a number of large sheets of paper fastened together. You can write or draw with crayon or black or colored felt pens, being sure to select ones that do not bleed through the paper. Writing should be large and bold to be seen—at least 1 inch high or more for every 20 to 30 feet of audience space. Inexperienced presenters may want to ask someone to do the writing for them.

Each sheet is turned at the top after completion. Finished sheets can also be torn off and attached to a wall. When you need a record of points made by the audience, a flip chart is preferable to a chalkboard because the sheets can be carried from the meeting. Alternately, one can prepare the sheets in advance and reveal them sequentially while standing facing the audience. This allows for the creative use of color, clip-art, glitter, fabric and, other materials. It is advisable to leave a blank page when the audience focus should be on the presenter.

Advantages

Informal and inexpensive.

Limitations

Awkward to carry very far.

Cannot be seen in larger groups.

Requires legible handwriting.

Requires practice to write quickly while speaking.

May be too informal for some purposes.

Overhead Transparencies

When an overhead projector is available, transparencies are a great visual comple-ment to a presentation. The speaker stands, not sits, beside the projector facing the audience, being careful not to block the view of the screen. Correct font size is essential.

The dietetics professional may ask someone else to change the transparencies while talking from a position elsewhere in the room. You may point to items while talking or progressively disclose the contents by covering with paper or cardboard the portions that you do not want seen yet. Some speakers like to have a title or other visu-al on the projector as the audience assembles. To assist the audience, number the points on the transparency in the order in which you are discussing them and in order of importance. If all items are of equal importance, bullets (•) are more generic. When not in use, the projector should be turned off so that people are not staring into a bright, blank screen.

It is possible to mark on the clear or colored plastic film while talking, such as underlining items or checking them off. Felt-tipped pens designed for transparencies come in various colors. Marks from water-based pens can be removed later with a damp cloth; the permanent markings can be removed with lighter fluid.

Keep in mind that the average projector surface is 10 × 10 inches, transparencies are 10 × 12, and most paper is 8.5 × 11, so the actual message areas is about 7.5 × 9.0 to 9.5 inches.(3,7) A border needs to be left around all the edges. Write legibly and large enough so that material can be seen at the rear of the room.

A more professional look may be obtained by typing the information. Large type size must be used. About 30 points or ¼ inch is good, but you need to check the room size to be sure.(7) See Table 15-1 for samples of font and type sizes. When the page is prepared, there are certain transparencies that can be placed in a photocopier to pro-duce the transparency. Some computer programs can prepare them also. Special trans-parency film is available for the printer, and color ink-jet or laser printers are capable of producing full-color transparencies.

Graphs or charts from scientific and professional journals, enlarged cartoons, and other data may be presented easily in this form. Photographs do not reproduce well except with a digital camera that will place pictures into a computer graphics file to be printed on a transparency. For repeated use, mount the transparencies in cardboard frames. This prevents static electricity, which makes the transparencies stick to one another.

Advantages

Easy to use and inexpensive.

Can maintain eye contact with the audience, which helps to control attention.

Uses normal room lighting.

Can write on them while talking.

Limitations

In a large, deep room, may not be seen in the back.

Easy to overcrowd information.

Bulb may burn out (carry an extra).

Print Handouts

Health care professionals tend to give patients and clients a great deal of information verbally. By the time they get home, most have probably forgotten at least half of the information. Trainers may do the same with new employees.

Putting things in writing that clients, patients, employees, and other audiences can refer to later solves this problem. For modified diets, for example, oral counseling is frequently supplemented with written materials including the foods to eat and those to limit, recipes suggestions, and websites to visit. Printed materials are effective in reinforcing individual counseling sessions and group classes. When planning employee training, the presenter may consider giving an outline of the content with space for note taking or a list of the main points to be remembered. When using an overhead transparency with lots of information, listeners will be writing instead of listening unless you distribute copies of the information on the transparency.

In teaching about normal nutrition, for example, the Food Guide Pyramid and/or the Dietary Guidelines for Americans may be distributed. Government agencies and private organizations produce printed materials for wide-ranging audiences, or you can make your own. If you are using materials produced by others, determine the right to reproduce the materials. If the material is copyright-free, just acknowledge the owner. If the material is copyrighted, obtain permission to reproduce the material. There may be a charge for this based on the number being used. Some materials may need to be purchased for distribution.

One-page instructional sheets written in short, simple words in active voice assist all clients, even when you are also giving out more detailed materials. These sheets can be posted on the refrigerator or hung at the office to remind clients of what to do and when to do it. Small give-aways such as pens, magnets, puzzles, and games may also be useful to remind the person of your message.

For written materials, assess the readability or grade level, since some adults have low literacy skills. It is estimated that as many as 20% of adults are functionally illiterate.(1) About 24.8% of adults are not high school graduates.(14) Some are recent immigrants with limited ability in English. Printed materials in other languages may be needed. Educational materials must be understandable to the people for whom they are intended. Therefore, nutrition educators need to select or develop printed materials that are easily comprehended.

Several readability formulas are available to help assess the audience's readability or grade level both as software programs and in print. The SMOG, FOG, Flesch, Raygor, and Fry tests are examples. The SMOG criteria are in Table 15-3. Readability tests examine the linguistic and structural qualities of written materials. Because of the scientific and technical nature of health communications, vocabulary and wording of patient education materials may be incomprehensible to many adults. Readability for-

---

TABLE 15-3 SMOG Readability Formula

1. Count off 10 consecutive sentences near the beginning, in the middle, and near the end of the text. If the text has fewer than 30 sentences, use as many as are provided.
2. Count the number of words containing 3 or more syllables (polysyllabic) including repetitions of the same words.
a. Hyphenated words are considered as one word.
b. Numbers that are written out should be counted. If written in numerical form, they should be pronounced to determine if they are polysyllabic.
c. Proper nouns, if polysyllabic, should be counted.
d. Abbreviations should be read as though unabbreviated to determine if they are polysyllabic. However, abbreviations should be avoided unless commonly known.
3. Look up the approximate grade level on the SMOG Conversion Table below:

Total Polysyllabic Word Count	Approx. Grade Level (+1.5 Grades)
0-2	4
3-6	5
7-12	6
13-20	7
21-30	8
31-42	9
43-55	10
56-72	11
73-90	12
91-110	13
111-132	14
133-156	15
157-182	16
183-210	17
211-240	18

From "SMOG grading: A new readability formula" by G. McLaughlin, 1969, *Journal of Reading*, 12(8), pp. 639-646. Adapted with permission.

mulas should be used to assess the approximate educational level a person must have to understand the material.

A study of WIC participants with a self-reported educational level of 11.8 years found a mismatch between reading and comprehension skills levels on the 1990 Dietary Guidelines for Americans, portions of which were written at the college level according to a computerized readability analysis program. It is well to consider that a person's reading skill level may be as many as five grades below the highest grade completed in school.(15)

In a study of the readability levels of 38 printed materials on cholesterol education available from various sources, both the SMOG and Fog Grading formulas were used. They revealed that the average reading grade level was close to grade 11, a difficult level.(18) Another study surveyed 209 nutrition education pamphlets that might be used with low-literacy adults. Using the Flesch, Raygor, and Fry tests, results showed that there were few materials for those with limited literacy skills. Sixty-eight percent of the materials were written at the ninth grade level or higher, and only 11% were at the sixth grade level or lower.(16)

Materials in print may be personalized using word processing and desktop publishing software. If writing a longer pamphlet, focus groups are a valuable tool in planning, pretesting, and evaluating printed materials.(17)

Advantages

Audience can refer to it later at home or at work.

Good when information has to be remembered.

Helps the person to focus attention and follow points.

Limitations

People may never look at it again.

Time spent in preparing materials.

Literacy level varies by users.

Audio Recordings

Cassette tapes, CD-ROMs, and DVDs can be prerecorded to illustrate communication techniques. Long recordings may be more appropriate for individual listening than for a group presentation, but short audios can be very effective in a large group. Testimonials, several sentences from a key leader, or a commercial or radio segment can be used as a springboard for many messages. If preparing your own recording, an informal, conversational tone of voice with slow, clear enunciation is needed. Listen to the recording before using it to assess whether the sound quality is acceptable. Background noise on the recording can be very distracting.

Advantages

Inexpensive and easy to use.

Portable.

Allows repetition and reinforcement.

Good for low-literacy groups.

Limitations

No guarantee of retention or learning.

No guarantee that hearing includes careful listening or comprehension.

Slides/Computer-Based Presentations

Slides may be computer-generated using such programs as Microsoft's PowerPoint or Corel or produced through traditional photography. A 35-mm camera of your own will make satisfactory 35-mm slides of a standard 2- by 2-inch dimension. Computer generation is the often common method of producing slides. Most word-processing software packages have a presentation program that assists you in producing slides. Typed-in words and pictures, graphs, and animations are cut and pasted into the presentation. Graphics, animations, and pictures use a considerable amount of space on a disk, so if you are using a standard computer diskette rather than a zip drive or a CD-ROM, limiting graphics may be necessary. In some cases, slides are available for purchase; generally these are on CD-ROMs.

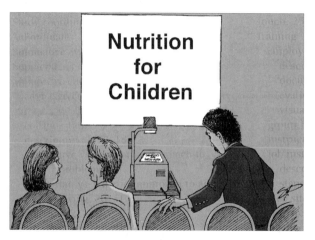

The title of one's presentation may be displayed as the audience gathers.

With a remote-control projector or computer, the presenter can advance the slides/presentation while talking and turn off the projector at appropriate times so that the audience focus returns to the presenter. Professionals begin and end with a black slide or a title/logo slide to avoid the white glare of the screen without a slide. If a very short part of the presentation does not include a slide, a black slide can be inserted there instead of turning the projector or computer off and on.

If you are using traditional slides, number and label them and mark the upper right-hand corner with a dot where the thumb drops the slide into the tray correctly, which is upside down and backward.(10)

Computer-based presentations connect the computer, generally a laptop, to a projection device. An LCD projector (liquid crystal display) or an LMD, which uses mirrors, displays the images on a screen.

Advantages

Small and easy to carry along in trays or as diskette.

Can change the sequence as appropriate.

Good for both large and small groups.

Limitations

May be out of order if not checked.

May be projected upside down or backwards if not checked.

Equipment may malfunction.

Need to dim room lighting; the better the projection the less dimming needed.

Videotapes or Video CDs

The combinations of sights and sounds from videos are pleasing to most people. Purchased or rented videos should be previewed to check for appropriateness. Many groups, such as the American Dietetic Association, American Heart Association, American Diabetes Association, National Dairy Council, Educational Foundation of the National Restaurant Association, drug companies, government agencies, and private media companies offer visual materials. A video cassette recorder (VCR) or an LCD projector and monitor are necessary for audience viewing. Because audiences tend to view passively, they should be told what to look for before viewing, and preplanned activities or discussion questions should follow. A video or CD may be viewed alone at the learner's own pace or viewed repeatedly to enhance learning. The presenter may put a video on pause to stop for discussion. Short video clips can highlight key points and help segment the talk.

Many employee programs for orientation and training use video formats, sometimes with printed workbooks or learner's guides. If the employee views a video alone, discussions with the instructor should follow to explain the relationship of the video to the job. Videos can be placed on a CD ROM or a video server and connected to a web-based site, where demonstrations of learning can occur. The learner watches the video and periodically or at the end is asked questions about the content to assess learning. Many employee education and orientation programs are moving to web-based training as a portion of their training because it is convenient and available to all employees rather than those available on a particular day; also, competencies can be documented. Customized unit-based training is also easier to facilitate via technology-based training. The employee or client can be directed to complete only the modules pertinent to the current role providing training on-demand or "just-in-time" training.(20)

You may be able to make videotapes with a video camera, but keep in mind that today's audiences are sophisticated viewers, who may not respond well to amateur productions. The time, money, and professional staff available will determine your ability to develop high-quality videos. If you have an idea for a video, you may use a storyboard to outline the shots for each scene in roughly sketched pictures.(3) It should include the audio and production techniques for each shot, the director, camera person, actors, behind-the-scenes crew, props, costumes, makeup, and lighting. If taping clients or employees, you should obtain a written release of use without limitations.

Videos should be short and to the point. Fifteen to 20 minutes is ideal; over 30 minutes may be too long for most audiences.(1) Videos should augment the learning. Teacher-facilitated discussion after the video should reinforce the concepts and promote active discussion. Short videos to take home after the presentation or counseling reinforce learning. This is especially useful for procedures such as preparing baby formula or conducting self-care.

Advantages

Realistic, enjoyable, and dramatic.

Includes both sight and sound stimulation.

If it tells a story, people retain it better.

For learning, someone can view it repeatedly and "just in time."

Can have an emotional impact and help to change attitudes.

Limitations

May not fit the purpose and objectives.

May be expensive to buy or produce.

Requires equipment at production site and at user's site.

Complex issues may be misinterpreted unless discussed.

Mixed Media

The dietetics professional should consider using more than one of the previously discussed visuals in a presentation, such as a combination of handouts along with overhead transparencies or slides. Alternatively, you may use actual foods, handouts, and the chalkboard. Music to illustrate a point and a brief video may help. Many combinations are possible. Think of the message, and select the visual media best for the session. The focus is on the learners' needs.(18)

PURCHASING PREPARED MEDIA MATERIALS

The question often arises about whether to prepare your own media materials or use existing materials. The most basic answer is to use the least expensive media to accomplish the goals with the best quality possible.(18) The anticipated longevity of the material before it is outdated and the number of times you will use the material should influence the decision. The cost to purchase media versus the cost to make your own media need to be considered in terms of time, quality, and expertise. The availability of technical expertise in design and production are essential, especially for audio and video production. The availability of prepared pamphlets or videos to meet the objectives is also important. In addition, the cost to reproduce the material is a consideration.

Regardless of who produces the media, the materials should be assessed for readability, first impressions, content, and format. Is the content accurate? Does it address the needs of the audience? Is the material legible and readable? Have you pilot-tested the material on the target audience? Table 15-4 lists some questions to use to evaluate materials.(19)

It is important to evaluate media as you use them. Eventually, you want to know what proves most effective in the shortest time frame in learning and retention, thus providing efficiency.

TABLE 15-4 Evaluating Nutrition Education Materials (n = 142).

General evaluation practices

Distribute nutrition education materials to clients

Use a variety of printed nutrition education materials

Thoroughly preview nutrition education materials

Use a formal checklist to evaluate nutrition education materials

Develop new nutrition education materials

Pilot test modified or new nutrition education materials

Use nutrition education materials provided by a reputable source

Request feedback relative to nutrition education materials from clients

Conduct a client assessment before providing dietary guidance

Consider the client's age

Consider the client's gender

Assess the client's education level

Consider the client's ethnicity/cultural background

Consider the client's lifestyle

Consider the client's socioeconomic status

Assess the client's reading ability

Readability criteria

Readability level

Length of sentences

Length of paragraphs

Number of syllables per word

Use of examples

Use of jargon, cliches, idioms

Word appropriateness

Legibility

Style and typeface

Size of print

Highlighting of specific information

Active or passive words

First, second or third person

Typographical errors

Content criteria

Addresses the needs of the client

Age appropriateness

Applicability of information

Consistency of information

Objectivity of information

Gender appropriateness

Implications of information

Motivational messages

Accuracy of information

Summarizes information

Credibility of information

Number of of content errors

Date of publication

Flow of concepts

Ethnicity or cultural appropriateness

Scientific basis of information

Practicality of information

Focuses on behavioral change

Continuity of information

Format criteria

Color scheme

Photographs

Layouts

Use of white space

Use of higlighting techniques

Quality of copy

Captures attention

Interactive

Complexity of details

Illustrations

Illustrations that support messages

Attractiveness

Quality of paper

Use of charts, graphs, and tables

Margin justification

GIVING PRESENTATIONS

After preparing both the presentation and the visuals, several practices are critical to success. During practice, you may find that a few changes need to be made. Can the writing on charts or transparencies, for example, be seen from all areas in the room? If not, modifications are needed.

The presenter needs to practice with the slides, overheads, or other media. You may practice at home with a friend or colleague to obtain feedback. If no one is available, practicing in front of a mirror is a possibility, although not as effective. Videotaping yourself using a video camera on a tripod is a great method of seeing yourself and identifying how to enhance the presentation. Preferably, you should practice in the actual setting of the presentation. As a presenter, you should also arrive 30 minutes in advance to check on things and give instructions to anyone assisting. You need to know, for example, how to run the equipment and lower the lights in the room.

EVALUATING RESULTS

Educational evaluation is treated in detail in Chapter 12. It is important to obtain feedback not only on your presentation. Some educational programs use written evaluation forms. Figure 15-2 provides a sample evaluation form to assess the quality of a group teaching session. If a written form is not used, you may inquire about audience reactions afterward. Any suggestions may be used as a basis for revising and improving the materials. Although it is probably not possible for novices, experienced presenters can watch the audience for nonverbal reactions during the presentation.

There is no doubt that media enhance learning and retention from presentations and educational sessions as well as having the potential to enhance the speaker's professional image. If you are not using at least five to eight visuals, you may be 5000 to 8000 words short.

THE FUTURE GENERATION

Today's audiences grew up with television and tend to relate more quickly to pictures than words. The data show that 98.3% of households own television sets, with an average of 2.2 sets per home.(14) According to one estimate, the average American family spends 7.5 hours daily watching television, more time than any other activity except sleep and work.(21) They also rent videos. Visual images bombard us daily in everything from media advertising to Tee shirts with messages and pictures.

Today about two-thirds (64%) of family households with children have a computer at home for personal use. We are becoming a cyber-nation. This is especially true among children. Sixty-one percent of 9- to 17-year-olds use the internet, whereas 52% of their parents do not. "In general, and fairly consistently, a higher percentage of children surveyed aged nine to 17 in every demographic group report that they are online than did parents we interviewed" (National Schools Board Foundation: Safe and Smart. http://www.nsbf.org/). Computers and the internet are having a profound impact on education and teaching in the current decade. People read fewer books and newspapers

GROUP TEACHING EVALUATION FORM

Name _____   **Signature** _____

Date _____   **Rotation Site:** _____

Evaluated by: _____

Topic _____   **Audience: Pt/Staff/RDs/Other**

CRITERIA	RATING 5 4 3 2 1	COMMENTS

1. Observes social amenities: introduces self; ensures that audience is comfortable
2. Explains purpose of "class" to group
3. Speaks clearly and loudly
4. Uses grammar/language properly
5. Holds interest of group
6. Adjusts content of talk to educational level of group
7. Incorporates group participation as part of lesson
8. Follows a logical order in imparting information
9. Emphasizes key points
10. Summarizes at end of presentation
11. Allows time for questions
12. Encourages questions
13. Answers questions
14. Presents lessons appropriate to time allotment
15. Is familiar with space and equipment
16. Prepares visuals/other aids to enhance presentation
17. Uses visual aids large enough to see clearly
18. Uses visual aids effectively
19. Plans and uses some method to evaluate learning
20. Provides resource/handout information for those who want further information
21. Content: thoroughness of lesson
22. Accuracy of lesson
23. Overall effectiveness of lesson

KEY

5 = Consistently demonstrates skill
4 = Demonstrates majority of skill
3 = Adequately progressing with skill development
2 = Needs emphasis
1 = Unable to demonstrate skill

TOTAL AUDIENCE COMMENTS

AUDIENCE INITIALS

Used with permission of UMDNJ-SHRP Department of Primary Care.

Figure 15.2 GROUP TEACHING EVALUATION FORM

CASE STUDY 1

At 9:00 AM, Julie gathered her flip chart and magic markers and headed for her office door. She was conducting an employee training session that began at 9:00 AM. As she entered the training room, she said to the 20 participants, "Oh well, I'm here. Let's begin by watching a short video."

As Julie inserted the video into the VCR, she realized that the carriage was broken and she would not be able to show it. Frustrated and embarrassed, Julie said, "Nothing in this company works right. I guess I'll have to ask them to bring me another VCR."

After calling Media Services to obtain another VCR, Julie turned to the group and said, "I was in a hurry this morning, and I forgot my handouts for the session. It will just take me a few minutes to go back to my office to get them."

1. What should Julie have done to create a more positive image of herself and to improve this training session?

CASE STUDY 2

Doris Burns, RD, works for a large corporation in their corporate wellness center. Recently, the center nurse mentioned that a number of employees have high blood pressure. She asks Doris to join her in planning a health education program for them. In considering various approaches, they decide to have a booth for a week in the employee cafeteria, where they can display information and answer questions over the lunch break (11:00 am–1:00 pm).

1. Write an objective for nutrition education in hypertension.
2. Based on the objective, what should Doris have at the booth as far as nutrition education media materials?

and may dislike the concentrated effort that reading requires. News events are instantaneously available on the internet or on television. People want information right away, in small segments, and in easy-to-use formats. The availability of educational materials on the internet will continue to accelerate in the 2000s.

Projecting to the future, computer-based education will become the norm for learning techniques and testing. High-quality videos of cooking demonstrations, exercises, and procedures such as inserting a feeding tube will assist in group and individual educational sessions. As more animations and video clips become available, the computer will become more of an integral part of most counseling. A videotape, CD-ROM, or website will augment handouts so that clients or employees can review techniques, such as insulin administration, "just in time" for use in their home or office. Computerized testing is the norm for professional credentialing and is becoming common in higher education because of ease, better ability to create pools of examination questions, and the ability to analyze the quality of the questions. The impact of instrumental media will grow in the next decade.

REVIEW AND DISCUSSION QUESTIONS

1. What benefits does the use of visual media provide in presentations?
2. What should be considered in planning visuals?
3. Why should the readability of printed materials be assessed?
4. Why is it important to evaluate visual media as one uses it?
5. When training employees, why is it preferable to train them using the real object, such as meat slicer, dish machine, cash register, or other equipment?
6. What are some advantages of using computer-assisted formats for training and education?
7. What is the "rule of six?"
8. Why should a presenter arrive at the presentation 30 minutes before it starts?
9. List 15 criteria for evaluating a presentation.
10. When would you use synchronous versus asynchronous learning? What is the value of each method?

SUGGESTED ACTIVITIES

1. Think about your earliest experiences in school. Can you remember any visual materials used by a teacher? Describe as much as you can remember and your age at the time.
2. Prepare a chart or poster depicting one idea. Write a description of your objectives and intended audience. Write a critique of your visual explaining how you used art and design principles to enhance quality.
3. Prepare overhead transparencies by hand by using a photocopier machine and by using a computer program. Assess the cost and quality differences.
4. If a video camera is available, plan a media presentation using the storyboarding technique. Prepare a video of a new employee process or something the employee needs to learn about, such as kitchen sanitation, food handling, hand washing, and the like. Or, tape a recipe preparation for a modified diet or a session on normal nutrition.
5. Create a computerized slide presentation, inserting at least one graphic.
6. Assign one student or a group of students to learn to use various types of equipment (overhead projector, slide projector, videocassette recorder (VCR), LCD projector, etc) Each should write a task analysis (see Chapter 12) for the equipment and then train others in its use.
7. Select a commercially prepared video. Evaluate it in terms of its intended audience, objectives, effectiveness, art and design principles, and cost.
8. View an educational program on television. Evaluate it using an evaluation form from the instructor.
9. Find two food labels. Describe how one could use the labels in testing.
10. Select two educational pamphlets. Critique the content using a readability formula, if available. Critique the visuals as well. Determine whether the pamphlets can be reproduced and find out what the cost will be.

WEB SITES

http://www.ala.org/work/copyright.html or http://www.loc.gov/copyright / information about copyright

http://www.readability-software.com / information about measuring readability
http://www.premier-presentation.co.uk / information about media equipment
http://www.osha.gov or www.powerfulpresentations.net / information about visuals for presentations
http://www.microsoft.com/office/powerpoint/default.asp / information about PowerPoint

Sources of NIH-based copy free educational materials can be found at the following sites:

http:///www.niddk.nih.gov/federal/dnr.html
http://www.cc.nih.gov/ccc/supplements/intro.html
http://www.nci.nih.gov
http://www.nhlbi.nih.gov/health/pubs/index.htm
http://www.nih.gov.nia/health/
http://www.nichd.nih.gov/publications/pubs.cfm
http://www.niddk.nih.gov/health/diabetes/diabetes.htm
http://www.niddk.nih.gov/health/digest/digest.htm

REFERENCES

1. Rankin SH, Stallings KD. Patient education: principles & practice. Philadelphia: Lippincott Williams & Wilkins, 2001.
2. Johnson V. Picture-perfect presentations. Train Dev 1989;43:45.
3. Heinich R, Molenda M, Russell JD, Smeldino SE Instructional media and technologies for learning, 5th ed. Englewood Cliffs, NJ: Prentice Hall, 1996.
4. Bjerkness S. The next step: making sense of education. DCE newsflash. Diabetes Care Educ Newsletter 2002;23:15.
5. Brandao JJ, Brademan GM, Moore CE, et al. Effectiveness of videotaped dietary instruction for patients hospitalized with cardiovascular disease. J Am Diet Assoc 1992;92:1268.
6. King WL. Training by design. Train Dev 1994;48:52.
7. Raines C, Williamson L. Using visual aids: a guide for effective presentations, rev ed. Menlo Park, CA: Crisp Publishers, 1995.
8. Glanz K, Rudd J. Readability and content analysis of print cholesterol education materials. Pt Educ Counsel 1990;16:109.
9. Brock T. How to make your tech work in their home. Training 2000;37:S9.
10. Hernandez J. A recipe for food safety training. Food Mgt 2002;36:87.
11. Carroll JM, Stein C, Byron M, Dutram K. Using interactive media to deliver nutrition education to Maine's WIC clients. J Nutr Educ 1996;28:19.
12. Carson CA, Hassel CA. Educating high-risk Minnesotans about dietary fats, blood cholesterol, and heart disease. J Am Diet Assoc 1994;94:659.
13. Coulston AM, Stivers M. A poster worth a thousand words: How to design effective poster session displays. J Am Diet Assoc 1993;93:865.
14. The American Almanac: Statistical Abstract of the United States, 1995-1996. Austin, TX: Reference Press, 1996.
15. Busselman KM, Holcomb CA. Reading skill and comprehension of the Dietary Guidelines by WIC participants. J Am Diet Assoc 1994;94:622.
16. Dollahite J, Thompson C, McNew R. Readability of printed sources of diet and health information. Pt Educ Counsel 1996;27:123.

17. Trenkner LL, Achtenberg L. Use of focus groups in evaluating nutrition education materials. J Am Diet Assoc 1991;91:1577.
18. Turmel WW. Technology in the classroom: velcro for the mind. In: Piskurich GM, Beckschi P, Hall B, eds. The ASTD handbook of training design and delivery. New York: McGraw-Hill, 2000.
19. Tagtow AM, Amos RJ. Extent to which dietitians evaluate nutrition education materials. J Nutr Educ 2000;32:161.
20. Moore E. Technology-based training methods. Food Mgt 1998;32:57.
21. Kamalipour Y. The brain drain: what television is doing to us. Chicago Tribune, May 2, l994.
22. Pennington J, Hubbard V. Nutrition education materials from the National Institutes of Health: development, review and availability. J Nutr Educ 2002;34:53.

Page numbers in *italics* denote figures; those followed by a "t" denote tables